New 5th Edition!
Updated, Revised, &
Greatly Expanded!

The *GREAT* LIQUID DIET

Diet Integrity / Life Equanimity

Practicing Higher Ways of Life

Leonard Mehlmauer, ND
A *Grand Medicine* Book

The *GREAT* LIQUID DIET©

Original manuscript 1 March 2002
1st Edition 6 July 2006
2nd edition 2 December 2007
3rd edition 4 March 2010
4th edition 16 September 2013
5th ed. 1 January 2020

Written by Leonard Mehlmauer, ND (ret.)
Art and Graphics by Nenita Sarmiento, BS, CPA
Grand Medicine Press • ISBN #9781710671247
San Marcos CA USA • 619-240-3711 • Copyright 1 January 2020
gm@grandmedicine.com / www.eyology.com

Note: The opinions in this book are solely those of the author and are not intended as an official representation of the views of Avatar Adi Da Samraj and Adidam.

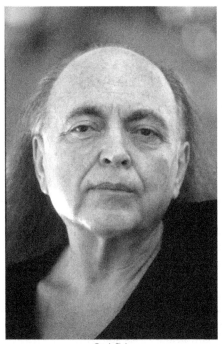

© ASA

Dedication

Most Beloved Avatar Adi Da Samraj, Giver of Wisdom, Divine Blessings, and Grace, Your devotees turn again and again—and always—to You, in constant gratitude for Your Many Gifts. You Inspire us to grow in Real Understanding toward the Great Awakening of the Heart. This Understanding includes all we know of any real value of how to rightly care for the body-mind. You Provide us with whatever we need to bring balance and equanimity, thus enabling the foundation for Real Spiritual practice and to be Healed at the heart. Your Great Wisdom shines in the lives of Your devotees as well as in all who would approach You with the open heart for Your Blessing. May we be ever more responsive, sensitive and attentive to You, practicing the disciplines You've Given us, in loving remembrance of You. This is our gift to You—and, by Your Grace, our Awakening. (Ref. www.adidam.org)

Acknowledgements

Not long after the release of the fourth edition, the need for new inclusions became obvious. People were asking for more recipes. Other questions arose. But, before even thinking of the creating the full fifth version of *The GREAT Liquid Diet*, whole pages of recipes, ideas, and concepts that would help others use this book came pouring in. As the new edition neared completion, we received a call from a long and trusted friend, Jefferson Nunn.

Our conversation focused on health—his, mine, how so many others have been helped by the GLD, and how we might spread the word on this simple and yet profound concept. Speaking ad and marketing language and I hear what sounds like Martian. I'm at home with health, Anthropology, world culture and events, music, and an assortment of other subjects related to Eyology, Anatomy and Physiology, macro-civilization, and Spirituality.

Jefferson, on the other hand, excels in qualities related to the computer and the Internet—for which I have counted on him any number of times over the years. Experiencing the GLD up front and personal, and then on hearing of some of the difficult health cases solved by the GLD over the years, Jeff agreed to help tell others. Soon, he invited Esther Kacmar to join the team.

In this edition, we take the opportunity to provide access to a great number of life-positive lifestyle factors learned over these several decades. This enables us to reach out and offer them as part of the higher way of life so sorely needed in our world at this time. Finally, I am deeply grateful to the Divine Person of Love for this opportunity and to have these talented people, including my intimate partner, Nenita, supporting and assisting in this process.

Special Note on Language and Spelling

Certain unusual spellings of words in this book are done on purpose. E.g., English words with suffixes like "gh" are often changed, so that "enough" becomes "enuf," "although" becomes "altho," and "tough" becomes "tuff". These and similar spellings are for the sake of logic, streamlining, ease of understanding, improved visual recognition, and finally, represent the author's humorous play with language.

The spelling of some words involving the actions and activities of the sacred, or the esoteric, including the Spiritual Masters, may begin with capital letters. Examples: the Truth of God, the Divine Person; Jesus Said (instead of Jesus said); the esoteric Teachings; Adi Da Samraj has Spoken of the body as…etc. These capitalizations are done purposely to honor That Which Is sacred in life.

Guidance on Your GLD

IMPORTANT!

Besides this book, two more modes of guidance are available to you on your *GREAT Liquid Diet* (GLD):

> **Your GLD Notes**. Go to www.GLDiet.co for a free page of **GLD Notes** for each day of your recommended 30 Day GLD. Each page inspires and guides you with tips, recipes, suggestions, or other descriptions, pictures, and illustrations.

> **Your GLD Lifestyle**. To power your GLD with a mighty foundation— all the details of this superior way of life—go to www.GLDiet.co for membership in **GLDLifestyle**. (More details below)

CONTENTS

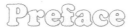

Preface

Sickness, Health, and *The GREAT Liquid Diet* (GLD)

Sickness is a pain in the ass! Or the stomach, heart, back, or some other organ or system of the body. No one really likes it. I sure don't. Some years ago, I was confronted, as a physician, with a situation that demanded a revision of my thinking about how to deal with disease. These raw liquids seemed to be suggested, an easy answer to a very difficult health circumstance—namely, cancer. Where fasting or all-raw diet wouldn't help, it worked!

Over the years since it was discovered (in 1975), the GLD was applied to the widest variety of health and disease conditions. Not only did it come thru, many other associated considerations about disease, health, diet, and lifestyle appeared. Now, how was I going to get this information out to benefit others? That's what this book is about!

Our Basic Human Needs—*Exoteric*

A check of many common sources on the Net brought the following eight basic human needs. In some sense, as when compared to the *esoteric* or sacred, we can think of these as being on the *exoteric* or secular level:

- Air
- Water
- Sleep
- Safety / Security

- Food
- Clothing
- Shelter
- Belonging

"Belonging" includes social acceptance, warmth, love and connection with others, social interaction and affiliation, acknowledgement, esteem, self-worth, having one's skills and competence appreciated, recognition, respect, significance, self-actualization, growth, a feeling of bringing a positive contribution to one's community.

Our Basic Human Needs—*Esoteric*

We must live our lives based on recognition of our True (Divine) Condition, the Great Consciousness, or the Context within Which all forms, conditional realms and beings appear. Rest in It. To do this best, beyond the basic mostly gross physical needs of air, food, water, clothing, shelter, etc. (above), to be fully human we also need:

1 – Peace and quiet
2 – A natural, human-size environment
3 – Ordinary intimacies

1

4 – A few people to see regularly
5 – A place, an occasion in which to be private

"All these things are your obligations if you are to fulfill the true Condition of our Meeting. All of these are required. All of these should be accommodated. So, we will all see one another and we will all live our privacy, as well. Because if we are not 'in private', if we are not given up, our meeting has no opportunity to grow, to represent a new adaptation, and we'll simply be struggling, striving here anxiously, never really being released from this mess, this world here."

—Avatar Adi Da Samraj, from middle of the Talk, ***Our Unlimited Capacity for Delusion***

Questions arise in this regard, including...
1 – Are these needs being rightly and most fully met by most Americans? In our local community?
2 – Are there community designs that can allow them to be met more completely, effectively, and efficiently?
3 – What other means might be employed that could more effectively meet these needs?

The answer to #1 is "No!" For #2, yes, we discuss this interesting and important question here, especially in Appendix G. For item #3, and for many other sensitive and even currently crucial reasons, we highly recommended the book, ***Prior Unity*** (Amazon, $14.95).

Both of these lists (above), exoteric and esoteric, are real human needs. We at Grand Medicine are not alone in feeling that our world already has the wherewithal to provide them—all of them—for every single human being on the planet. These are essential for real human growth. We want to see this happen—and it absolutely can.

Idealistic? Not at all. It is entirely realistic and achievable. We touch on it in this book and via www.gldiet.co. The whole world circumstance and how to help turn it around to a higher way of life, a higher consciousness, is described in the book, ***Not-Two Is Peace*** (4th edition, Amazon, $14.95).

Conditional and Unconditional Life
Bodily life depends on many *conditions*—air, water, food, clothing, shelter, etc. Our universe (one among countless others) and all the many planes of existence—gross physical, etheric, emotional, brain-mind, higher mental, astral, mystical, causal—all are in the *conditional* domain, influenced by and dependent on all manner of *forces*. Of course, there is one "Force" the conditional domain—and everything in it—depends on utterly and absolutely.

The Force that the *conditional* domain and everything in it appear *within* and entirely depends on is the *Unconditional*, the Great Consciousness-Energy of Reality, The Divine Person of Love. We live within Its Great Body. It is everywhere and pervades everything—including "us," "we," who feel like separate beings but are, in Reality, not at all separate from anything or anyone. "We" are a unity in the Great Starry Body of God.

So, how does this connect with **The GREAT Liquid Diet**, the "GLD"?

A Difficult World—and its Remedy

It doesn't take a genius to see that these are very difficult times. The human world is ego-mad, the inevitable result from being based in the secular—instead of in the sacred. In secular societies, power corrupts. The wealthy and powerful demonstrate this madness most obviously. Without the sacred as our firm cultural foundation, we are subhuman, less than human. These truths are mentioned occasionally in this book—for reasons that should be obvious.

While we cannot change this situation overnite, there are things we can do right now, both severally and individually, to help righten it. The purpose of this book is to provide many tips and references on how to serve the Absolute Reality by serving our fellow humans. Caring for our own body, we broadcast positive messages, like ripples in a stream, outward to everyone. This is the GLD!

Life as Purification

Here's how. The GLD is essentially about **purification**. Yes, it's about weight control, youthfulness, longevity, and a lot more. But *the GLD's bottom line* is **purification**. Interestingly, *life itself* is also essentially about **purification**. Purification is what we are here for—at every level of our being.

- The GLD approaches **purification** via the physical body.
- The "life" approach to purification is via the Divine Reality.
- In the GLD, we address both levels of approach.

How does it work, then?

The GLD shows how to purify *the gross "FOOD" body*—from toxics and toxins that enter thru many channels, especially diet. Meanwhile, we are often not even aware of how we get all junked up thru *the other energy systems*. So, to deal with and prevent further encumbrance from those *other kinds of toxicity*, we mention their leading causes, their one source, and ways of understanding them. Then, we refer to the *higher means of purification*, the most profound means. This way, for fullest purification, we cover all the bases.

Ready?

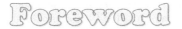

After sacred practice, **taking care of your health** is the most important thing you can do in your life. Yet today, everything we see and hear about our health has been monetized. One out of every five dollars in the U.S. economy goes to so-called "healthcare."

As consumers in and of this information economy, we now think of health as exercising regularly, drinking sugary energy drinks, and eating at fast food restaurants. This lifestyle, which includes toxins from environmental sources including the air and water, leads to a malnourished body straining under an eventually impossible load.

As we get sickened by this exhausting pollution of our bodies, we turn to our "healthcare" providers for help. These providers are funded by the same folks sponsoring the advertisements that got us sick in the first place! Medical prescriptions are largely ineffective at remedying this situation. They wind up leading to further disease and, ultimately, death.

What do our bodies truly need? Our minds have been preconditioned by the mainstream media to consider various ads designed to trigger the desire of foods made tasty by dangerous chemicals. Meanwhile, our bodies only need naturally nutritious foods in order to function properly.

What if there was a way to directly infuse the body with the highest quality nutrients? Our author, Leonard Mehlmauer ("Dr. Leonard"), has uncovered something truly remarkable with *The Great Liquid Diet*. Since I have known him over the past 25 years, I have watched as he helped people via the GLD to be completely cured of diabetes, to have heart problems 'go away', so that all of these patients now lead healthier lives.

Here's another thing. Our current medical science is not designed to recognize environmental problems of our bodies. Ingestion of our air, water, and food, largely determines our health. Early in his career, Dr. Leonard ingeniously discovered a most amazing method of accelerating the healing process. By infusing the body with pure liquefied nutrients, he found that the healing process is sped up and greatly improved.

Then, by surrounding the body with life-activity elements designed to promote well-being—namely, The BIG 7 and GLDLifestyle—he observed the healing process magnify to that degree, as well. This GLD method can and has worked for a wide variety of ailments—pretty much every disorder that came his way.

So then, one might ask, why isn't this promoted by regular doctors? I asked a similar question to my doctor in September of this year, 2019. I also asked, *"Why are there no tests for these types of bacteria, viruses, and other problematic pathogens?"* The doctor replied simply, *"Because the pharmaceutical companies do not test for things for which they do not have products (namely, drugs)."*

The body wants to be healthy. It is designed to absorb nutrients from the environment and use them in whatever ways it can to make itself healthy. Modern chemicals in our food and environment did not exist even 100 years ago, so our body has not yet adapted to properly processing them—if, indeed, it even can.

Infusing our bodies with pure living nutrients for a period of time in an exclusively liquid "delivery system" form (blended and/or juiced) is the quickest way to enable our bodies to clean out the garbage and to resume being healthy. In the following pages, Dr. Leonard describes exactly how to do just this.

Jefferson Nunn
Plano, Texas
November 20, 2019

Introduction

The GLD Notes

The GREAT Liquid Diet ("GLD") concept developed out of a situation with a patient where neither fasting nor the taking of solid foods seemed tenable. It worked so well, in fact, that it was used subsequently in many other health and disease situations, including as the author's yearly prophylaxis and general purification. More recently, on mentioning it at a science class, the idea arose to invite class members to join in. Surprise! Most of them did.

With thirty persons onboard, it seemed appropriate to provide daily notes of inspiration, encouragement, and direction. This seemed to work. The next idea was to offer the "Notes" to all and sundry so that everyone could benefit. The GLD Notes are available free online from www.GLDiet.co.

The GLD Lifestyle

Out of that idea grew the notion that some of those enjoying this unique kind of purification might also like learning the higher way of life gleaned from personal experiences since 1940 and professional office practice since 1972. The selection of topics is quite wide-ranging, each designed to enhance one's life by making it simpler, healthier, less expensive, longer-lasting, happier, freer, more balanced, more creative, and more exciting (or peaceful). For a sample and the current list of topics, go to www.GLDiet.co and click on *GLDLifestyle*.

Motivation

As you might expect, folks are variously motivated to do the GLD. Some have a possibly painful or otherwise irritating disorder that they'd like to eliminate. Some want to lose excess weight. Some wish to detoxify years or even decades of toxins from a lifetime of poor dietary and life-negative lifestyle habits. Some have been given a death sentence by their MDs and hope to prove them wrong—and thus live to enjoy their grandchildren.

Whatever their motivation, they will find—thru GLD connections—sympathetic others with whom they can share (or not) their personal stories. Along the way, they will have an excellent opportunity to grow, not just in their understanding of their personal habits and patterns of diet and lifestyle but also in real higher human terms. And this, regardless of their religious background, practices, training, or lack of any of these. We are all brothers and sisters.

The Four Basic Human Motivations

Before we even become ready for higher (religious, Spiritual) life, we all participate in any one or more of four basic motivations shared by 99.999999% of humanity:

- Food
- Money
- Sex
- Social egoity

While the religion and Spirituality are not the focus of the GLD, GLDiet.co, or of *GLDLifestyle*, they are an inherent part of life, and therefore are worthy of consideration in the midst of learning about bodily purification, Moreover, such purification, at every level of our being (not just the gross physical), is considered a prerequisite to entrance into even the preparatory levels of genuine religious life and practice—much less the Spiritual.

Money, food, and sex have traditionally been required to be dealt with and priorly mastered in these higher human pursuits. Avatar Adi Da Samraj has added social egoity since it also needs to be considered, understood, and mastered before taking on the higher stages of real Spiritual practice. Regarding the GLD, we are essentially—certainly at the beginning—involved with purifying the gross level vehicle. In later 30-Day GLDs, we get into more subtlety in this regard for those who wish to do so.

Justification

In the past few years (2016-2018), as reported by the USA Centers for Disease Control (CDC), the life expectancy for American men and women has been in decline. Men can expect to live no longer than (on average) 76.1 years and women 81.1 years. Why the decline? Experts list such *causes* as increasing suicide, and drug and alcohol addiction and abuse, with the underlying *source* as **despair**. This book discusses ways of turning this picture around—including via *The GREAT Liquid Diet*.

We are told (in late 2019) that Type 2 diabetes is and has been on the rise worldwide. The International Diabetes Federation reports that more than 400 million people were living with diabetes as of 2015. The World Health Organization (WHO) estimates that 90 percent of people around the world who have diabetes have type 2. Type 1 diabetes is also on the rise. Why? Diet! All symptoms of this disorder are easily eliminated via the GLD.

Every chronic degenerative disorder we encountered clinically— unless already well into the terminal stage—was either significantly improved or the symptoms were variously and even completely eliminated via the GLD. This includes cancer and even ALS. We are also told that most adult

Americans are overweight. You don't have to be told this to believe it. Just go into almost any public place to see it for yourself.

Why are so many people getting sick, including with disorders that never even existed before? Why don't they know how to get well? Why isn't it in the media? We will discuss and elaborate on this. People are struggling in life at every economic level—not just the poor and the (ever-shrinking) middle classes. Most people are confused, fearful, frustrated, disoriented, and even desperate in life. There are many reasons for this. Unfortunately, some go mad and go on a shooting spree.

Among the causes cited by some of our top philosophers (e.g., Gregg Braden) is the persistence of concepts of Charles Darwin propounded in the late 1800s and recently debunked and otherwise proven false. His concepts of evolution—especially of macro-evolution, where humans evolved from apes—has clearly and emphatically been debunked. Meanwhile, some of Darwin's concepts have become deeply embedded in Western cultures ever since.

Perhaps most important was his claim of "survival of the strongest", which became "survival of the fittest", where we all, as countries, states, counties, local organizations, family, and even as individuals, must compete and struggle against each other and alone in a hostile world against all odds. If we "fail" to succeed or even flounder or come up short somehow (whatever any of that means), we "flunk life's test," we are seen as weak, "guilty" of an untold crime, and deserve to die.

The unfortunate part of this concept is that it is deeply imbued in our psyche now, in our levels of consciousness, in our outlook on life. It has us continuing to believe the total bullshit that we must "win" a superior and commanding position in life at all these levels, from our "tribe" country down to us as individuals. This has us waving flags, spouting emotional patriotic nonsense, and even killing others for no damn good reason.

Where is the tolerance of personal differences in all of this? Where is the compassion for the suffering of others, the empathy, the sympathy, the loving cooperation taught to us by our Great Saints, seers, Yogis, sages, and Avatars? Where does that come into this picture? This is what we have to see, to understand, so we can get beyond this petty competitiveness, this divisiveness, the bickering, and non-cooperation we see and hear in the daily news.

Beyond the societal aspect of social Darwinism, we have to understand ourselves at the deepest level, what makes us feel separate from others, from each other, what keeps us from truly and consistently tolerating our differences, and cooperating with and loving each other. We have to learn about *egoity*—the bottom-line most fundamental source of our sense of separateness—and how to transcend it.

So, we don't survive by competing with each other. Competition in friendly sports games is one thing, but what about nations against nations? For military dominance? For resources that other countries have more of than "us"? Hell no! We must first see ourselves as one human family, a unity, which "one family" unity is, in fact, inherently and intrinsically so. United we stand, divided we fall? Yes, in this case. Absolutely! So, let's get the word out!

On the GLD, we share our approach, our feelings, our failures, our challenges, and our successes, with family and friends, with naybors, with colleagues. We email and skype each other, keep up with each other, form groups that support each other—not for money but simply because we want to, because this is what real humans do. In this way, we do something that is missing from so many levels of our present world.

Why "Religion" in a Book about Diet?

Spirituality is a part of life (Chapter 13 – *The BIG 7*) and thus a part of health. A crucial role we must all play. The most important role there is. It's why we're here. Of course, in some sense, you wouldn't know it by the history of religion. But all the religious killing, wars, book burning, people burning, persecution, beheadings, Crusades, destruction of whole cultures, etc.—we're talking about bullcrap downtown silly religion—not Real religion, which is about spirit, and Spirituality.

In writing this book, the author speaks from the heart, from valid knowledge gained thru direct experience, reasoning from facts, and competent testimony. Human history is littered with the bodies of innocents, the destruction (and attempted destruction) of whole cultures, at the hands of influential institutionalized "religious" organizations and no doubt well-meaning individuals seeking to gain and maintain their power over people "in the name of God." They're still doing it. Such is the current ego-insanity of our divided-and-conquered my-people-are-superior world.

But it was their god, the god of their believed or conceived righteousness, the god of their mind. No mortally conceived god (meaning necessarily limited by the human mind) is Real God or Reality Itself. Thru millennia, we have invented all manner of gods and ideas about multiple gods or the "one god," and justified all kinds of activities based on those concepts. Meanwhile, there have been, in our history, genuine Realizers of "God," the Divine Reality.

These Divine Realizers of various levels—as Saints, Sages, and Wisdom practitioners—have appeared among us to Teach us the way of love, cooperation, and tolerance thru submission to, surrender to, and identification with Them, or the Divine Person. But because of our egoity, our sense of separateness from Reality—*especially the egoity of those in power*—They were rarely treated kindly—as witness the heartbreaking murder of Beloved Jesus. In our current world, the truthful are rarely appreciated.

Meanwhile, this ego insanity continues with a modern twist, our current version. This is not human nature. Egoity is **sub**human nature. The Great Realizers didn't teach us to kill or to hate one another. That's just something the followers of silly religion do—or silly science, too, for that matter. So, I am not advocating for anything these two groups do or have done. I offer only my best understanding of health, Spirituality, and life, from the best sources (and capital "S" Sources) I can find. What you do with it is up to you.

What The Ego Does

The Ego Typically…

(1) **Objectifies**—always finds everything separate from itself, which is frightening to its false sense of separateness

(2) **Surrounds**—attempts to understand "the object(s)," figure them out toward gaining an advantage

(3) **Controls**—or at least attempts to gain control over the "thing," the "other," even all "others."

(4) **Destroys**—winds up destroying whatever it controls, or even that which it feels it cannot control

---

In some real sense, "egoity" is likely what in Christianity is called "sin"—forgetting the Holy Spirit, The Divine Reality. Its epitome is not just simply forgetting, but actual denial that The Great One or Person of Love even exists. That would be "Unforgivable"—not because The Divine is Unforgiving but because the "sinner" or ego would not even accept such Forgiveness. It would be Forgiven as soon as submission to (remembering) God occurred. Immediately.

It is not hard to find the dark work of egoity in this world. It is not hard to see it in ourselves! It is the "sin" of separation from the Divine Reality, forgetting The Great One. One cannot separate from "It," The Support, Source, The Very Substance and Ultimate Destiny of existence. But the ego (sense of separateness) can and does—all the time. We have lost sympathy with The Spirit, The Spiritual, The Great One, "God," The Divine Person of Reality.

In earlier Earth civilizations—of which there have been several—and peaceful, we had this connection. We honored it, cherished and practiced it, but we've since lost it. After the great flood or other natural catastrophes? Perhaps. Somehow, in any case, we have to get it back. In the recent writings of many of the most brilliant philosophers, this is the one and most important item missing from their prognostications—and the very most important thing in life: our connection with Reality, our sympathy with The Divine, with Real God!

Purification and Our Life Purpose

There are only four things you can do with your life:

(1) get better
(2) get worse
(3) stay the same
(4) transcend the whole damn thing in Happiness!
        —Avatar Adi Da Samraj

In our egoity, we all tend to fall into any of the first three of these categories—which are essentially about ways of *becoming* happy. Only the Perfect Help of a true Spiritual Master can accomplish the last—which is about the way of *practicing* Happiness (notice the difference between "becoming" and "practicing"—and also the capital "H"). We *practice* Happiness simply by communing with The Divine.

Since life in this realm is all about **purification**, this book focusses on the first of these options—*getting better*. The fourth option is our connection with (submission to or communion with) the Spiritual Master. That's your call. However, *The GREAT Liquid Diet* (GLD) book and lifestyle can, in specific ways, prepare us for the fourth option. How? Essentially by means of pure liquefied foods and life-positive lifestyle. We show you how these can help you *enjoy food, eat less, manage weight, gain health, and live longer*—thru this essential purification.

Disease, pain, suffering, rapid aging, hi stress—no fun! We've all suffered these common, mediocre achievements, for which no congratulations are deserved! Look at our present health situation. One health modality (Rockefeller-Big Pharma allopathic medicine) dominates all others. And yet, powerful as it is, there is more disease and suffering than ever in human history.

In our rapidly world-spreading "crazy random" Western culture, we're not instructed by government or Big Pharma in the principles of radiant health, which is our birthright. Nor even in simple means of body-mind balance. We may live a bit longer than in many former times, but we're sicker—and at many levels of being.

Technology notwithstanding, we suffer hi stress, hi anxiety. These pages offer simple means of eliminating the symptoms or at least alleviating the distress of virtually any chronic degenerative disease—and how to prevent further suffering. Here, we find *seven diet and lifestyle practices* that, when used intelligently and strategically, can be most effective against stress, aging, and disease. Get ready for a pleasant surprise!

The "Great Liquid Diet" ("GLD," "GLDiet") was accidentally stumbled upon in 1975 as a means of dealing with two specific diseases: a case of "arthritis" and (especially) a malignant tumor. The quotes around the term arthritis point to the fact that many diseases, medically named or not, often involve far more than just the expressed symptoms: show us any ten medically diagnosed arthritis patients and, while there are similarities, we'll show you significant differences, one person to the next.

Many additional diseases the patient may currently suffer—along with any already named/diagnosed—often go unrecognized. Eyology (the Iridologies and Sclerology—www.eyology.com), can help us see these disease conditions coming—a big advantage that allows us to prevent approaching or potential disaster. Combine these with (1) right use of all types of medicine (modern, conventional, ancient, Natural and Traditional), plus (2) life-positive lifestyle—and throw in (3) pure dietary liquids, and you have the future of medicine—at least a good possibility one.

Which Treatment to Choose?
OK, say the patient is already suffering a long-term disease. Do we rely exclusively on drugs, radiation, and surgery to deal with chronic degenerative circumstances? Do we trust completely in Natural Remedies? How about right use of both? Which of these two avenues to choose isn't always simple. Healing is an art as well as a science. Sometimes we need to have a tumor surgically removed.

Short-term medication can be justified in those willing to change dietary and lifestyle habits—unless they're at the end of life, in which case certain medications—especially pain killers—can be appropriate to the end. Certain other highly dangerous and invasive medical practices, like chemo and radiation "therapies," as currently practiced, are (in the opinion of many) rarely if ever justified. *"Only a fool takes a cure that kills!"*

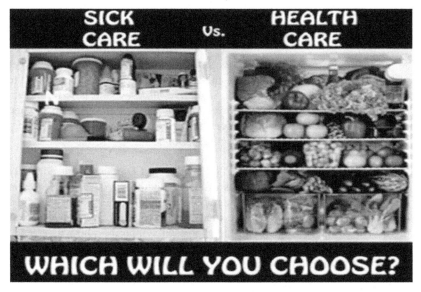

In our egoity, we all tend to fall into any of the first three of these categories—which are essentially about ways of *becoming* happy. Only the Perfect Help of a true Spiritual Master can accomplish the last—which is about the way of *practicing* Happiness (notice the difference between "becoming" and "practicing"—and also the capital "H"). We *practice* Happiness simply by communing with The Divine.

Since life in this realm is all about **purification**, this book focusses on the first of these options—*getting better*. The fourth option is our connection with (submission to or communion with) the Spiritual Master. That's your call. However, *The GREAT Liquid Diet* (GLD) book and lifestyle can, in specific ways, prepare us for the fourth option. How? Essentially by means of pure liquefied foods and life-positive lifestyle. We show you how these can help you *enjoy food, eat less, manage weight, gain health, and live longer*—thru this essential purification.

Disease, pain, suffering, rapid aging, hi stress—no fun! We've all suffered these common, mediocre achievements, for which <u>no congratulations are deserved</u>! Look at our present health situation. One health modality (Rockefeller-Big Pharma allopathic medicine) dominates all others. And yet, powerful as it is, there is more disease and suffering than ever in human history.

In our rapidly world-spreading "crazy random" Western culture, we're not instructed by government or Big Pharma in the principles of radiant health, which is our birthright. Nor even in simple means of body-mind balance. We may live a bit longer than in many former times, but we're sicker—and at many levels of being.

Technology notwithstanding, we suffer hi stress, hi anxiety. These pages offer simple means of eliminating the symptoms or at least alleviating the distress of virtually any chronic degenerative disease—and how to prevent further suffering. Here, we find *seven diet and lifestyle practices* that, when used intelligently and strategically, can be most effective against stress, aging, and disease. Get ready for a pleasant surprise!

The "Great Liquid Diet" ("GLD," "GLDiet") was accidentally stumbled upon in 1975 as a means of dealing with two specific diseases: a case of "arthritis" and (especially) a malignant tumor. The quotes around the term arthritis point to the fact that many diseases, medically named or not, often involve far more than just the expressed symptoms: show us any ten medically diagnosed arthritis patients and, while there are similarities, we'll show you significant differences, one person to the next.

Many additional diseases the patient may currently suffer—along with any already named/diagnosed—often go unrecognized. Eyology (the Iridologies and Sclerology—www.eyology.com), can help us see these disease conditions coming—a big advantage that allows us to prevent approaching or potential disaster. Combine these with (1) right use of all types of medicine (modern, conventional, ancient, Natural and Traditional), plus (2) life-positive lifestyle—and throw in (3) pure dietary liquids, and you have the future of medicine—at least a good possibility one.

Which Treatment to Choose?
OK, say the patient is already suffering a long-term disease. Do we rely exclusively on drugs, radiation, and surgery to deal with chronic degenerative circumstances? Do we trust completely in Natural Remedies? How about right use of both? Which of these two avenues to choose isn't always simple. Healing is an art as well as a science. Sometimes we need to have a tumor surgically removed.

Short-term medication can be justified in those willing to change dietary and lifestyle habits—unless they're at the end of life, in which case certain medications—especially pain killers—can be appropriate to the end. Certain other highly dangerous and invasive medical practices, like chemo and radiation "therapies," as currently practiced, are (in the opinion of many) rarely if ever justified. *"Only a fool takes a cure that kills!"*

Simple Definitions of Purifying Diets

Solid food diet – Any diet consisting essentially of pure solid foods (preferably hi-raw or all-raw Vegetarian)

Mono diet – Any diet consisting of one solid food only (e.g., only grapes, or only oranges, or only avocados)

Modified liquid diet – Any diet consisting of mostly pure liquids + a few solids (perhaps one solid food meal daily)

Liquid diet – Any diet consisting of essentially and preferably only pure liquefied fruits, veggies, nuts & seeds

Juice diet – Any diet consisting of the juices of fruits and vegetables (preferably natural fresh-squeezed)

Juice fast – Any diet consisting of fresh raw fruit & veggy juices thinned 50:50 with water; also possible herb tea

Water fast – Any diet consisting of pure water and herb teas sweetened with a few drops of honey + fresh lemon

Total fast – A diet consisting of no food or water

Health Responsibility

We at GranMed, of course, cannot be responsible for your health situation before, during, or after the GLD. We don't know how you'll apply it. Enter the healer. The healer is rightly a teacher, a coach, the one to help and guide you to improved health. But even the healer—unless they're practicing hands-on-the-body techniques—can never be responsible for anything more than instruction—and/or, otherwise, at best, helping bring energy down the frontal line of your body to promote healing (see the book, *Conductivity Healing*).

The same is so with this information. Health responsibility is in your hands, the hands of the patient—and/or those capable persons around you if you can no longer make health decisions on your own or manage your personal health care. With the GLD, it's up to you and your health practitioner, then, as to how you apply the instruction here. You may need to add a few days of fasting now and then—like, e.g., to speed up the purification.

You may need to increase the viscosity (thickness) of your liquids to keep weight on or to provide more concentrated nutrition for specific periods—maybe even during the entire course of your GLD. Special healing herbs or certain nutritional supplements could help your condition. Your qualified health practitioner should guide you in this. If it's very late in the disease process, and the end of the body's useful life is near (terminal illness), the GLD can still be helpful in relieving pain and suffering and otherwise bringing some general bodily comfort.

The GLD, in and of itself, is no miracle, altho it can seem as such in many cases. It is merely *a dietary delivery system*—and a very efficient one, at that. It is a very conservative approach to cleansing and healing in that it actively conserves bodily energies for detoxification, cleansing, energy balancing, tissue rebuilding, and the general healing processes.

Take Your Time and Do it Right
We've seen people apply the GLD in a wide variety of ways. Some have been strict about the basics (*fruits, veggies, and nuts/seeds*), keeping what others told them is a balance of these items daily (about 33% of each group)—and getting excellent results. Some have quit after three or four days, insisting the GLD didn't work for them. Some have exaggeratedly emphasized one food group over the other two.

Others have neglected a whole group—the nuts/seeds, or the veggies, or the fruits—altogether, only to suffer lack of energy, prolonged irritation from their disease, and slowed progress. Still others have decided to "fudge" here and there—even, in some cases, a lot!—adding silly foods. Result: their weight stayed on far longer than desired or expected—even tho their body enjoyed significant purification. Some blended cheeses and meats into soups, again slowing the process of healing by adding these highly acid foods.

So, how long do you do your GLD? With disease conditions, it's usually until symptoms adequately abate or disappear entirely. With chronic degenerative disease conditions, it's usually 30 days as the first general cleanse. Usually, you'll know when to quit. You'll feel it. But, you must *give the GLD a chance to do its work*. Do your GLD for 30 days. This is what we recommend. If you want or need longs, do longer. So, what is the truly "right" radio of fruits to veggies to nuts/seeds? On average, it's fruits about 30%, veggies (especially greens) about 45%, and nuts/seeds about 25%.

A Community of Help
The GLD is a way of cooperating with the body in its constant attempt to rid itself of disease processes, which means toxics and toxins of all kinds—even mental, emotional, and psychic ones. The gross physical body is, in some real sense, a community of organisms working together as individuals, groups, and whole systems working on getting and keeping itself (as a unit) well.

There are various ways we can help in this wellness process—and multiple ways we can impede it, slow it down, and even make things impossible for this inner community of help. The immune system of the body is only one body system working to protect and keep it well. All other body systems play their role in this. The GLD is a way of giving these systems, organs, and tissues what they want—and what they need!

GLD Buddies, GLD Groups

Having done the GLD for many years, your author can say for a certainty that altho one can easily do the 30-Day GLD "alone," or by oneself, it is generally even easier and more fun when doing it in the company of others. The more, the merrier! Even with one other person, there is that sense of support, helping each other along, the encouragement of someone who cares about you and how well you do—not just on the GLD but in life.

It is easier to "cheat" when "alone" (and thereby slow your progress!) than when with someone joining your GLD, someone to confess to, confide in, and share the challenge of something new and different. The child and adolescent in us want to "hide out" and be secret, while the adult in us is open and confessed. Moreover, those who are suffering chronic disease states need the support of a buddy who is right there doing the GLD, drink-for-drink.

It is thus recommended to call and tell your friends, your mate, your relatives, and colleagues about your upcoming GLD adventure. Invite them to join you in your GLD. You never know who among them will want to join you. You might be surprised! The GLD is for the open minded, those who at least sense the fundamental and even crucial importance of bodily and self-purification in life. The website www.GLDiet.co has more—thru *GLDLifestyle*—on GLD Buddies and GLD Groups.

Disease as Motivator

Yes, pain and disease can be great motivators. In this sense, disease can be a good thing. So, in pain and disease situations, you should ask yourself how much you want to be well, to be the right weight, to feel good in the body, and to like what you see in the mirror?

Some go to great lengths and spend enormous sums of money to achieve a certain appearance—via plastic surgery and other extreme means. Of course, those suffering from genetic defects and disfiguring accidents can be justified in such measures and expenditures. But, one wonders how much pure diet and life-positive lifestyle can help in so many of those cases as well as in chronic disease situations.

We at GranMed feel that in many cases, time spent on the GLD alone would bring the desired change. But then, there's our powerfully embedded social, cultural, and otherwise learned attachment to our favorite foods—and the fact that drug and surgery remedies are so strongly recommended, thru the corporate-controlled media, for our ills. Some of our dietary habits come just from imitating others, including from TV ads. Time for something new!

How Much Food do we Need to be Healthy?

Another thing most people notice on the GLD is how very little food we **actually need** to be healthy. Look at this: *most of the food on the GLD is* *raw produce*. By taking raw natural foods, our body is nourished the way it was originally meant to be by Nature. The cells of the body are getting what they need, so cravings fall away.

We start to enjoy these raw liquids. We notice that we need no big breakfast—unless we're athletes or laborers expending enormous amounts of energy. In older age, we need no breakfast at all. We no longer need our coffee to feel awake (awake-ness and energy should not have to be stimulated—except perhaps in emergencies).

We feel contented with our Green Smoothie (the GLD's main drink), our delicious other smoothies (blended fruits and nuts), RMVJ, and our blended soups, raw or even perhaps cooked. Our body starts taking the shape it was meant to have by Nature, and our diseases disappear. We have the knowledge and satisfaction of having done this ourselves—a powerful tool we can always use—and share with others. BTW, it has been said that if you want to see what your body is supposed to look like by Nature, you should do all raw foods for at least 90 days!

The Era of Instant Gratification

Egoic Western Culture has developed in us an attitude of immediate gratification, a desire for convenience and quick satisfaction. It's so strong that we don't want to bother with anything that "takes time." Standing in lines makes us crazy. Reading is going out of fashion. We fully expect to get what we want right away, to be pleasurably stimulated thru money, food, sex, social and visual and aural stimulations and gratifications.

We feel we should be able to lose weight overnite—by taking a pill or a shot, or perhaps via stomach stapling, liposuction, or other invasive (but quick) surgical procedure. And if it's herbs or diet, these should work equally fast.
Interestingly, when combined with right lifestyle, the GLD will work quicker than probably any other natural health therapy to eliminate excess weight and heal diseases of the physical body   naturally and without undue side-effects, allowing the body to take a normal, natural shape. It may even teach us patience! Maybe.

People have so many different health circumstances. Some who do the GLD have fairly good general health and do the GLD for periodic cleansing. Others are in dangerous waters, having been medically diagnosed with severe chronic degenerative diseases—even to the point where their doctors have given up on them. The rest of us are everywhere in between. And when we do have a chronic degenerative disorder, and we take a longer GLD, we are going to experience some symptoms of purification—whether during or after the GLD. This is normal.

18

Your experience on the GLD, then, will be your own. Essentially, you could think of your GLD as a lifeline, a saving grace, an insurance policy that you can always depend on to help you get and be well. To many who've done it, one of its best merits is the fact that, if necessary, we can eat one or more solid food meals during some celebratory occasion (Holiday, family event, marriage, social or business occasion) right in the middle of our GLD, and then go right back onto it.

Of course, this can be abused—e.g., by overdoing alcohol, or spending a day or two eating junk or otherwise rich foods—thus retarding your progress toward eliminating the disease process you've been suffering. Intelligently applied, however, the right use of solid food can be a significant asset or aspect of an excellent health promotion tool. But, when it comes to purification and dealing with chronic degenerative diseases, we at GranMed can't think of a better, faster, gentler, and safer way than ***The GREAT Liquid Diet***.

The GLD's First Application

In the early 1970s in San Diego, your author and GranMed director, Leonard Mehlmauer, ND, was in the developing stages of his professional clinical practice as a Traditional Naturopath. A tall and obese woman in her mid-thirties named Ina Ball [*fictitious name*] called my office with a request that would change both of our lives. She suffered a cancerous tumor in her leg and multiple forms of painful arthritis. Her medical doctors had told her the tumor must be removed. The leg could be saved, but it would be stiff for the rest of her life. She sought a less frightening alternative.

We considered the options. Generally, in Natural Health practice, such cancers would not be treated by <u>fasting</u>, since the body would need a constant supply of high-quality nutrients for maximum immune capability and optimum organ functioning. <u>Solid foods</u>, even all raw, might be too slow, diverting energy to the jaws for chewing and to the stomach for digestion, energies very much needed for purification—and for fighting the cancer.

What else would work? During silent prayer, the idea came that a balance could be achieved with maximum cleansing—on a "liquid diet." It should work, since the principle of fasting would be employed. And yet, unlike fasting, with the quality, viscosity, and intensity of the essentially raw liquid nutrients—including nuts and seeds (which are never taken on a fast)—the client could, at least theoretically, continue the diet for months—or otherwise as long as necessary. This is because all the crucial-to-health food items—fruits, veggies, and nuts/seeds—would be included. So, it should work. Theoretically.

GLD's History: the Experiment Begins

So, we decided to try this "liquid diet" on Ina. She should begin, and I would monitor her progress. In the initial weeks, things seemed to be going well. And then, suddenly…Ina was nowhere to be found! She had moved and changed her phone number.

We kept hoping she would call. Six months later, our paths crossed at Ocean Beach People's Food, an excellent natural food market in a coastal San Diego suburb. Her weight had gone down from the original 323 pounds to 161. She looked radiant! She was wearing a green dress. On recognizing her, I blurted out, "Ina! Is that you? You look like a beautiful green vegetable!"

Amidst hugs, Ina recounted an amazing story of 6 months on the GLD. Twice, her friends frightened her with the possibility that she was hurting herself. Both times, on submitting herself to a local hospital for tests, she left with negative pathology, 100% scores, and pre-med students crowding around and questioning this woman who seemed perfect in every category!

"*Let me outa here!*" she exclaimed. She went on to describe how the arthritis had quickly vanished, and how the tumor had shrunk down to nothing, being destroyed by the greatly empowered immune system, and then completely eliminated by the body as waste. It was a happy ending—and reunion.

In the ensuing years, The GLD was employed at Grand Medicine— very occasionally, at first, and later with greater frequency, in the more difficult cases. More recently, in these times of great stress, multiple diseases, obesity, and overweight, it seems to have a particularly useful, more urgent, and wider-ranging application.

Attitude

Illness is no fun. There are so many things you can't do when you're sick. It can make almost any life activity difficult—including Spiritual practice, which is most important of all. So, how motivated are you to be well? How important is it for you to feel really good, to be healthy again, to be the rite weight, strong and vibrant? Attitude is crucial to your success on the GLD.

The right, successful attitude on the GLD comes from a careful, feeling assessment of your situation altogether. This is not magic. It's work. It can be a happy ordeal of increasing improvement toward radiant health, or it can be a nightmare of struggle. It's really up to you. We strongly urge you to take the GLD on *like a hobby*. In 30 days, you will learn a treasure trove of data about yourself, your body, the effects of food, and much more. You will learn about how Mother Nature cures. She is slow—but she is sure!

If your attitude is, *"Oh, hell, what am I getting myself into here?"*, you're already shooting yourself in the foot. That attitude sets you up for failure. Doubt-mind will wreck your plans every time. Put a positive spin on this adventure. It is an adventure in eating, in understanding, and in health.

It's more fun when we make this GLD event into a hobby with positive statements such as:

> *"I'm going to do this right!"*
> *"I'm getting well."*
> *"I can feel the improvement as each day goes by."*
> *"I'm so happy to have a plan that works."*
> *"I'm happy to be on my GLD."*
> *"I'll stay with it as long as it takes."*
> *"My goal is always already happening by God's Grace."*
> *"I'm doing my part to make it happen with positive actions."*
> *"Success is assured."*
> *"Real vibrant health now comes to me."*
> *"I have everything it takes to be well."*
> *"Yahoo!"*

Diet and Spirituality

Is there a connection between diet and Spiritual life? Everyone knows the health nut—the one with the orange skin from drinking a gallon of carrot juice every day! He's going to achieve Paradise or break thru Heaven's Gates by eating a sandwich! He's a vegetarian, or a vegan, maybe even an all-raw-foodist, so he's "better than you!" Or so he thinks!

We at Grand Medicine have listened, seen, practiced, and learned from long, hard experience, and from the Wisdom of Adi Da, that *diet has nothing whatsoever to do with Real Happiness or Spiritual life*. The very best that diet can do is bring some level of equanimity to the gross body-mind, some form of balance, which can help provide a gross foundation for real Spiritual practice.

That's a lot, actually. And, that's fine. We should not expect food to do more than this. In and of itself, diet and food are not Spiritual. We can "Spiritualize" food by asking God's Blessing on it. That's as close as gross food can get to being Spiritual—the health nut's idealism notwithstanding. Food can do a lot to help bring balance to the body, but beyond that, we need The Divine Person, the Spiritual Master, Divine Grace.

"The real disease to be healed is egoity. You can deal with some physical things [via the flow of energies in the body, but]...*you cannot deal with all karma, and you cannot deal with ego, which is the real dis-ease. The*

'world' is a complex pattern of karmic design, and the 'root' of it is separateness, ego. Thus, true healing is, ultimately, a Transcendental Spiritual matter." —Adi Da Samraj, in <u>*Conductivity Healing*</u>

BTW, our references to "God" and "The Lord" are not meant to direct anyone to any particular religion. These religious and Spiritual references are all meant as non-denominational. Everyone is urged to follow the dictates of his and her own heart when it comes to religion, Spirituality, diet, lifestyle, politics, and everything else in life.

Curing Chronic Degenerative Disease via Raw Liquids
In the many years of our clinical work at Grand Medicine (since 1972), and since retiring from the office (2003), we've seen and worked with thousands of patients who suffered a wide variety of disorders. In those years, we learned that virtually all chronic degenerative disease could be cured via raw liquids, as long as the patient (1) believes in the natural health procedures, (2) is willing to participate in the protocol, and (3) is not terminally ill.

What this means is that while many patients were already well into the disease process, suffering symptoms and taking their prescribed medications, they were able to eliminate the symptoms and the pharmaceuticals *to the degree that they applied themselves to the natural GLD protocol*. This is to say that while some walked away totally free from symptoms and drugs, others achieved various levels of purification and improved health according to how they applied themselves to the program developed for them.

Of course, we had a few "failures," too, essentially involving miscommunications with patients in terms of what was necessary for them to get well. For example, some, thinking they'd be well within just a few days, were disappointed and quit the program. Others moved away or were otherwise unavailable to our calls. These were the ones that we felt "fell thru the cracks." And with few exceptions, we never heard from them again. These were rare.

Then, there were the ones who "reappeared" years later, begging for another chance. *"Will Dr. Leonard see me?"* Of course, this was an opportunity to help someone who was now really ready to make the change from life-*negative* diet and lifestyle to life-*positive*. We happily received them and gave them lots of encouragement.

The big-name diseases such as diabetes, cancer, heart disease, and arthritis, e.g., are all curable—even such diseases as ALS—again, as long as they haven't progressed too far, and that the patient is willing to dig in and do his or her part. And each case must be considered individually, since altho you can have ten people lined up with the same diagnosis, each will need to be given a protocol that fits his or her specific circumstance—albeit with ***The GREAT Liquid Diet*** (GLD) as the center-post of the protocol.

Transitioning to Raw Liquids

We're saying that virtually all of these chronic degenerative disorders would involve, as part of their protocol, certain periods of all raw liquids—meaning the GLD. This is because the GLD offers a most effective and efficient "delivery system" of the highest quality nutrients—the gross physical basis of health improvement. Why food? Because the gross physical body is a FOOD body, the quality and quantity of which food largely determine physical bodily health. This has been known since ancient times—and yet is somehow lost in this current era.

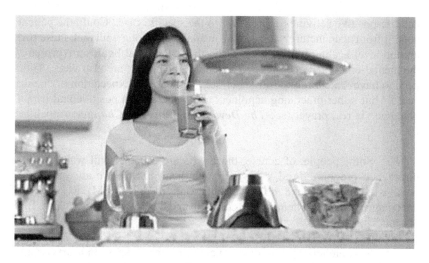

In most cases of chronic degenerative disease, the best way to proceed is to have the patient prepare for two days of transition prior to the all raw liquids: the first day with 50% raw food and 50% steamed or cooked pure natural foods (no junk food!). The second day would be about 80% raw, with a salad and a green smoothie and perhaps one small cooked natural food meal.

The choice of whether to engage a certain level of intensity of the GLD would depend on the severity of the case as decided by the attending natural health professional. At this time in history (2019), very few MDs have the understanding and experience needed to manage the natural health purification regimes necessary in chronic degenerative diseases. Their training and focus are, essentially, treating disease symptoms with pharma drugs.

For that matter, only somewhere around 20% of Naturopathic physicians (NDs) in the USA at this time could accomplish significant management of a 30-60-day-or-longer GLD—with enemas or colemas or colonic irrigation, appropriate herbs and nutrition supplements, hydrotherapy, and other natural therapy protocols as may be needed. The *Traditional* Naturopath, on the other hand, would likely be the most experienced and capable in such cases.

However that may be, we're not likely talking about the use of sophisticated hospital machines and devices—altho a working relationship with MD's managing the more advanced disease cases could be developed and work out quite successfully. Usually, it's going to be pretty much a simple understanding of the importance of moving the vital force (etheric energy) down the frontal line of the body. When that happens, healing is imminent.

The healer is merely the guide to protocol, the teacher of right health and life-positive activities appropriate to the specific case. Could the patient benefit from acupuncture? Is massage available? (Along with diet, these two are top-level healing modalities.) Altho the raw natural liquids are primary, the mental-emotional energies and moods of the patient are also vital. They need to have an entirely positive outlook, without any expectation of "being cured," but rather practicing happiness and visualizing a positive and happy outcome via real prayer (see *The Devotional Prayer of Changes*, Appendix E).

Some people, of course, those who are capable, will want to self-direct their program. And, can you blame them? While we all want to be well, we cannot depend on the mainstream media (MSM) to teach or encourage wellness. Their money comes from Big Corporate, especially Big Pharma.

Rockefeller-Big Pharma medicine runs the sickness industry world-wide. It is essentially a for-profit cartel. It is about disease treatment, not wellness. It wants everyone on drugs—for life. Big Food / Agriculture / Chemical, including Bayer-Monsanto, want everyone on prepared, packaged, processed, GMO, pesticide-laden, and commercial fertilizer-grown foods. No wonder people everywhere are creating backyard gardens, growing their own!

Likewise, peoples' medicine. We're learning how to care for ourselves and our loved ones by these natural means—and using the Internet to locate the needed resources—like www.NextWorldTV.com and www.theRealFoodChannel.com. In most cases, one can do a GLD oneself and eliminate the symptoms of chronic degenerative disease. In general, it is only those who feel they cannot do this without expert help that actually need that assistance. And they should get it accordingly.

The old, the infirm, the very young, and those who are otherwise not competent to guide themselves thru the purification process, should seek the help of those practiced in natural health and the natural healing modalities. At the least, those who desire to be self-directed in their work to regain their health, these can be in contact with nearby trusted natural health professionals who can occasionally or periodically monitor their progress.

Easy on the Body

Moreover, as noted elsewhere in this book, the GLD, unlike a fast, is not harsh. It is so gentle that virtually anyone can do it—including the pregnant, the elderly, and the very young. Children naturally "fast" when sick. Otherwise, fasting can interfere with their growth process. However, not so with the GLD. The rich, thick smoothies contain everything their growing bodies need—fresh raw fruits, veggies, and nuts and seeds.

The elderly and the very sick can also benefit from the GLD—and without the strong healing crises common to true fasts. Those on dialysis and those taking pharmaceutical medications for years on end may find themselves moving away from the machines and the meds. These cases, of course, will need careful supervision on their GLD.

Trigger Factors

There is usually a "trigger" factor that starts disease symptoms. Most diseases of the gross physical body involve dietary abuses or insults. Exercise abuse (lack of it, usually, or too much of the wrong kind, etc.) is another symptom trigger. Lack of adequate rest and sleep is yet another (see "*The BIG 7*"). General unhappiness, along with other negative-reactive emotions (the NRE's), are also (and often *the*) major players in disease.

One ALS patient was doing 3-4 hours daily of extreme Mixed Martial Arts and eating at least one meal per day at Burger King. This was his recipe, his symptom "trigger," for health disaster—these two activities. (Subsequently, however, he beat the disease via 5½ weeks on the GLD! (Yes, that's Amyotrophic Lateral Sclerosis.)

The patient needs to be aware of how they got into the difficulty they're in and to be willing to take responsibility for this process of purification now required. Adi Da Samraj describes disease as "*the wrong practice of life*"—which, of course, is true. In diabetes, e.g., the person was usually eating processed foods and not getting enuf exercise. They usually have a genetic tendency to pancreas metabolism dysfunction—which genetic tendency, BTW, is easily seen in the eyes (Eyology science—see www.eyology.com).

How Long Should I Stay on the GLD?

The length of the GLD is to be determined by you or your health professional based on such factors as your age, the degree of body tissue health, relative immune strength, your attitude (positive or negative), your home support system, how long it takes to eliminate or significantly diminish symptoms, and so on. A 30-day GLD is usually an excellent place to start the healing process. If I, your author, were diagnosed with a chronic degenerative disease, or otherwise if there were some significantly irritating symptoms, I'd get onto a GLD immediately. I do a 30-day GLD starting 3 January every year as a powerful <u>health promotive</u> (<u>not</u> as a disease preventive). Therefore, it is not about <u>disease</u>—it is about <u>health</u>!

The Four Levels of Healing Practice

Consider four levels of healing practice:

(1) The lowest form of medicine is **treatment**—which, of course, is sometimes necessary.

(2) Higher than that is disease **prevention**. But, notice that both treatment and prevention are about <u>disease</u>!

(3) Above prevention is **health promotion**, which deals strictly with engaging life-positive activities. It is not about disease. It is about health. Done rightly, health promotive activities help relieve and eliminate disease.

(4) However, the highest form of medicine is *health beyond cure*, or **Radical Healing**

Radical Healing—a term used by Adi Da Samraj to refer to submission to the Very Divine, and the prior presumption of radiant health as our birthright. It is about taking full responsibility (to the extent one is able) for one's health circumstance.

This fully responsible and accountable participation in the healing process must occur on the part of both healer and healee. It involves (1) turning to the Divine Reality, (2) right breathing, (3) right practice of conductivity, and (4) the counter-egoic use of the Devotional Prayer of Changes (Appendix E).

1—What IS the GREAT Liquid Diet?

What is its purpose?

The dietary process now known as **The GREAT Liquid Diet** (GLD, or GLDiet) was discovered and named by Traditional Naturopath Leonard Mehlmauer (ND, ret.) in 1975. It has since been used to help many patients, friends, students, colleagues, and family members. The basic principle: "less is more," in the sense that by reducing the food processing work needed by the mouth and GI tract, bodily energy is freed up for **purification**. And, BTW, in the case of health, and in life altogether, **purification** is the name of the game.

It's long been known that pure raw foods, with their high natural nutrient content, are healthier than cooked ones, where many nutrients are lost. But, raw or cooked, solid foods of most kinds take much energy for the mouth and stomach to break down (and for the rest of the GI tract to process). By blending the (mostly) raw foods, we get the nutrients—while *the blender (and juicer) do the chewing*—which helps both mouth and stomach.

But the good stuff doesn't end there. Most of us don't eat all-raw—or even <u>hi</u>-raw (like 80% raw). Many aren't even aware of the dangers of GMOs and pesticides. The fact that the GLD takes these into account is a major part of its success. And it gets better. The experience of nearly five decades (since 1972) of clinical and personal work provides the practical, realistic details of how the GLD applies in your life.

After seeing hundreds of cases of chronic disease healed or helped, we know the power of the GLD to change lives for the better. Weight loss, pain elimination, getting off drugs, increased longevity, and a more youthful appearance, are just side-effects of this gentle and amazing purification program. Children, the elderly—virtually anyone can do the GLD. Are you ready? Welcome!

The Pleasures of Eating

The poet said, "*You are locked into your suffering, and your pleasures are the seal.*" If you had to choose between eating whatever you wanted and eating in a way that brot health and freedom from disease, which would you choose? These two are not mutually exclusive, but there is a principle here that has to be carefully considered by those wishing to be healthy. Within our current "crazy random culture," the foods that we've learned to eat—and that are tasty—have been killing us by degrees, destroying our health.

Face it, some of us will choose to keep on eating whatever we want and whatever we like, even when we know very well that they are powerfully negatively affecting our health. We see this with cigarette and alcohol addicts, and it's basically the same with food. People with gross addictions of any kind may even be measured "geniuses," but they are singularly lacking in the wisdom needed in bringing discipline to the body-mind. We have to, at some point, admit a food addiction—and deal with it in a truly adult fashion, man or woman.

No need to belabor the fact that food-taking—along with sex—is among the most pleasurable activities in life. There are certain of us for whom eating is the single most enjoyable life event. So much the worse for them—especially if—because of their food addiction—they find themselves in a situation in which they must do without food for some period of time…like being fed thru an NG tube in a hospital!

No problem for those rare few who deeply understand the real function of food, and therefore enjoy the play of their relationship with it. No problem with them enjoying food "to the fullest." *Appropriate use and intelligent abstinence*—that's the rule—**if** we are going to enjoy good health while eating gross food. No need to necessarily totally eliminate lower quality foods. There's a time to eat otherwise "unhealthful" (celebratory) food, and a time to avoid it. Everything in its season.

Taste or Quality?
The trouble is, we Westerners, or otherwise those of us in this world who have plenty to eat, wind up eating plenty—and plenty of what our bodies don't need to be healthy. Plenty of what is difficult for the body to manage, with wastes that are polluting to the body, with hollow or missing nutrients, all with toxifying, disease-producing, and even (eventually) deadly results.

The infantile, childish, and adolescent approaches to food (see below) most often result in disease. Whereas, the adult approach allows balance, clarity, and purity. There is an allowance for the enjoyment of what others abuse. There is freedom instead of license. Intelligently applied (the adult approach), our diets can include almost anything, while—as a general rule—consciously and essentially (and at least most of the time) choosing that which brings real nourishment. There's nothing inherently wrong with enjoying tasty cooked and prepared food. But to indulge taste as a first principle over nourishment is often disastrous.

Creating a Foundation for That Which is Great
We will only take on a diet if it tastes good or otherwise makes us feel good. The GREAT Liquid Diet (GLD) does both. The GLD came about not as a carefully conceived plan to lose weight, cure disease, or to accomplish anything at all. It was more like an act of desperation to help a desperate

patient. It worked! And worked again and again, both for patients and for your author—who is now on some version of it frequently. And it can work for you.

However, since that first time, we've learned that there is a higher purpose for the GLD: true bodily equanimity. Bringing balance and longevity to the body allows for more easeful and effective religious and Spiritual practice. When the body is disease-free and lives longer, we have more clarity and focus in what is most important in life, in the real purpose of life: Blissfulness, Freedom, and Happiness—and more time to be effective in its realization: *We can love God better, longer, and more intimately when we don't have to deal with problems in the body!*

Food, as suggested, has nothing to do with spirit. Spirit is beyond body and mind. Food, then, in and of itself, is not Spiritual. But, food can certainly help provide a practical foundation for real Spiritual practice by eliminating those troublesome irritations referred to as our various bodily diseases. And, diet strongly influences the <u>etheric</u> body, the energy field that powers our nervous system and feeds the gross physical body thru our <u>emotions</u>. The <u>lower sense mind</u> is also powerfully affected by diet. This is easily proven: eat six candy bars for breakfast tomorrow morning and watch what happens with the mind and emotions!

The GLD is a way of eating, a "dietary delivery system" that enhances many healthful qualities, such as…

- Digestion (since liquids are generally more easily broken down in mouth and stomach)
- The efficiency of nutrient uptake (via "live" enzymes in raw natural liquids)
- More energy available to boost the Lymphatic-Immune
- The removal of burdensome wastes that ordinarily plague the body in the various forms of disease
- Nutrient quality (since most or all GLD food is raw natural)
- Overall greater purification than most diets by far
- The opportunity to observe one's dietary habits in a relaxed manner, and understand and transcend them

What You're Getting Into

Taking on the GLD means abandoning old habits of eating—at least for 30 days. (Yes, you can do this gradually.) It means moving into pure diet, a diet that includes increasingly higher percentages of raw foods. It means getting healthier, yes, and facing and overcoming negative patterns and tendencies of food taking. This is an important step in diet and life, and <u>necessarily a gradual process</u>—unless there is a chronic disease that demands immediate access to the benefits of the liquids (in which case, let's just get busy, waste no time, get right into the higher aspects of the 30-Day GLD—Level One—and get the job done!).

For most of us, it is going to be a gradual process of moving to increasingly higher percentages of raw foods—*as liquids*. It takes the average adult 2½ years to phase off the typical North American junked-up diet and into the pure foods hi-raw or all raw veggy diet. Therefore, don't be in a hurry. On the other hand, why wait and get sicker? Why put off the great rewards of the GLD? One doesn't <u>have</u> to take 2½ years! You can accomplish an all-raw diet in 4 weeks—either thru solid foods or thru the 30-Day GLD.

The GLD, Raw Solid Foods, and the Principle of Fasting
The GLD is <u>not</u> a fast. A fast is thin juices and water—or just water and herb tea. But, the GLD works on the same principle as a fast: when the body is denied solid foods, it goes into a **purification** mode. Of course, the body will go into a generally purifying mode by simply eating all raw foods <u>as solids</u>. With fasting, the body purifies itself far more rapidly than on raw or any other <u>solids</u>. The length of the fast depends on several factors, most of them specific to the faster's case (age, relative health, immune strength, willingness to participate, etc.).

When solid foods enter the body, at each meal, <u>an average of **25%**</u> of the body's total energy comes to bear on the stomach—to digest the food. Compare that to <u>an average of **5%**</u> for a juice fast, and you'll see why a fast is so "fast" at cleansing the body.

Mainly, that extra 20% of energy that would have gone to digestion is now freed up for cleansing and **purification**. And please note: the body knows exactly what to do when it doesn't have to work on digesting solid food! Out prance the tiny guys with the "brooms" (the white blood cells) to do their amazing work.

Fasting is a wonderful, tried-and-true means of cleansing the body. Jesus Christ is reputed to have fasted for 40 days. Many historical figures have written about their fasting experiences. Fasting is simply an intelligent means of periodically cleansing accumulating junk that invariably finds its way into the body—whether intentionally or not. And fasting will definitely lengthen life. Trouble is, most people are either afraid of fasting, believe it to be unnecessary or harmful, lack the needed discipline for it, or for other reasons just won't do it.

The GLD, however, is much easier to do—and much more fun—than either whole raw foods or fasting. A fast is not fun. And you can do many things on the GLD that you cannot do on a fast. Like a snack! You can accomplish just as much and more on the GLD as on a fast, altho purification will take longer on the GLD.

Not everyone can fast, but upwards of 98% of human adults can do the GLD. And most children. The typical 30-Day GLD requires <u>an average of only *8%*</u> of total body energy per full meal. That leaves a lot of energy for cleansing and purification.

How the GLD Works

There are *four basic principles* that make the GLD effective:

VEGETAL Vegetable foods are superior to animal foods for human health. They contain energy directly from the sun and Earth. Killed animal flesh, and animal by-products, while useable as food, are second-hand nutrition.

RAW *Live* vegetal foods are better for our health than are any cooked foods. Generally, the higher the percentage of raw vegetal foods we eat (various portions of fruits, veggies, and nuts/seeds), the healthier we are.

LIQUID If we take raw vegetal foods *as liquids*, we lessen the stress on bodily systems. Careful chewing of raw vegetal (or any) food is important for many reasons. But on the GLD, machines do most of this chewing for us. This means less food processing stress on the body, thus increasing available energy for the crucial **purification**.

FULL NUTRIENT RANGE Fasting is taking thin liquids for maximum bodily purification. But, we can fast only for so many days before the body begins to starve, to self-digest. With the full nutrient range of the GLD's blended and juices liquids (fruits, veggies, nuts and seeds), plus the bulk and ruffage, we can take these tasty liquids indefinitely and thus sustain the health and life of the body optimally.

The fact that liquids are being taken simplifies the process of eating quite significantly—and cuts way back on the kinds of foods taken, including all those "goodies" that corrupt the body. We don't blend or juice hamburgers, fries, pizza, or fried chicken on the GLD. And there's no need to count calories, either. The food taken on the GLD is essentially pure, natural, and mostly (or even all) raw: blended and juiced fruits, veggies and nuts/seeds, and perhaps even blended cooked and/or hot raw veggy soups.

There are other blender and juicer drinks, and even some purchased liquids like amazake and home-prepared hot raw carob and raw cocoa drinks and herb teas. Deliciously rich coconut-avo-banana smoothies. And many others that are possible. And the snacks, and the fact that when it's time to celebrate someone's birthday or wedding one can, if necessary, take a solid food meal and get right back onto the GLD. You can't do these things on a fast.

The GLD can, of course, be used effectively for weight loss—a huge plus for many people these days. But perhaps its greatest general public appeal and effectiveness is with alleviating or eliminating chronic degenerative disease—if not for the gaining and maintaining of good, balanced health. And, the GLD shines as a steady and ongoing dietary practice for older age and longevity. Many use it to just stay healthy—by doing a 30 Day GLD yearly.

For dealing with anything from arthritis to zinc deficiency, from colds to cancer, the GLD as a diet excels. As a healing mode, it's quick when compared to solid food diets, even all-raw veggie diets, and yet it's mild and relatively easy on the body when compared to fasting. The GLD is using our technology (especially the blender, but also the juicer, citrus juice extractor, water distiller, and even food dehydrator) intelligently.

Wave Good-bye to Hospitals, Doctors, and Dentists
The GLD is basically all liquids. No chewing required. Well, OK, a little, to get oral enzymes going. So, how hard is that on your teeth!? Yes, continue to brush your teeth after "meals." Your teeth can continue to grow and enamelize, hard and clean, unimpeded. The GLD's prime recipe, *the Green Smoothie*, is most important.

Then, there's the RMVJ (it's the deep red juice pictured below), involving juicing 3 carrots, 2 apples, half a cucumber (or zucchini), 1/3rd of a lemon with peel, 1/3rd of beet, a garlic bud the size of the last digit of your thumb, and two sticks of celery (see Recipes chapter). How quickly could you eat all that produce in solid form? Jaws getting tired yet? You get tired thinking about it. In juice form, you can get it down in a few minutes—and it's delicious!

All that nutrition-dense power speeding to your cells! Later, add a green smoothie (a fruit-veggy-nut blender drink) and you've got all the daily nutrition bases covered. Soon, your health problems are gone, gone, gone! *Note*: The photo here includes, from top L to R: fresh real orange juice, RMVJ, coconut-almond milk, a spirulina smoothie; 2nd row: blueberry smoothie, strawberry smoothie; bottom row: mango smoothie.

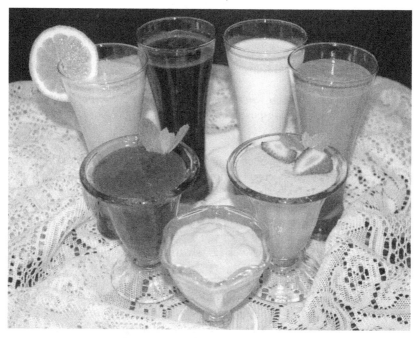

Allopathic medicine is good at acute care, emergency care, like when we break an arm or leg, or otherwise are in pain. And it can be good at certain diagnostics. But when it comes to treating chronic or degenerative disease processes, or even the common cold, it's lost. It just wants to throw drugs at them. This is where Traditional, Natural, and the so-called Complementary medicines shine.

Some even suggest that 90% or more of Allopathic medicine is bogus, harmful, wasteful, and dangerous. Mainly, because drugs don't cure disease. They are not designed to cure. Cure isn't desirable to Big Pharma. That would cut into their profits—from selling drugs. Drugs can take away pain and dilate tissues, but otherwise—and even in those cases—they actually contribute to disease by toxifying the body.

OK, so how long will this process of getting well take us while on the GLD? Ask yourself this: How long did it take for you to get into this diseased state!? Using your GLD, it won't take anywhere near that long to get out of it. Nature can seem slow to work, but given the right tools, she'll get the job done. Enter pure raw foods—especially in liquefied form. These are her tools, along with *The BIG 7.*

- early bedtime
- daily exercise
- natural sunshine

- positive thinking
- clean, orderly and positive environments
- right activity
- Spiritual study

What can happen when everything you do is life-positive? What are the logical results? Life-positive!

The On-going Diet Experiment

Correct diet depends on so many things: genetic inheritance factors, environmental changes, age, and various other social, cultural, emotional, and other influences. It takes much observation by self and others—especially expert others, at least initially—to do it right. It needs to be designed and developed against various imbalances and symptoms that occur within our current Western culture. Imbalances can appear from eating any kind of food, including raw foods. One can over-eat raw fruit bars, e.g., and get symptoms of imbalance.

Certain of us can feel too cold on raw foods, or move too strongly into the etheric and away from the vital physical to where we feel like we're floating above the body. ***A raw diet has to be adapted to gradually and intelligently***. This whole process takes <u>conscious awareness</u>—on our part as well as that of our health practitioner. We learn by adaptation and experiment. But, we must stay with this process of adaptation to hi raw or all raw to see how this diet thing works. The GLD can make this simple.

Diet will necessarily change over time, anyway—at least thru bodily aging. The stomach does not work as well after age 45 or so. The influences of life come to bear. We travel and cannot get the food we are used to or have learned is best for us. But, **raw natural veggy diet is the primary way to get and stay well** because <u>the gross physical body is a *food body*</u> designed by Nature to receive food as it comes in Nature (which means <u>not</u> cooked).

Raw diet maintains health, vitality, and energy. When some of us—because of our specific genetic makeup—get into too many sweet foods, our blood sugar can spike and dip, swinging wildly. If we get too cold while eating raw foods, we may need heat-producing substances like cayenne (capsicum) or ginger to add to the diet, both of which bring heat to the body. Or simply have some hot cacao. Too much raw garlic—altho it may keep the vampires at bay(!), and is excellent for lowering blood pressure and killing parasites—can over-stimulate the immune system and slow signal transmission in the corpus callosum of the brain.

So, imbalances can occur even on a raw diet, and we need to be conscious and mindful of these changes. We shouldn't let deficiencies and imbalances continue. Nuts and seeds, e.g., and also chilies and hot peppers, are stimulating—including to the sex drive and sex impulse. But, without nuts and seeds, the body can become depleted. We must learn to use them rightly. Raw foods serve both *thin*-body types, who tend to lose weight rapidly, and also *thick*-body types, who seem to gain weight merely by thinking about food. We need only apply the hi-raw or all-raw diet <u>rightly</u>, noting what works for us and what doesn't <u>as individuals</u>. This way, we have everything to gain.

So, what does all this discussion of raw solids have to do with the GLD? First, it helps to know why we're using such a hi percentage of raw food on the GLD. Second, it helps prepare us for the solid food meals we'll be eating when we're not taking the GLD. You get a clearer sense of the how and the why of raw foods as you proceed along on your GLD—and how it all applies in your case. It gets clearer and easier as you go along.

The GLD as a Life Monitor

Amidst your practice of the GLD, you'll come across many signs and patterns in yourself—physical, mental, and emotional, some of which you won't particularly like. You'll see certain life-negative habits you've developed and adapted to regarding food, like using it exclusively to pleasurize or entertain yourself—even when you're not hungry—instead of just rightly nourishing the body. Such habits are part of the reason we suffer our physical diseases.

We will see that doing the GLD and *The BIG 7* are not merely about physical issues, but also about <u>how we approach life altogether</u>. We will see our tendencies just by taking on the disciplines of the GLD in the context of *The BIG 7*. Therefore, the GLD offers us an educational opportunity. We can use it to grow in our understanding—of ourselves and our culture. Meanwhile, done rightly, thoughtfully, and with proper guidance, most of us will be helped on all levels, even quite significantly.

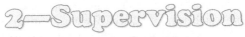

2—Supervision

The importance of right guidance

Whenever a highly purifying dietary process is engaged (e.g., fasting and liquid dieting), particular possibilities arise. There can be (and eventually is, with true cleansing practices) a ***reversal of symptoms*** in those who have developed chronic diseases. This will especially be so if a drug suppressed the symptoms of the original disorder. This means that the disease you had before the one you're currently suffering may well appear—**briefly**, if your GLD Program is being done correctly.

Some of these <u>purification / toxic elimination events</u>, altho relatively brief when compared to the suffering of the original <u>disease</u> symptoms, can be irritating. And then, of course, there is the initial and occasional displeasure of hunger pangs (see below). As you'll learn on the GLD, it's OK to feel hunger. Truly. To some, however, this is unacceptable—especially when they have plenty of tasty food in the house and otherwise available to them. And, because our crazy random culture has little knowledge of or sympathy for fasting and purifying regimes, all of this can be frightening to the beginner.

Hunger Pangs

The economy and purity of the food (as raw liquids) on the GLD allows the body to last far longer without the hunger pangs common to fasting. When they do occur, the pangs are not as strident and irritating as are those that occur when many hours pass between solid food meals. Additionally, the body requires an overall smaller volume of food intake (the liquids) since much of the ruffage has been broken down by the blender. BTW, here's a tip on dealing with hunger pangs: wait a few minutes—they'll pass!

In the excellent book on diet, <u>*Green Gorilla*</u>, we learn that fasting or otherwise missing regular meals is actually our normal and natural situation. (What? Did I read that right? Yes!) In Anthropology, we learn that hunter-gatherers lived this way for hundreds of thousands of years. We wandered from place to place, the young men out looking for an animal to kill while the women, children, and elders foraged for fruits, nuts, seeds, berries, and edible herbs. When the young men came back without an animal, and we otherwise couldn't find food, we went without.

Yes, we learned to carry extra food for those in the most need—the growing young and the feeble old. But, without refrigeration of some kind, available food stashes can spoil. They must be continually replenished. Therefore, fasting was common. Not because we wanted to, of course. We went hungry a lot of the time. Fasting, then—not eating—was, for most of our existence as human beings, normal to us.

However this may be, we're not suggesting you go around starving yourself on your GLD! Of course not. What we are saying, however, is that you will get hungry more often than when on solid foods. You will feel what could be called a "low-grade" hunger. Even lots of that. It comes and goes. What we're suggesting is that you take some liquids when you are clearly and definitely hungry—and not every few minutes that you feel a desire for food!

So, don't be afraid of being hungry on your GLD. It's a sure sign of purification—at least at some level. When you're doing your GLD right, the purification is occurring at <u>every</u> level! And that's a lot of levels—gross physical, vital, etheric, emotional, lower mind, higher mind, psyche, astral, and even causal. Getting hungry, feeling hungry—this is good! This is normal on your GLD. When you learn what is actually happening within the body during them, you'll look forward to the hunger pangs. You'll welcome them and be very glad for them!

Choosing the Right Guide

Altho quite safe when done rightly (and it's so easy to do rightly), engaging the Great Liquid Diet requires not only instruction (as described here in this book), but also at least (at first) some expert guidance. Such guidance is necessary with certain chronic degenerative disorders or otherwise difficult disease circumstances are present—and also with those who lose weight rapidly (see below). Among the practitioners to look for are the Traditional and Modern Naturopaths, those with "ND" after their name.

Many of the old-fashioned Nutritionists and holistic practitioners can also be helpful, <u>especially those experienced in fasting and raw diet</u>. You want someone with experience in fasting, both with patients and with themselves, personally. Meanwhile, times are changing in medicine, and more MDs are becoming aware of the importance of learning about holistic and natural procedures. But, with MDs, <u>they must have the experience</u>. You should consult only those who do. This is one of the first questions you'll ask them to qualify them.

The chances of someone developing a real problem on the GLD, when following directions as given, are estimated at less than 2%. Therefore, the likelihood of success is 98+%! But, just to be completely safe, for insurance against that small percentage of negative possibility, hedge your bets: always have your Natural Health Practitioner's fone number and email address handy for guidance and reference. If you have any doubts or concerns about your health condition during a GLD, that's a sign you need guidance.

The healer you <u>don't</u> want is one who looks at you merely as a body to put drugs (or even herbs!) into, who says, "Well, you have this disease, so let's give you this drug (or herb)." You want the one who treats you holistically, as a body of energy, as a part of Nature, a creature of this Earth—like birds and trees, dependent on pure air and water, pure food, and loving energy.

You want a healer who (in other words) treats *the whole person*, one who understands the importance of the emotional component, and one who will require you to be responsible for these qualities. The real healer will (1) get to the bottom of how you got the disease, (2) make sure you understand this and what to do about it, and (3) *demand that you do it!* S/he will be practiced in the use of natural therapies.

> *In Western Culture, our minds are typically full of doubt. There is so little trust. We are so often lacking in faith, having lost our connection with Sacred Tradition. But every heart wants the Guidance of True Authority from Those Who Have Awakened. With that Guidance, we can create a Wisdom Culture. We can, and we must!*

This expert guidance and counseling can help you feel safe and secure during the initial days and weeks of your GLD. Some dietary and herb supplements may be needed according to your health situation. Chronic diseases usually require the use of such supplemental aids. This is the domain of Natural Health professionals. As your GLD—and your health—progresses, and you clearly notice improvements, your need for such supplements will necessarily diminish in number and kind.

Your Natural Health professional will assist you in cutting back on such supplements. If you are on pharma drugs or medications, your prescribing physician should lower the dose or eliminate the drug as you get well and symptoms are eliminated. If s/he doesn't, and you are feeling great and know very well you don't need a drug in this or that amount, or even at all, fire him/her. Go only to medical professionals you trust.

Avatar Adi Da Suggests that…

(1) minor health problems can be managed one-on-one by local healers
(2) health ailments of moderate significance should be dealt with within a community setting, and
(3) disorders of major importance need medical diagnosis and appropriate treatment
We at Grand Medicine feel that such appropriate treatment can surely include the GLD.

Length of Time Needed to be on the GLD
The length of time needed to see these positive changes varies according to several factors, such as age, relative immune strength (which always rises on the GLD), attitude, will and desire to be well, severity and

current state of the disease, the support (or lack thereof) of those around you, materials availability, and so forth. Health improvement is usually faster on the GLD than on any other diet. Bear in mind that it usually takes years of diet and lifestyle abuse to develop chronic degenerative diseases (no praise, no blame).

With Natural Health practices like the GLD, however, the time of the needed purification, harmonization, and regeneration is far less than on most other health regimes. Be content to remain in place and practice patience on your GLD. Be grateful that you now have a program that works! All you need do is follow it—one day at a time—to the best of your ability. So you're going to miss some solid food meals. Big deal! Considering the potentially enormous benefits, it's worth it.

A seasoned healer will understand that when the irritation of some disease purification arises on the GLD, you should simply persist, perhaps with a special technique (herb poultice, oral pain reliever, hot bath) being added to alleviate the situation. Sometimes, simple bed rest is all that's needed. It may even be appropriate to take a pharmaceutical pain medication temporarily. Again, those on various prescription medications are encouraged to check with their prescribing physicians periodically to allow for the elimination of such drugs.

The intensity of purification on the GLD is modified by the quality and viscosity of the liquids taken in. Natural fruits and veggies are essential to the GLD, as are fresh raw nuts and/or seeds. (Incidentally, were you aware that before food chemicals came into being, all produce was natural?) The percentage of raw vs. cooked liquids makes a difference, too, in the level of purification and tissue rebuilding. Your Natural Health practitioner is responsible for guiding you thru these determinations—especially if you have a chronic degenerative disease.

"Fundamentally, [I recommend] the practice of assuming that you do not have a 'problem' of health. Rather, you have an obligation for health, and not a 'problem' to be corrected. When the body's functioning is limited in any way, yield the body to the lawful situation in which the condition may be set right, rather than presuming a 'problem' and seeking a solution. When the systems-based approach is applied, healing is straightforward.

"Part of the process is time—one establishes the lawful practice and then allows the body time to show its signs. If there is to be well-being, the body must be yielded to its unified circumstance in the unity of its natural domain. How is that yielding accomplished? Simply by establishing the lawfulness of bodily discipline. The body is a food process. Fundamentally, it does not need to be cured. One needs simply to stop bothering the body with "self"-

indulgent habits of life, stop throwing it out of balance, stop maintaining it unlawfully.

"In reality, you are your own 'problem', and that is why you are always functioning as if you have one. The problem-free or searchless approach to discipline, rather than the search for a solution to a 'problem', is the principle of right-life practice. When you accept the discipline of lawfulness that I describe, healing is a spontaneous manifestation of the bodily life. Fundamentally, you leave the body alone. You observe its signs, rather than trying to manipulate it into well-being."
—Avatar Adi Da Samraj

In these passages, Avatar Adi Da is not suggesting we do nothing and allow whatever disease condition to go its way. No. There are positive things we can do toward helping in the health-giving process—including the GLD. Here, he is pointing to the great importance of doing right life disciplines—*The BIG 7*, e.g., He is talking about us moving away from our wrong use of the LQFs and of any and all other life-negative habits and patterns.

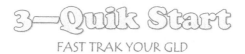

FAST TRAK YOUR GLD

Here's the quick way to get started on your GLD.

For details, check the appropriate chapters, including the Materials and Products List and Recipes at the end of this book. For more, go to <u>www.GLDiet.co</u> and sign up free for the full 30-Day GLD Notes. Once there, get access to the whole higher-way-of-life by clicking on GLDLifestyle.

How Long Does it Take to Make Liquids?

Whether you make them yourself or have someone prepare them for you, it takes about <u>6 minutes to prepare the average daily Green Smoothie</u>, start to finish—a handful of greens, a piece of fruit or two, and some water into the blender, blend, pour, then rinse the blender. More elaborate liquids with multiple ingredients require more time. If you can afford 5-10 minutes or so, you're set.

Setting up Your GLD Kitchen

1 – *Purchase a blender, a juicer, and an enema bottle* (see Appendix B). There are *cheaper* blenders and juicers, and there are *pricier* ones, but those listed here are for people serious about a lifetime of diet purity and improved health.

JUICER = *Omega®, e.g., J8000HDS* ($292) *or NC900HDC* ($395); it's called a *VitalMax® Oscar 300* in Australia

BLENDER = *VitaMix® 5000* or later model (USA and Canada; about $300USD, www.vitamix.com; in Australia, the *Breville® Optiva* is OK; in Iceland, choose the *VitaPrep* which is by *VitaMix*.

ENEMA BOTTLE = *Faultless*® or equivalent (at drug and department stores) Get the full kit with accessories—bag, tube, nozzle, etc. (not the fleet enema)—about $20.

2 – *Buy pure natural produce (or grow your own).* Check out the recipes (Appendix A), then go to the nearest natural foods market or farmer's market and purchase natural unsprayed produce for your recipes, such as carrots, celery, chard, broccoli, kale, baby spinach, beets, lemons, apples, avocadoes, unsweetened shredded coconut, bananas, almonds, pure coconut sugar, dates, oranges, and pure water. Nothing chemical/pesticide sprayed or GMO.

Getting into the GLD Lifestyle

3 – *Make your Green Smoothie*. The Green Smoothie recipes are in Appendix A. The Green Smoothie is meant to be the first drink of the day, or otherwise your most important drink, it tastes OK-to-good-to-REALLY-good, depending on how you make it, and it satisfies your basic nutrition requirement for vegetables, fruits, and even nuts.

4 – *Make another drink*. Perhaps your RMVJ (a juice) or an avocado smoothie (see Recipes)—both favorites. Some drinks satisfy all three nutrition requirements—veggies, fruits, and nuts/seeds—and can be especially tasty.

5 – *Read* Chapter 13 on *The BIG 7*. It describes the practices we urge everyone to be doing on the GLD—and into the future—practices that help free your body from disease and harmonize your life:

The BIG 7

- Diet purity via hi-raw or all-raw natural food
- Regular appropriate exercise
- Early bedtime—adequate rest and sleep
- Daily hygiene—keeping the body clean
- Clean and wholesome environments
- Right occupation—using your time wisely
- Spiritual—cultivating the Divine

BOTTOM LINE on the GLD: The GLD, in the context of *The BIG 7,* is likely the quickest way to get and stay whole-bodily healthy—short of fasting (which not everyone can do). It's a clever and exciting way of getting raw foods into the body and a gentle and conservative way to eliminate disease conditions. It's really all about **purification**—the most important thing in life (as you'll see, not just for the body).

Raw foods aren't as tasty as the great cuisines of the Chinese or the French, but are tasty enuf and far better for us. And remember, it's likely essentially life-negative (junk) food that gets most of us into problems with the body, and it's these raw liquids that'll go the longest way to get us out! *The BIG 7* is a complete and truly adult life-positive way of living. (Don't think about it another minute. *Just do it!*)

It is thru our association with The Divine that we transform the world.

4—Basic Rules to Follow
Guidelines for Success

- **Rule #1** – *Gross body equanimity* or balance thru **purification** is the *basic purpose* of the Great Liquid Diet (GLD). Genuine equanimity of body and mind supports preparation for (and actual practice of) real Spiritual life. Improved health is merely a result or side-issue that occurs thru right use of the GLD, and is not rightly its primary goal or purpose.

- **Rule #2** – *Do your GLD under the supervision or guidance* of a trained and experienced professional—especially if you have a chronic degenerative disease (and also if you've never fasted or taken a hi-raw diet). When your health is regained, and you've had sufficient experience on your GLD, you may continue to use it on your own.

- **Rule #3** – *Take only liquids* while on the GLD. Generally avoid eating solid foods during the GLD, as these will slow the progress of purification and balance essential to its work at the gross level. Exceptions and guidelines are noted below, that may include certain snacks, but these instances generally include holidays and other celebratory occasions—however, even then, only as appropriate.

- **Rule #4** – *Eat from the three basic food groups daily*:

    —Fresh raw ripe in-season preferably locally-grown natural unsprayed fruits
    —Raw natural unsprayed veggies
    —Raw fresh nuts and/or seeds
    —Certain grasses (wheatgrass/barley grass) and sprouts may also be taken in juice or blended form, plus soups and other liquids.

- **Rule #5** – *Bowel cleansing* is important (altho not crucial) on your GLD. Toxic waste builds up in the bowel during the GLD, in addition to embedded wastes that have been in there for years. BMs (bowel movements) usually (will, in certain cases) slow down on the GLD. For good health, the bowels must move. If and as necessary, employ entero lavage (bowel washing) as enema, colema, or colonic irrigation, self-administered or by others (bowel cleansing procedure described below).

- **Rule #6** – *Chew Your Liquids* The great nutritionists of the past and present all agree: careful chewing before swallowing—even of liquids—significantly aides in breaking down and preparing the food factors for further processing by introducing special enzymes for improved nutrient digestion, absorption, and assimilation.

- Rule #7 – **Do *the BIG 7*** while on your GLD, including right use of the Low Quality Foods (LQFs—see Ch. 12). What you avoid is as important as what you do. Doing everything life-positive assures your success. Right diet and lifestyle are keys to positive health progress. Establish this *BIG 7* foundation for longer life in better health.

- Rule #8 – **Attitude** You now have a plan for good health and balance in life. An *attitude of gratitude* is appropriate. The continuous heartfelt chant, *"Thank you, Lord!"* is not only intelligent; it dramatically boosts immunity. Stay positive about your GLD. The company of positive people, too, will help keep your spirits up.

- Rule #9 – **Quantity,** The average time between intakes of your GLD liquids is two to three hours. This will vary with several factors (age, energy output, specific health condition, the viscosity of liquids, etc.).

Breaking the Rules

Rules, they say, are made to be broken. Another saying, however, is, "Break the rules at your peril!" Both of these apply to the GLD. Ask yourself (or your trained health practitioner), "How much leeway do I have?"

If you are in relatively good health, with no symptoms as such, no clinically treatable disorders, then you have more room to "play around" with natural-style snacks and maybe even a solid food meal—certainly more than those with chronic disease circumstances. Everyone taking on the GLD does so for his and her own reasons, and you will see results according to your application of the above "Basic Rules."

The GLD is an opportunity to learn about yourself, your tendencies and patterns, some of which are of very long standing—even from past lifetimes. As you go along in your GLD, you will learn your strengths and weaknesses, where your will power starts and where it ends. There is no praise or blame in this. Meanwhile, as you do more GLDs, you will learn and grow, you will improve. And everyone around you will benefit!

The GLD is not fun. It is not meant to be fun. There are all manner of things we'd rather do than drink raw liquids for a whole month. HOWEVER, it's the growth factor that's most important here. To grow for real as a human being, by whatever means, is always important. The GLD presents this opportunity. Going thru it to the finish brings a sense of accomplishment. But that is only one of many benefits, most of which are hidden from easy view.

Five Qualities, Limitations, Orientations, or in some sense
Roadblocks to Correct Dieting and Purifying Practices*

1 – *Egoity* (our constant activity and sense of separation from people, things, life, God, etc.)

2 – *Seeking* (in our egoity, engaging the GLD—and anything else—as a strategy to <u>accomplish</u> something to extract ourselves from some real or imagined dilemma, rather than simply doing it as something appropriate to the body's periodic cleansing, purification, and balance)

3 – *Yes / No Extremes* (being caught in the paradoxical nature of this conditional realm: what's good, what's bad, and going to one extreme or another in that regard)

4 – *Stages of Life Prejudices and Illusions* (engaging or avoiding the GLD according to the ideas and concepts characteristic of your current stage of life)

5 – *Great Tradition Orientation* (engaging the GLD according to the various cultural, ethnic, racial, economic, political, social and other qualities of the background or tradition you were raised in)

*Adapted from Avatar Adi Da's Teachings by your author to in some way apply in the GLD context.

Vis-à-vis the above, our recommendation is…just do it!

You may jump into the GLD for the best of reasons. Cleansing, purification, weight loss. Then, in the midst of it, you find yourself "playing around," getting into the snacks—especially late at nite, after a hard day's work, and feeling the need for some "entertainment." Who could blame you for that? Food, of course, is helpless. The refrigerator doesn't have a voice that says, "*Hey, wait a minute. You don't need anything in here.*" So, you go for some cheese. You go to the pantry for a few crackers. You grab a beer. And a few pretzels.

"We ARE what we EAT!"

Next day, you step on the scale and learn you've **gained** a pound, not lost it! What the hell!? Hey, no one did this to you. You did it. Fess up. Are you ready to take this challenge? Are you ready to go beyond this tendency in yourself? It's completely your call. And it will be easier if you have a GLD buddy you can make this confession to, describing what happened to a sympathetic ear. If your buddy encourages you to turn to the Divine for Help while you are right in the midst of your craving, you've got a real friend. You'll grow accordingly!

5—The Basic GLD Outline

Getting Into the Groove

The Great Liquid Diet (GLD) is a dietary concept developed by Leonard Mehlmauer of Grand Medicine in the mid-1970s. It was conceived as a means of allowing significant purification, balance, and regeneration in clients who were grossly overweight, obese, and/or otherwise challenged by chronic degenerative disease circumstances.

Such people often cannot be helped by fasting, since either (1) prolonged fasting would not likely be followed or would be otherwise exceedingly difficult—as in the obese/overweight—or (2) they need a continuous supply of rich, high-quality nutrients in a most efficient delivery system—as in those with cancer and other such disease situations, which fasting would not provide. Done rightly, the GLD can be engaged under the widest variety of health circumstances, especially in the high-stress environments so prevalent today. For this, the GLD is perfect!

The GLD is called "GREAT" because it is like a "trump card" that we can pull out to deal with health situations that are particularly difficult—and when other means of handling physical diseases and disorders aren't working. Over time, it just seems to manage everything. The longer one is on the GLD, the more problems get resolved—and the healthier one becomes! In fact, as long as you are doing it correctly (and therefore getting the basic daily requirements), you can remain on it indefinitely—meaning years and years—even for the rest of your life!

On your GLD, it is quite important to get *the three basic requirements* daily: (1) fresh raw <u>fruits,</u> (2) fresh raw <u>veggies</u>, and (3) fresh raw <u>nuts</u> and/or <u>seeds</u>. There are numerous ways of accomplishing this (see Recipes), especially by getting just one type of drink daily—the green *smoothie,* which includes fruit, veggies, & nuts/seeds.

For **extra weight loss**, emphasize juices, and also smoothies with thinner viscosity. Especially try the delicious *RMVJ*, which includes both fruits and veggies. Other liquids may include herb teas, various fresh fruit and veggy juices, and cooked and raw soups. Also, be strict with the raw liquids, and avoid snacks and any solid foods.

For **weight gain**—even while getting significant purification—emphasize the thicker liquids, those with higher viscosity. The avocado-banana-coconut smoothie is an example. Focus on drinks containing nuts and seeds, which are rich in healthy natural fats and oils (for more on fats and oils, see Ch 11). Also, drink more, of course.

In getting the daily basic nutrition requirements on the GLD, be sure to *try to get fresh, raw, in-season, locally-grown natural non-GMO produce whenever possible*. Best of all, of course, would be natural unsprayed fruits and veggies grown in your own garden *with natural compost*. Do whatever it takes to get natural unsprayed and non-GMO, usually available at your local farmer's market.

VERY IMPORTANT: *CHEW ALL OF YOUR LIQUIDS THOROUGHLY!* Even though your diet will consist of virtually 100% liquids, for optimum nourishment it needs to be predigested in your mouth before entering your stomach. (For those with weak stomachs, this is crucial!) Chewing accomplishes this nicely. Further breakdown of your food—and therefore enhanced digestion, absorption, and assimilation—is thus assured.

GLD Basic Daily Nutrition Requirements
- *Daily fresh fruit* (as ripe, preferably natural, in-season juices and smoothies)
- *Daily fresh veggies* (as liquids—especially the Green Smoothie—and also as broths, and raw and cooked soups)
- *Daily fresh raw nuts &/or seeds* (as blended into smoothies)

You may also take other liquids, of course—even healthy "entertaining" ones. Typically, your GLD day will include at least one green smoothie—a blender drink containing a handful of green veggies, one or more pieces of fruit, and sufficient pure water or home-made nut-seed milk. Also, there may well be some type of raw veggy drink—like RMVJ (Raw Mixed Veggy Juice). The Green Smoothie is the most important drink on your GLD. It covers the daily nutritional requirements. And there are many (and delicious) ways to make a green smoothie!

Why 30 Days?
Thirty days allows for a significant break from our daily intake of solid foods—most of which, unfortunately, include cooked, processed, chemicalized, and otherwise less-than-healthy preparations. Missing 90-odd such meals (@ 3 per day)...

— (1) provides real purification at all energetic levels of our being

— (2) allows us time to observe and consider the often deeply embedded life-negative habits and patterns of eating and lifestyle activities we have developed over the years of our life

— (3) affords us a genuine and rare opportunity to adapt to new and life-positive forms of eating and living so we can grow in real human terms

The Smoothie's Liquid Medium
Altho there are several possible pure liquids one could use for a smoothie (e.g., raw juice, nut milk, seed milk, pure cold or hot water, RMVJ),

the most common are water and nut-seed milk. An average-sized adult will likely use about 12 oz. (300 gm) of liquid. Use water for something quick and not so rich. Use (always homemade) nutmilk for a richer taste (see Raw Almond-Cashew Milk). The recipe for Extra Rich Nutmilk can be used 50:50 with water or even straight for those feeling the need for a very rich taste. Your best water is steam distilled.

A Typical Day on the GLD
Of course, there is no such thing as a "typical day." Every day is different in this Earth realm. But, on the GLD there are certain items in everyone's day that are necessarily similar:

- Taking liquid meals
- Getting the three nutrition basics—fruits, veggies, nuts &/or seeds
- Our individualized and creative use of *The BIG 7* life-positive lifestyle

Let's plot a day that includes certain *BIG 7* lifestyle features that could happen fairly regularly for us. Here (below) are some suggestions among the many creative possibilities. You can arrange your daily routine or schedule according to your personal circumstance. Be realistic, but consider adding at least one item per week that you don't currently do but that you know will help round out a good, strong, balanced lifestyle.

Rising early, we hit the **restroom** (bathroom, lavatory, loo), go directly to the communion hall for prayer and **meditation** (see Appendix F), then snuggle into a comfortable chair and do our **Spiritual study**. **Exercise** comes next, perhaps a 20-30 minute Power Walk, calisthenics, or exercise machine. **Dry brush** all over, then a nice hot **shower** follows. Next, as hunger starts, we begin our **dietary** day with a cup of herb tea, or a green smoothie, or RMVJ, or a glass of fresh-squeezed orange juice. Breakfast is the way we "break-the-fast" of last nite's sleep.

If we're going to **work**, we then take the opportunity to prepare thermoses of liquids for work. Perhaps we **lunch** on (1) a peanut butter smoothie, (2) our RMVJ, and (3) a hot raw veggy broth. At the office, these keep us going thru our breaks and lunchtime, all the way 'til quitting time. Back at home, we may check out the evening **news** on the Net to keep up with what's happening in the world. We do our **yoga**, and then a special treat. We fix ourselves a nice **hot chocolate drink**, using raw carob powder, raw cacao powder, sweetened with coconut sugar.

If we need extra weight, or if we're going crazy for something non-liquid, we might take a Tbsp. of sesame butter ("tahini") or raw almond butter. Our menu is always changing, always fresh, with new items rotating around the basics: fruits, veggies, and nuts/seeds. Then **dinner**: an avocado smoothie provides the fruit and nut/seed requirement, while a Green Smoothie or raw veggy broth (or RMVJ) handles the needed (and most important) raw vegetables. We relax into some **entertainment** with a hot cup of **herb tea**, finishing the day with **prayers**, perhaps meditation, and early **bedtime**.

Some Suggested Typical Daily Liquids (see Recipes)
- Herb tea (e.g., mint, fresh ginger root)
- Green Smoothie (greens, peach, nutmilk)
- Raw almond butter smoothie
- Orange coconut mint smoothie
- RMVJ (or other fresh-made veggy juice)
- Avocado Smoothie
- Hot cocoa drink
- Strawberry kale apple smoothie

There will necessarily be differences in your day on the GLD, depending on your circumstances, both specifically and generally. Bed-ridden and wheelchair people will not be doing the kinds of exercise as those who are ambulatory. You won't take the same liquids day in and day out, week in and week out. There will be other variations in your schedule.

Eventually, you may drop the soup from your routine—IF you began it in the first place. To lose weight more rapidly, you will avoid the snacks, get into thinner liquids, and take only herb teas within 2 hours of bedtime. Nonetheless, there are certain qualities and routines currently above your paygrade that you can aspire to, and some you should try to do daily—perhaps a new one per week. That said, this whole practice of the GLD—and of life— is not about perfection. It is rightly a humorous and happy process dedicated to the Divine.

The Daily Program: Establishing a Foundation of Health
Creating a pattern of daily practice requires us to notice the timing of our daily activities, those we do regularly. We can either stay with that pattern or make adjustments as needed to keep as many of our life-positive disciplines going daily as we can. This doesn't mean we have to slavishly maintain the exact pattern every single day of our lives. That is not the point of having such a disciplined program. The various changes in the conditions of life will necessarily interrupt our pattern of healthy habit practice.

The perfection of such a pattern is not the goal. This process is not about goals. It is about purification, balance, equanimity in psychophysical life and living. Rightly establishing this process is a matter of bringing it all into conscious awareness. This "enforces" our Happiness. Remember Adi Da's Admonition about discipline: *"Discipline is difficult enough! Why should we burden it with the requirement to make us happy? The only way to tolerate discipline is to be already Happy!*" (The capital "H" Happiness he's referring to is Divine-Communion.) This is the great secret of doing the discipline called the 30-Day GLD, of making the desired life-positive changes in diet and lifestyle.

On the simple, practical level, observe the timing of the events of your daily routines. If you do your grocery shopping once weekly, note when you go, the time of day. Let's say it is around noon on Saturday. If you leave at (say) 3 PM instead of noon, you may not return home in time to do your yoga. So, make sure you leave around noon. Get into a rhythm with these disciplines. (BTW, a short video of the exact yoga postures we recommend is available thru www.GLDiet.co by clicking on GLDLifestyle. You can learn the routine and do your yoga right along with us.)

Strange as it may sound, it all starts with getting to bed as close to 10PM as possible—but no later than midnight. This regular bedtime rhythm will help fix the pattern of your whole daily routine in place, creating a strong foundation of daily life-positive health habits (*The BIG 7*). If you can do this for 30 days in a row, your foundation will tend to be set, fixed in place. Sometimes, your "program" of daily disciplines will look ragged. Anyone watching may wonder if you have a program at all. On other days, it'll be "perfect," with everything in place. Ragged and perfect are both fine. Remember, tho, the body greatly enjoys a regular routine—especially bedtime!

Let's take another look at an outline that provides us with a foundation from which to work with our GLD. The liquids are *italicized*, and *The BIG 7* activities are in **bolded black**.

Possible *BIG 7* Day Outline on the GLD

- Arise early
- Meditation / prayer / **Spiritual study**
- Rapid Movement **Exercise** (a Power Walk? Namaskars? Exercycle?)
- **Dry brush massage, shower,** *herb tea*
- *Green Smoothie*; chew liquids thoroughly; **pray**, asking the Divine to Enter your food
- Do **work** you enjoy and feel entirely right about, serving God and humankind
- *RMVJ* or other fresh-squeezed fruit or veggy juice
- Tend to your **environments**, keeping them clean and orderly
- Do your **yoga** to help the body stay youthful, supple and flexible
- Hot raw veggy *soup, hot cocoa,* or blended cooked veggy soup
- **Entertainment** with moral, intelligent and responsible friends and family
- **Meditation, prayer**
- **Early bedtime**

Egoity is the <u>source</u> of disease; the <u>cause</u> is failure to practice *The BIG 7.*

What Makes the GLD so Effective?

The GLD is effective because

- Machine liquefying of food makes it easier on the stomach to digest
- This also makes things easier on the small intestine to absorb and assimilate
- You're eating purer foods than you normally would—it's essentially a raw diet
- You'll eat (drink!) less than usual, but your meals have greater nutrient density
- The overall effect is like fasting: **greater purification**
- You can take a solid food meal if necessary—even certain snacks (if appropriate)
- You'll learn many things about yourself, your levels of restraint and will power—so you can grow
- Everyone around you will benefit from your experience

One Sample GLD Practice

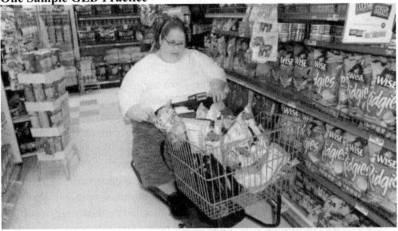

Here is what one friend of ours currently did (mid-2007) on his GLD: Orange Juice recipe for breakfast (blended OJ with garlic and coconut), Green Smoothie for lunch, avocado smoothie as 3rd meal, and guacamole with a few chips or natural-style crackers for dinner. Sometimes he had a few soaked raw almonds and dried fruit.

A Sample GLD Weight Loss Plan

Those of us with a large bone structure and a slow metabolism seem cursed! It is almost like we gain weight merely thinking about food! Folks with this combination in middle-age (starting at 45) and older age (old age starts at 70) are even worse off. These ages only complicate the weight control picture because the body wants to hold onto fat against possible dearth of food and starvation. Regardless, here's a sure way to beat the weight control problem.

Once you've gotten into the GLD for a day or two, settle into a routine of the following liquids, the actual amounts of which vary according to your size and general health condition. A standard green smoothie, RMVJ, herb tea of choice (or need), hot cocoa, and choice of hot raw soup &/or sip from a small cup of Spicy Salty Sipping Beverage. Avoid all snacks, emphasize raw liquids, drink only when actually hungry, and get daily exercise appropriate to your age and health situation. Tried, true, and proven to work! Wt. loss: ½ to 1 lb. or more daily.

How Much Liquid Should I Take Per Day On My GLD?

The amount of liquid taken on any given day varies by several factors, such as your age, sex, height, weight, energy output, climate, state of health, and liquid quality. If, for example, you are a 5' 8" 15-year-old girl practicing to be a golf pro, you will obviously need more and varied liquids than a 5' 3" 93-year-old man who slowly shuffles from bed to armchair to bathroom and back.

These factors considered, we can only make relative guesses. The basic rule is to try to get a sense of stomach satisfaction—neither ravished with hunger nor stuffed so full that it hurts. Something in between is best. You want to be hungry but not to the point of pain. (The "general state of health" factor can also be used to determine whether you will use *Level 1*, *Level 2*, or *Level 3* of the GLD—see below.) Let's take these factors one-at-a-time.

AGE – Altho we don't fast children, they can get along fine (when sick, e.g.) on the GLD. So, let's talk about adults. Younger people (late teens, 20s, and 30s) generally move the body around more than those who are older. This means more energy output, which translates into more liquids needed. No problem. Drink!

SEX – This factor has more to do with the simple general difference in body size, with more intake going to males than females—again, in general.

HEIGHT – Taller people generally need more food intake, especially if they're younger adults, male, more active, have a slower metabolism, and are a large-boned body type.

WEIGHT – Heavier folks usually need more food intake to accommodate their bulk, whether they are overweight, obese, or simply large-boned. This is a generalization, of course, but usually the case.

ENERGY OUTPUT – This is often the most telling factor in most cases regarding the question of how much liquid to intake. A 45-year-old man sitting behind a desk all day has far less need than a stevedore or athlete.

CLIMATE AND ENVIRONMENT – Extreme environments typically require more food—and thus liquid—intake. Tropical environments have us sucking down more juices, where very cold climates require more energy output to deal with the freeze. Moderate environments, of course, are easier on the body, and so require less food intake than climates of greater extremes in temperature.

GENERAL STATE OF HEALTH – A sick person consumes less, on average, than a person of the same age and sex who is well and active. Being bed-ridden, e.g., means far less caloric (or, generally, energy) consumption than moving one's body around all day.

LIQUID QUALITY – This factor involves such items as the relative viscosity of the liquid, nutrient density, percentage raw, amount of ruffage, and freshness. Nutrient-dense liquids such as the Green Smoothie with wheatgrass, other SuperFoods (see below), and an avocado smoothie containing spirulina, pack such enormous power that very little other nutrition or volume may be needed.

Note that all of these can be skewed by *mind-set*, attitude, emotional stress, life events that cause us to recoil into reactivity, self-reverie, and sadness, however temporarily. As noted in *The BIG 7* consideration, the attitude of gratitude and a generally positive outlook on life—including the "positive disillusionment" described by Avatar Adi Da—will serve to keep us balanced—and thus can make a huge difference.

Summarizing, taking all of these factors into account, it can be quite difficult to create a chart that shows us just how much liquid to take in daily as a specific individual. We can, however, make an estimate based on averages. The following includes the full range of viscosity, including an average of 12 oz. of herb tea or water, and the rest of the liquids no thinner than the RMVJ or thicker than an avocado smoothie as described in the recipe section at the end of this book.

Keep in mind, now, that most of these liquids are nutrient-dense, like an avocado smoothie or other drinks containing such as wheatgrass, spirulina, chlorella, and/or blue-green algae, &/or any other SuperFoods—thus minimizing the overall amount of liquid intake needed for optimum health. Also note that **the common recommendation for eight glasses of water (8x8 oz.) daily is total nonsense**. Only extreme athletes MAY need that much. That Rx is silly because there are too many factors involved in deciding the average human need for water.

Therefore, the estimated right GLD liquid intake will be different for each person. Not only that, it will change for each person—even on a daily basis. The most basic rule for drinking liquids is if you're thirsty, drink! The trouble with this is that people eat so much cooked and teased-up crap food that the body is almost always thirsty—often in an attempt to dilute the toxins. So, when you are back on solids after your GLD, maintain 80%+ raw.

However, on your GLD, your liquids count for what would otherwise be your solid food meals. Therefore, you'll be drinking liquids more often than usual—i.e., more often than when you are not on your GLD. We suggest, then, taking water only if you want to, only if you're actually thirsty for it, because there is so much water in your liquids, especially your fruit and veggy juices, like your RMVJ, and so much is raw, you won't likely feel much thirst.

If you start your day with 8 oz. of tea or hot cocoa, then later 10 oz. of RMVJ, plus 10-20 oz. of green smoothie, and then later on another 8 oz. of a smoothie or juice or such, we're looking at some 46 or so oz. of pure liquids. More is OK, and less is OK. Basic rule: if you're hungry or thirsty, DRINK!

The GLD in Cold Weather

Those in colder climes often wonder how to keep the body warm on raw foods. The fact is that cooked foods do not provide genuine natural heat for the body. Yes, hot foods can and will warm the tummy. They can be very comforting. But that "heat" is coming from without the body. Raw food, on the other hand, provides "heat" from within the body by giving the body the pure nutrients it was designed by Nature to have in the first place.

On your GLD, there are some hot liquids that can be used to provide that comforting outside "heat," liquids that are not harmful to the body like most cooked foods are. These include herb teas, hot raw cacao, and hot "raw" drinks. Some such drinks are made by placing heated pure water into the blender and adding chopped raw veggies and perhaps some natural veggie broth powder. Blend and serve!

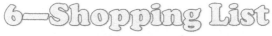

6—Shopping List

Food and Equipment Needed for the Kitchen

On your GLD, you will need (see Appendix B for more details on equipment):

Critical
- Blender
- Juicer
- Enema Bottle
- Sharp knife
- Fine mesh strainer
- Tea kettle

Variously Useful but Not Critical
- Steam Distiller (Appendix B)
- Nut-Seed Grinder ("coffee mill")
- Large marble cutting board
- Citrus juicer
- Food dehydrator
- Hot air popcorn popper

Juicers and Blenders

These two items are quite important to your GLD. Basically, you cannot effectively do your GLD without them—especially the blender. A wide variety of **juicers** is available for use on the GLD. If you're going to buy one at all, get a good one (see below). When veggy residuals build up on the insides of the plastic parts, just soak those parts in a sink full of water with 3-4 Tbsp. of liquid bleach overnight and the residues come right off.

Likely the overall best juicer is the Omega (see Chapter 3 and Appendix B for other suggestions on juicers and blenders). This juicer does everything you'll need from this kind of appliance: fruit, veggy, leaf and grass juices, and nut/seed butters—even wheatgrass. Our recommendation for the juicer is the *Vitamix*.

Other machines that are useful on your GLD—but especially for your GLD Lifestyle—include a small **nut-seed grinder** (a.k.a. "coffee grinder" & "coffee mill") for grinding hard items like almonds and pumpkin seeds. These typically sell for about $20. You may wish to also have a **water distiller**, a **citrus juicer**, and a **food dehydrator**. This should pretty much complete your kitchen device needs for decades to come.

MOST IMPORTANT ITEM: However, for those who want the very best in blending, the choice is clearly a "power blender" such as the VitaMix 5200 or later model ($350-600). Power blenders (see Appendix B) can make all your soups, raw or cooked, and all smoothies, better and in a fraction of the time of regular blenders. It's highly recommended on the GLD, and will likely become the most used (and important) appliance in your kitchen.

Juicers and Blenders

Avatar Adi Da has stated plainly that *the blender is the most important machine that human beings have yet created regarding food—* more important than the refrigerator, the stove, or any other such device. Yes, that is quite a statement! We're talking a power blender, now, not something cheap and weak. The reason for its importance is simple: it takes far too much chewing to break down the nutritional and structural materials in living greens—which are the most important of all foods for humans.

Gorillas, e.g., as other primates, spend many hours of the day collecting and munching on and otherwise grinding up such greens—the staple of their diet. We can't be doing that, not given our current needs for time. And even if we took the time, we'd be grinding our teeth down, wearing them out, trying to chew all those greens. So, we let the blender do it—and not just any blender. It has to be a strong one—fast and powerful.

The main differences between a juicer and a blender are (1) the viscosity of the liquid, and (2) the question of pulp (bulk and ruffage). Juicers remove most of the pulp, a bulking and roughage factor normally occurring in raw foods and needed for bowel movements (BMs) and general bowel health.

During fasting, such removal is important: the bulk requires more processing energy, so that its removal means that purification is maximized. However, bulk removal limits the length of time (about 40 days) one may continue the purification process. In other words, you can only fast for so long before the body starts digesting itself—which is starvation.

Regarding viscosity, the inclusion of such items as blended bananas, avocados, nuts and seeds on the GLD—items that are never used on a fast— on the one hand slows the purification process, but on the other hand provides a rich supply of essential nutrients, allowing purification to continue **indefinitely**.

The juicer and blender you purchase may well be decided by how serious you are about getting well and being well over time. If you intend merely to achieve some purpose that will take 14 days or so on your GLD, you may be satisfied with inexpensive equipment.

However, **if this is going to be your way of life**, with at least periodic (or even daily) juicing and blending of pure foods, you are well to consider getting into the higher-end hardware. It will be entirely worth the money. If you suffer from a chronic degenerative disease and wish to conquer it and move onward and upward, then take this whole thing on as a "happy"-serious hobby! Get the best equipment.

Fasting doesn't provide enuf sustenance to allow the purification to continue more than perhaps 40 days or so. After that, as we're saying here, the body begins to self-digest, which is "starvation." The GLD, however, provides plenty of sustenance. Fasting is about a "faster," more aggressive form of purification, with (necessarily) minimal sustenance, whereas the GLD is about speeded up purification (compared to solid food diets) with enuf sustenance for indefinite lengths of time.

IMPORTANT: *absolute* purification is not possible. The body is inherently imperfect—in the sense that there's always something wrong with it, something irritating or off somehow. Therefore, use both fasting and the GLD rightly—for basic purification and body-mind equanimity. This intelligent approach supports the most important use of (and basic reason for the very existence of) the body-mind: **purification**—toward Divine Awakening.

Basic Recipe Ideas: Variety
Variety, they say, is the spice of life, and this applies to the GLD. Get a variety of fresh fruits (as available), veggies—especially, and nuts &/or seeds into your diet over the span of a week for continuously good health. It's not hard to do. At a local farmer's market, or from the garden, watch what is in season and locally grown. What grows well in your area of the world?

Can you grow all season long via a greenhouse? (With the right greenhouse, you actually can! See Appendix G) Prefer in-season, local-grown, and natural, over the common randomly GMO, environment destroying, pesticide-sprayed, chemical fertilizer-grown produce. In other words, do not use commercial-industrially farmed foods! If you do, we assure you, it will be at your peril!

If you have a strawberry smoothie one day, have a pineapple smoothie the next. Then, an avocado smoothie. Then, a carob-coconut (chocolaty) one. BUT, **always try to have your green smoothie first!** It's the most important drink on your GLD. Invent smoothies by rotating fruits and nuts—and always throw in at least some leafy greens, even fresh mint. Of course, if you have several ripe avocadoes and you like avocado smoothies, have avo smoothies for the duration, no problem. The varieties are virtually limitless.

Play with different veggies in your RMVJ. Be careful, however, to use plenty of carrots and/or apples in RMVJ, since these keep the more pungent and angular-tasting veggies from overwhelming your drinks. You will notice early on, for example—if you are making your own drinks like the RMVJ—that if you add too much beet to the mix, the taste will be too strong. The same will happen when adding too much celery, or too much of many other green veggies. Fix this by adding more carrots and/or apples.

A little extra lemon (with peel) can also be used to mask the flavor of too much beet in your RMVJ. Bring different nuts into your smoothies, and also use seeds—like sunflower, sesame, and pumpkin. If you have the right kind of juicer, you can make nut and seed butters, and these can be taken— very sparingly—as a special treat on your GLD. And don't forget berries and melons on your GLD.

Melons—like cantaloupe, muskmelon, honeydew, and, of course, watermelon—can each be blended alone and drunk as a delicious beverage. Chilled or room temperature, it's your choice. The berries are typically used in combination smoothies. One of our favorites is blackberry.

Try 6 or 8 plump fresh blackberries with a banana, 4 chopped dates, 2 tablespoons of shredded coconut, and 6 ounces of Extra Rich Nutmilk. Add 2 or 3 pure-water ice cubes to chill and extra water to make it thinner if desired. Then, there are blueberries (the only berry that freezes without losing its nutritional value), elderberries, and raspberries. Mix and match. Invent your own special blends. Have fun with all.

Type and Location of GLD Food

Most of the food you will be purchasing on your GLD should come from your own garden, a nayborhood garden, a farmer's market, or other trusted natural food source. Most communities in the USA and Canada have these sources. Some larger stores such as Whole Foods Market, Wild Oats, Trader Joe's, and Costco are increasingly including pure organic foods. San Diego (the health food capital of the world) has many choices: e.g., Jimbo's, Ocean Beach People's Food (best of them all), Whole Foods, and Boney's Bayside Market on Coronado Island.

In other chapters of this book, we describe why natural food sources are important—and, of course, why natural foods themselves are our choice. The recipe section in Appendix A provides ideas as to which groceries to buy for specific recipes. Here, we'll give you an idea, perhaps a typical shopping list.

A Starter GLD Shopping List

- VitaMix Blender
- Omega Juicer
- Almonds
- Apples
- Bananas
- Beets
- Berries
- Carrots
- Cashews*
- Celery
- Coconut Oil*
- Coconut*
- Cucumber
- Garlic
- Ginger root
- Herb teas (your choice)
- Kale
- Lemons
- Mint leaves*
- Oranges
- Papaya
- Raw cacao powder*
- Raw carob powder
- Swiss Chard

Notes*

The cacao (cocoa) should be free trade and non-alkali processed. The cashews should be raw unsalted. The coconut can be whole. If packaged, it can be shredded or flaked but must be dried raw and unsweetened. The coconut oil must be organic virgin and (if possible) expeller-pressed. The mint leaves may be "live" or in tea form. Costco has aa good coconut oil. The powders are available on the Net (Anthony's is good). The rest of the produce should be raw organic and (if possible) locally grown.

Other Helpful Accessories

The enema bottle consideration is presented in Appendix B—Helpful Devices. You will need a sharp knife or knives to cut produce. A good paring knife is helpful for removing the tops of carrots and the roots of beets. A larger knife will be needed to cut thru larger, thick, and dense produce such as apples, beets, and carrots. An ergonomic nutcracker can be useful.

Alternatively, and especially for nuts with very hard shells—like macadamias—a garage vice is excellent. A large marble cutting board is preferable to a wooden or plastic one since marble is easier to clean than plastic or wood, it doesn't hold bacteria like wood, and it doesn't shed like plastic. More details on this process, including videos, are available thru www.GLDiet.co.

Cleaning and Preparing Produce

Be sure to carefully clean all produce before liquefying it. If it is natural and unsprayed, it will need less cleansing. Berries can be simply rinsed in pure water. Firmer fruits and veggies may need to be scrubbed with a brush and soapy water. Produce purchased in regular markets and supermarkets where its handling is not known should be carefully cleaned—as with a dip in hot soapy water then rinsed in cold clear water.

Apples, cucumbers, and certain other items are often coated with wax—which is unfortunate because the skins of most fruits and veggies contain most of their nutrients. Scrub these carefully with hot soapy water. Nuts and seeds in the shell need no preparation more than shell removal.

Once out of the shell, they should be refrigerated prior to use since they'll go rancid over time. Almonds can be soaked for at least 3 hours or overnite before use, especially if blending. Remove peelings of pesticide-sprayed produce. Produce that is known to be completely natural and untainted need not be peeled—except for oranges, bananas, melons, and other produce whose peels we do not eat.

"Right life is the always practical life-demonstration of ego-renunciation."
—Adi Da Samraj

7—The Modified GLD

If and When to Interrupt, Change, Modify, Alter, or Break your GLD

Definitions Regarding the GLD

Breaking it temporarily / Interrupting it – stopping your GLD briefly, taking solids for a meal or two, as needed, then resuming it.

Changing / Modifying / Altering it – can mean either (1) using different rules, including arbitrary abuse of the LQFs, or (2) making appropriate changes to your GLD that apply to your personal health circumstance—especially in consultation with your health professional.

Ending it – means bringing it to an end by taking solid foods on an indefinite basis or until your next planned GLD (see Chapter 37, Ending Your GLD).

Breaking your GLD

First, let's separate the "breaking" of the GLD from the "breaking" of a fast. One cannot "break" a fast (which means ending it) and then, within hours or even a day or so, go back into it. This is a shock to the body, a big disruption of bodily energy, and can be quite painful. It's different with your GLD. One can stop taking liquids and resume solid food eating for several meals without any significant negative effect on the body.

This is not at all to suggest that, while on your GLD, you should arbitrarily have a solid food meal any time you take the notion. Altho it can happen by necessity, you should hope that it doesn't happen often, because it will significantly slow the purification fundamental to the purpose of the GLD. Not to mention weight loss—if that's an issue. If you are merely tempted to take a solid food meal without a specific need to do so, it's better to resist. Let your GLD buddy know. If that doesn't quell the action, use your Divine Resort. That always works!

For the average relatively healthy person, there are times when it can be necessary (for business and other reasons) that one will need to take solid food meals for longer periods of time. What then? Just resume your GLD whenever you are able. Pick up where you left off. The negative effects will depend on such items as the quality and quantity of the food you eat while on the solid foods diet. (Experience with your GLD will teach you to improve this quality.)

Let's say, hypothetically, that amid a prolonged GLD, a very important business lunch in which the CEO or other dignitary is present. It could be embarrassing or otherwise inappropriate for you to be taking juices and liquids only. On the other hand, it might be quite impressive for the dignitary to learn that you have the necessary restraint and discipline to take pure juices and liquids in the face of tasty solids that others are eating. This can place you in a very beneficial light. Such a decision—to stay on or go off the liquids—is one you'll have to make.

For those with chronic degenerative diseases, on your GLD, only in certain very special cases may you take a small high-quality solid food meal without significantly compromising your purification program or causing undue stress to the body. Your health practitioner will decide if this is appropriate in your case. (This is another of the advantages of the GLD over fasting.) Then, after the small meal, simply resume your GLD. For those in better health, a day of solid food meals may be acceptable.

Other occasions of breaking the GLD include special family occasions (birthdays, anniversaries), major Holidays, and other such celebratory events. These events should be relatively rare, like once monthly (if that), and celebrated with one meal only—if that. If you plan your 30-day GLD carefully in advance, you can usually bypass occasions that even tempt you to interrupt your GLD with a solid food meal.

Remember, the bigger and more low quality the meal, the more energy required by the body to process it—and therefore the less the purification. For the most part, one of the better ways to deal with these hunger pangs, desires, and other diversions that are driving you batty is to engage what is called the Divine Gourmet Principle (see below), which involves simply taking a teaspoonful of this or that food that is so tempting—and stopping right there.

Overeating

Whatever you do at such times (when eating cooked food), ***DO NOT OVEREAT! Overeating is the worst dietary habit of all***, and for reasons both exoteric and esoteric. Overeating is very hard on the systems of the body, and one of the primary reasons for heart disease, diabetes, kidney disease, and many other completely preventable disorders. Fortunately, it's hard to overeat on a rightly done GLD.

Finishing your GLD of 30 days or more, you'll find yourself naturally increasing the percentage of pure raw solids into your diet. You'll notice that now you naturally choose better quality foods than before you began your GLD—and you overeat less because you've lost weight, your stomach has shrunk, and you don't get as hungry as often. Besides, if you haven't learned your lesson yet re overeating, you will—with further GLDs.

OK, confession time: your author struggled with overeating for years, tending to conveniently forget the negative consequences of this habit when confronted by various tasty foods. The worst situations: <u>buffets</u>, where adolescent indulgence can—and usually does—run rampant. He had to suffer pain, illness, and overweight until the message finally came thru loud and clear! Overeat and you're gonna hurt! It's that simple.

Of course, again, we're talking about cooked and processed foods. One simply doesn't overeat on raw foods—because they're so satisfying to the body. Example: how many bananas do you think you can eat at one time? How many strawberries can you eat before your brain sends its natural signal to the stomach saying you've had enuf? They will stop tasting good when your body has had enuf. This will never happen with cooked and processed foods—because they are not our natural diet! They always taste good—even when you're stuffed full!

Esoterically, **etheric energy** passes down the frontal line of the body with every breath, bringing life and health. (Breath is the conductive means for Spirit to move in the body.) When the stomach is full—much less over-full—this etheric energy is stuck at the stomach level. But, that is just the beginning of trouble with overeating. Moderate eating must be mastered for us to be truly healthy, intelligently healthy, and the GLD is among the easiest ways to do this—mainly, because of the raw factor.

Raw foods satisfy the body's need for genuine nutrition, thus obviating the need to overeat. It's hard to overeat on the GLD for reasons we discuss later having to do with instinct. It's those rich, cooked, processed, prepared, and junk foods that we overeat on. Overeating these, or just eating them regularly, sooner or later there's a consequence involved. You're not going to like it: it's called "disease!" And all human adults, sooner or later, experience it. The disease began with the first bite of processed food.

Special Lifestyle Considerations
Certain people have lifestyles that have them frequently traveling, jetting all over the world. Others have work and business situations that otherwise make it difficult to stay on the GLD for significant lengths of time. Faced with business and other ceremonial dinners at which one must participate, it can be more appropriate to eat at least some amounts of solid foods. This could be disconcerting to one just starting a GLD.

It's best to begin your GLD when you have at least two clear weeks ahead of you, two weeks to get into it and learn how it feels altogether. Two weeks gives you time to get a real sense of it. Meanwhile, the lifestyle that requires occasional solid food meals can be managed on a *variation* of the GLD. On the GLD, it is far easier to go into and out of liquids and solids than it ever would be on a fast. This simply cannot be done on a fast. The fast would be ruined, and the body would be shocked by the come and go of solids and liquids.

However, this is not so with the GLD. This is not to encourage those on the GLD to eat solid foods whenever they like. Here, we're talking about situations that are beyond one's control. As long as you are not "under the gun" to eat a solid food meal, you should stay with your liquids. Some GLD'ers tote their blenders and juicers in their luggage and prepare their juices and smoothies in their hotel rooms! Sound strange? Hey, it's a way of life— and a very healthy one! Not that this is a requirement on your GLD. But, it does make sense.

So, what do you do in such a situation, faced with a solid food mealtime? Have some. Then, if at all possible, your next meal is right back into the liquids. If this has to happen even once weekly, it can work. Try, of course, to minimize the solid food meals. They slow the process of purification, cleansing, and weight management. And any significant number of back-and-forth liquid-to-solids-and-back irritates the body. So, when this needs to happen, always choose the purer foods, to whatever degree possible, like the salads and other raw produce.

Satisfying the Desire for Crunch

Initially, you will feel a need for "crunching" onto something. Liquids don't crunch, so now what do I do? Certain natural style snack crackers can be used. How many? Perhaps 1 or 2 per day, depending on your health circumstance. The healthier you are the more you can snack, but you don't, on the other hand, want to defeat the purpose of the GLD by over-snacking. A level teaspoon of crunchy raw nut butter is better than taking snack crackers.

Healthy snack crackers can be made in your food dehydrator. You may wish to use them with your veggy soup, or even take them with some salsa or nut butter. Certain natural-style chips can be used instead of the crackers. These should be baked instead of fried. Especially avoid deep-fried chips (or deep-fried anything!).

Snacks can also consist of soaked almonds and dried fruit— especially dried unsweetened banana chips. You can make up guacamole from avocado, chopped tomatoes, chopped onion, garlic, and cilantro—with a little squeeze of lemon juice. Other such natural ingredients are possible. You can crumble and mix a few chips into this.

As you progress on your GLD, you will feel better and better, and less and less likely to feel the need for snacks or other solid foods. Moreover, the fewer the solids (processed solids, especially—as opposed to raw food solids), the greater the purification, the higher the nourishment, the more rapid the weight loss, and the sooner you'll get well. Eventually, you may see the bodily need to let go of snacking altogether.

Over time, you'll notice how the body will reject impurity of all kinds, choosing instead only the purest food and drink. You'll then likely be already moved to either all raw solids, all raw liquids when on your GLD, or some combination of all raw solids and all raw liquids in between GLDs. Some even go to a diet of mostly all raw liquids, with perhaps occasional use of solids, no cooked foods at all, depending on the real needs of the body. Some people level off at around 80% raw and stay there. In any case, this is all an intelligent and conscious process.

Possible GLD Snacks

- Dried Fruits: dates, figs, raisins, dried apricots, dried cherries (sometimes dipped in nut butter)
- Soaked Nuts and Seeds: almonds, sunflower seeds, pumpkin seeds, other nuts and seeds
- Raw Nut and Seed Butters (except peanut butter)
- Humus—plain or with herbs and spices
- Guacamole (preferably self-prepared of pure raw natural produce)
- Salsas (natural-style, especially including home-made)
- Crackers, chips, pretzels (natural-style, best home-made in food dryer, up to a few per day—see Appendix A)

The Ultimate DIY

There is a movement in the world today back toward Do It Yourself—home gardening, composting, self-prep, growing your own, and sharing pure living produce with naybors and those living in the local community. This will be good to whatever extent that movement takes us in a positive direction, away from the mechanical-industrial-chemical food environments and production methods that have been leading us down the road to Shitsburg.

The GLD website, www.GLDiet.co, and its membership vehicle, **GLDLifestyle**, are both designed to bring you details of this higher way of life, one that not only encourages but also provides specifics—the recipes and videos that show you how this all happens. How to use these five kitchen devices, how to grow healthy food, how to compost, how to do yoga, exercise, meditate, make delicious and nutritious raw granola, green smoothies—the whole thing.

Can anyone do the GLD?

The GLD is especially effective for those of us who…

(1) have various weight control problems (overweight, obese, underweight)

(2) have chronic degenerative disease situations

(3) are above age 65 and otherwise simply need a diet that will work best to keep healthy

(4) suffer OCD (obsessive compulsive disorder)

(5) want to observe and overcome our negative health-related tendencies

(6) wish to reduce or eliminate certain pharma medications

(7) desire to learn right use of diet and lifestyle toward genuine balanced health

Most people can do the GLD. However, some are *psychologically* unprepared for the GLD, including those who abuse fasting, become very thin, and even enter starvation for sympathy or otherwise to draw attention to themselves—which is an emotional disorder. Rather than the GLD, they need psychological help.

Certain thin-body types who lose weight rapidly, and therefore need to be careful on the GLD, using richer and thicker drinks (emphasizing nuts and seeds, e.g.) accordingly and perhaps using the GLD for shorter lengths of time. They should check with their qualified Natural Health Provider, one who is experienced in fasting. Altho the GLD is not a fast, some thin body types may wind up struggling on the GLD, especially those with rapid metabolisms and who lose weight quickly and have trouble regaining it.

It may be more appropriate for them to instead do a few days of a mono-diet, like (e.g.) taking only avocadoes for 4-5 days. It is usually easier for these types to maintain their weight on an all-raw diet than on the GLD. These types can maintain weight on the GLD, but this involves real strategy on the part of the guiding health practitioner. Likely, nut and seed butters will play a more significant role in their GLD.

Variations on the GLD Theme

There are several ways to apply the GLD, ways to fit the desired circumstance. For those who need extreme cleansing—and yet must have regular intake of the three basic nutrient sources (fruits, veggies, nuts/seeds), a GLD that is closer to a fast is recommended: fresh juices, thin smoothies, herb teas as appropriate to their case, and pure water. Certain overweight and morbidly obese individuals would also benefit from such a GLD regimen.

The other extreme includes those who are already healthy and also thin body types who want the purification and balance of the GLD but without significant weight loss. For them, it's a matter of rich, thick avocado smoothies with coconut and coconut oil, other thick nut-seed smoothies, RMVJ, raw and cooked blended soups, and frequent snacks that could include nut and seed butters. The rest of us are in between these two.

So, what is "in between"? That could include such as ordinary green smoothies—perhaps even made with the Extra Rich Nutmilk; the Orange-Coconut-Mint smoothie (strained or unstrained); RMVJ; hot cacao; and maybe a nut butter smoothie. Always think in terms of an extra green smoothie variation if still hungry at day's end. But, in this case we're talking real hunger, not merely "entertainment level" hungry.

If you are not sure where you fit into this schema, consider the three "*LEVELS*" below. If you seem to fit into *LEVEL 2* or *LEVEL 3*, and you're still confused, try experimenting with viscosity (relative smoothie thickness) and the snacks. Try thinner juices, adding a little extra water to them. This moves you closer to fasting and greater weight loss, and it provides greater purification. You can also thin down the smoothies in the same way—with a little more water or more regular nut milk. Avoid the snacks altogether and notice the difference.

Alternatively, you may moderate your GLD by taking your RMVJ, one smoothie, and 3 or 4 snack crackers with a hummus dip. This is somewhere in the middle of possibilities. It may work well for those over 60, but younger people may need more in quantity. In any case, always get the three basics, and try to keep the every-3-hours rule in practice. This brings us to the "Three Basic Levels of Application" of the GLD.

Three Basic Levels of Application

We all have our personal health circumstances, and they are different in each case. So, how do you decide where to start in applying the GLD to you personally? There can be any number of arbitrary levels of application we could propose, but for the sake of simplicity we've created three basic levels:

—*LEVEL 1*: Chronic Disease
—*LEVEL 2*: Periodic Deep Cleanse
—*LEVEL 3*: Healthy Maintenance

Determining which level you should engage is up to you and your health professional. Age is not necessarily a factor in this consideration. If you have a chronic degenerative (clinically treatable) disease, we urge you to begin at *LEVEL 1*. If there are irritating symptoms that you've been living with but that are manageable without professional help (sub-clinical), you'll likely be better using *LEVEL 2*. If there are few or no symptoms, and you simply wish to maintain relatively good health and longevity (prophylaxis), *LEVEL 3* is likely just right for you.

GLD LEVEL 1 – Chronic Disease

This level of application of the GLD involves those who are suffering clinical symptoms of one or more disease processes and need regular health monitoring by a professional healer. This GLD level is the most intense form of application. In 97% of cases, there will be one green smoothie daily (fruit, green veggie, and nut/seed/oil requirement) and the RMVJ (fruit and veggy requirement). No snacks, no LQFs, no solid food meals. *The BIG 7* lifestyle practices are strictly applied as appropriate to the case.

Length of application: *indefinite*—continue until symptoms are entirely manageable or otherwise sufficiently diminished that your health professional releases you on your own recognizance.

GLD LEVEL 2 – Periodic Deep Cleanse

This level is for those who have some symptoms but have been managing them without clinical help—including moderate weight control. There are a lot of possibilities here, and many pathological circumstances are potential with GLD Level 2. Therefore, it's best to err on the side of caution and be in consultation with a sympathetic and experienced health professional. A daily natural-style snack is OK, but strictly avoid the LQFs (especially refined sugar). Also, observe your work schedule: try to avoid breaks (solid food meals) in your GLD.

Length of application: *30 days once or twice yearly*.

GLD LEVEL 3 – Healthy Maintenance

This level of application is for those who have no special symptoms and generally are (and act and feel) healthy. In this category, regular health and perhaps weight maintenance is the motivation, plus longevity. The length of time on the GLD could be any number of days, depending on various circumstances of work and leisure and whether you can engage your GLD without significant compromise. At GM, for this purpose, we would recommend a suggested annual GLD of one month.

Length of application: *30 days yearly*.

Prioritizing GLD Applications

There are a number of reasons people would take on the GLD. The more obvious reasons include eliminating a disease process, losing weight, longevity, and regaining a youthful appearance and quality in the body. Let's consider a few more, and how they might be prioritized in terms of the most and least appropriate applications. Of course, everyone has his and her priorities and ideas as to what is important and why. To us, the best motive of all is merely helping one toward true body-mind equanimity. Beyond that, here we go:

Appropriate Applications of the GLD

1 – Establish Equanimity

2 – Eliminate disease

3 – Regain former health

4 – Reduce disease

5 – Bring discipline to diet

6 – Help substance abuse withdrawal

7 – Maintain good health

8 – Detoxification

9 – Recuperation

10 – Purification

11 – Improve physical appearance

12 – Get off drugs

13 – Eliminate pain

14 – Rehabilitation

15 – Achieve nutritional balance

16 – Control / stabilize / lose weight

17 – Regain function

18 – Gain a more youthful appearance

19 – Reduce stress

20 – Eliminate irritation

If losing weight is your primary goal, be encouraged. You'll lose weight anyway on the GLD, depending on the GLD design used (e.g., thickness of liquids, use of snacks, exercise). As a bonus, you'll learn more about the dynamics of weight loss on the GLD than on any diet—just by staying with it!

Disease States Helped by the GLD

Most disease states, by far, can and will be reduced by the GLD. Virtually everyone can be helped, even people who are paralyzed, paraplegic, and otherwise disabled by accident and genetics. Of course, missing limbs cannot be re-grown on the GLD. Even nerve tissue, once *destroyed*, can be regenerated. (*Damaged* nerve tissue can be replaced, and the GLD will significantly aid this process).

Those near death can be helped by the GLD in the sense that the pure liquids will be more easily digested and therefore serve an easeful passing. Moreover, those near death tend to lose their appetite anyway. All the other common disease circumstances, notably including the chronic degenerative diseases that modern Allopathic medicine can only drug, irradiate, or cut out via surgery, are aided to one or another degree by the GLD. In any case, one must be patient and stay with the GLD. It works for you—more or less quickly.

Given the right circumstances, or given half a chance, the body is self-healing and self-repairing. The problem, these days, is that we don't do that. We tend to pile stress on stress, toxins on toxins, negative on negative. In such case, what can we expect of the body? To get well and heal in spite of our madness? To take a drug, and that's going to make it all better? Drugs are palliatives, useful for the short term—at best. We need a different strategy.

There are several ways we can assist in the healing and self-repairing process. The diet, the mind, the emotions, the lifestyle—these all these play a role in healing. Even tho there is always some silly thing or another wrong with the body—at least some little thing—the more difficult disease states can be overcome in various ways and by various means. While the GLD can handle most of the little things, it can also handle most of the big ones.

Below, we list the areas or categories of disease in which or with which the GLD is most effective. If the disease has progressed to a certain profound degree, and it is already "very late in the game," the GLD will be less effective. Progress will be slow to the degree that immunity is weak and the body's resources are diminished. Various factors are involved in the health and disease processes. All must be taken into account.

For example, what is the attitude of the person regarding their current health situation? What kind of energy do they demonstrate? Are they terrified of the possible outcome—of death, e.g.? Everyone dies, but are they ready? Are they in denial? Are they actually far from terminal but acting like it's all over for them—to get sympathy? If all the signs and symptoms point to a potential recovery, are they ready to give it their best shot?

Maria in a Different Universe
Once, Maria, a Mexican woman, entered our office as a patient, begging for relief. She was accompanied by her daughter, who interpreted for her since she spoke little English. She had some choice words in Spanish—that we won't repeat here—for the medications she was taking! She'd been diagnosed with five different kinds of arthritis, and the pain was so bad that

strong meds were prescribed—drugs that made her feel like she was in a different world.

It was easy to feel compassion for Maria. Her poor arms and legs were swollen twice their size with edema, and they were cold, wet, and purple. When she sat down, she needed help getting up. Her fingers were stiff as rakes, not able to flex much at all, and she was a good 30 lbs. overweight. But to her, all that was secondary to the bizarre mental plane she suffered from the pharmaceutical cocktail she was told to swallow daily.

Maria's doctors, with one hour of silly nutrition and no training in natural therapies, could only offer her relief in the form of drugs, which they informed her she would need to take for the rest of her life. OMG! How often we had heard such a "life sentence"! How often we had seen our patients, our clients, relieved of as many as (in one case) sixteen different drugs at one time! No tests have ever been done to learn what such a chemical combination was doing in the body. None! Never! Meanwhile, we got to see the adverse effects. Not "side effects." Effects!

Imagine her delight when we told her that she could be well and away from the medications altogether! She wanted to believe, but balked a bit when we informed her that her diet for the next 30 days was to be liquids. She asked if she could blend her tacos! We gave her the recipes for RMVJ and a few smoothies and sent her home to "self-medicate" on these—with the loving help of her daughter. Like a trouper, she got into it, knowing that this might be her last hope of feeling something like a human being again.

Returning a month later, Maria walked confidently and proudly in the door and took her seat. When we required her weight, she easily and *proudly* stood up—herself, without aide. Her limbs were no longer swollen. They were red—not purple—and they were warm and dry. Her fingers could flex at least 50% further.

Maria had managed to lose 30 lbs. in those 30 days, and she looked like a new woman. She was without pain and had no further need for her medications. Perhaps most importantly, she knew who had done this and how it was done. She had only herself to thank for this big change, but she praised us for the information.

What is Cure?
Consider this: "cure" is defined in different ways by different people. Many doctors consider a disease cured if the patient lives for six months after treatment—and then dies! To us, cure means the person:

(1) learns what caused their disease
(2) learns how to deal with it effectively, and…

(3) makes the needed changes toward both general and specific life improvement

In other words, they learn how they got the problem, what to do to get rid of it, and they do it. They make the changes necessary. That's cure. The healer absolutely MUST empower the patient in this regard. This is <u>the healer's</u> responsibility, then—to teach. Learning how they got the problem and what to do about it, the patient must then DO IT! It's now time for them to kick ass and get the job done—that's <u>their</u> responsibility.

A cured person has become health self-responsible, perhaps even health-unexploitable. As Avatar Adi Da has Said, ***cure isn't the goal,*** anyway. Most people who experience a "cure" go right back to their former habits and develop another disease, and yet another—until one of these diseases finally kills them! What's intelligent about that?

A "cure" isn't about walking around like a zombie, so drugged that the symptoms are not visible. Now you have <u>two</u> diseases: the one the drugs are *suppressing* and the one they're *causing*. Yes, there are times when drugs are needed, like against pain, in certain genetic conditions, and for those who <u>will not change</u>. For intelligent people, there's dietary purity and life-positive lifestyle. Drugs are supposed to be palliative, temporary. The real healer requires the patient to get their act together, understand this, and act accordingly, so they don't need drugs past a point.

Disorders Helped by the GLD

- Allergic
- Cardiovascular
- Dental and Oral
- Dermatologic
- Ear, Nose, and Throat
- Endocrine
- Gastro-Intestinal
- GenitoUrinary
- Hematologic
- Hepatic and Biliary
- Immunologic
- Infectious
- Metabolic
- Musculo-Skeletal
- Neurologic
- Nutritional
- Oncologic
- Ophthalmologic
- Pediatric
- Psychiatric
- Toxicity / Poisoning

GLD for the Dying /Terminally Ill

At some point, the body that is born and lives for a time eventually dies. We don't like to think about this because our crazy random culture does not rightly prepare us for the cycle of life—which necessarily includes death. Notwithstanding, unless we're faced with death, in some real sense there is no point in considering it. On the other hand, having a clear sense of our mortality can (and must!) keep us in constant remembrance of the Divine—Which Is Happiness, the very context Within Which we (and everything else) appear.

Meanwhile, in any case, those about us, our loved ones, are going to die—(i.e., technically, their *body* is going to die; "they" are capital "C" Consciousness, and as such cannot ever die). Thus, it's good to be prepared for these eventualities. Yes, there are cultural differences in the way we look at this process, but generally we are usually in a mood of fear relative to the death of the body. Certainly, sadness at our loss is called for. We obviously won't be able to interact with them as before. Missing their psycho-physical presence can hurt us very deeply.

As we grow Spiritually, this fear lessens and relaxes to one or another degree. Even mere aging can loosen fear's deadly grip on us relative to the end of bodily life. And as this end approaches, whether involving disease or the simple and noble wearing out of the gross physical, diet is usually economized, and we tend to be less terrorized by the prospect of bodily death. In some sense, we can even welcome it as a rest from *"life's fitful fever."*

Many of us, at least at some time in our life, will wind up spending time in a hospital (tonsillectomy, broken arm, etc.). Regrettably, hospital stays have become "normal" for most people near the end of their life. This "hi-tech death" is unfortunate for many reasons.

Consider the loss of dignity and intimacy with loved ones, the silly hospital / institutional diet provided to the dying and terminally ill, the imposition of drugs and other highly invasive medical procedures, the society of the sick and the strange, the lack of intelligent, sensitive preparation and organization for this transitional and ultimately sacred event, and so on.

The booklet *"**Death is a Living Process**"* (Dawn Horse Press; the Wisdom of Adi Da Samraj as collected by devotees), and especially the book _**EASY DEATH**_, by Avatar Adi Da Samraj, deal most directly and wonderfully with this whole process of the death transition. The passage of death truly is a sacred process and should be treated as such. The book, _**EASY DEATH**_, is entirely positive, showing how this occasion can be completely turned around.

In hospitals in the West and some other countries, and especially in the USA, there are specific FDA rules and regulations that obviate the use of pure liquids for those who are hospitalized. Instead, they have approved the use of liquid nutrition in cans that have been pasteurized and contain various chemical preservatives. These are used to feed those who cannot any longer eat solid foods, or in some cases even take foods orally. Such liquids are fed to patients thru nasogastric (NG) and gastric (G) tubes, tubes that enter the stomach thru the nose or directly thru a surgical opening in the upper abdomen that connects with the stomach.

Such feeding thru tubes can be appropriate enuf, but the liquids could undoubtedly be far more healthful. However, doctors may be constrained by these FDA rules to provide only these Registered Dietitian-approved junk liquids to patients—one of the many reasons we say that "institutional nourishment" is a mutual contradiction in terms!

Therefore, the best circumstance for the health of the patient in the hospital is to be released to home care as soon as possible, and to the extent possible, so that pure liquids can be provided by and in the company of loved ones. This applies to the terminally ill, as well as those who have a chance at bodily survival. (Please note that the so-called "terminally ill" have many times fooled their prognosticators, turned the corner, and lived long and healthy lives!)

The RMVJ and green smoothies can be prepared so that they can easily be transferred thru NG and G tubes for the feeding of the sick and dying. The dying who can take liquids and perhaps solid food orally, can also, of course, be fed these nourishing liquids that require the least energy for the body to work with. (Of course, if the dying person expresses the desire for a meal of bacon and eggs chased with Drambuie, it's usually well to honor that!)

With smoothies, the viscosity (relative thickness) may need to be reduced to pass easily thru these tubes. The RMVJ is already thin enuf for this process. Recovery for those whose bodies have hope will be given the best opportunity via these two liquids—perhaps with the addition of wheatgrass juice and the juices of other SuperFoods (see Appendix C). We at Grand Medicine, and other healers of our acquaintance, have experienced this process and seen very positive and encouraging results.

A Note on Toxics

Today's world exposes us to a wide variety of toxics and toxins. It's a chemical feast out there! Dentists still fill teeth with highly toxic mercury amalgams. Mercury is pumped into the atmosphere by coal production. Petrochemicals abound in commercial products of many kinds, from lipstick to paint—and, of course, their waste products, the hydrocarbons and other toxics from the burning of gasoline and oil, are altering our planet's weather.

Pesticides and chemical fertilizers pollute our food, rivers, streams, and underground aquifers. Antibiotics and other pharmaceuticals are abused by over-zealous or misinformed doctors. Food processing chemicals, pesticides, herbicides, fungicides, and genetically altered and irradiated foods abound and proliferate in supermarkets. What does this mean to our daily health? Can the GLD help against this onslaught of chemicals?

Some of the diseases now developing (new ones daily!) are quite complex, involving poisoning by a wider variety of toxic substances than ever. It is harder to discover the exact nature of some of these diseases, and more difficult still to come up with an effective treatment plan for each case. This can require some real creativity on the part of healers. While we cannot expect miracles from the GLD, it can certainly play a role in the healing process.

The efficiency with which the GLD manages cellular health, and the rapidity with which it works to restore function, make it a major tool in the healer's medicine kit. Still, some complicated cases will require the strategic use of various modalities, such as homeopathics, chelation therapy, hydrotherapy, Earthing, mega-vitamin / mineral therapies, SuperFoods, or more exotic means now being tested. The GLD may then be an adjunct to new and powerful modalities that involve the creative use of natural and human-made forces.

After all, only by being intelligent with food, by choosing pure foods as our basic diet, and by living *The BIG 7*, can we gain equanimity and remain healthy in such a world.

Allergic Reactions

By the way, if you do happen to sense that any food item within the RMVJ or smoothie recipe you've made causes a negative reaction in your body, like an allergic response—including making your heart suddenly beat faster after ingestion, for example, leave this item out entirely or replace it with another food item until your body can once again accept the food (via purification that will necessarily eventually occur). You can easily test for allergies yourself in this manner. Check your pulse with your fingers before and after a meal (or a single item) to see if something triggers a rapid heartbeat.

We dig our graves with our knives, forks, and spoons."

8—The Divine Gourmet Principle

Preventing the "Nutritional Jail" Feeling

Three Personalities of Bodily Being Inside Us

It's easy to see where people are with diet. Ask them what they eat. *"Well, my wife serves me..."* = a child! *"Well, I like..."* = an adolescent! *"I choose this because it makes me healthy..."* = an adult! How do we know this? It's easy. Children basically eat what they're fed. Adolescents tend to eat whatever they want. Adults (there actually are a very few in this world!) consciously choose essentially what brings nourishment to the body—even if it's not what their taste buds are highly tickled by.

Here is a summary of the childish, adolescent, and adult ways of eating and acting altogether, based on the Wisdom Teaching of Avatar Adi Da Samraj. See if you can easily spot yourself and your way of eating amidst these descriptions. (For a full description of right infant, child, and adolescent development, see the book, *The First Three Stages of Life*.)

CHILDISH, ADOLESCENT, AND ADULT STRATEGIES

Childish
- *Dependent:* and the desire to be so
- Weak, full of wanting, and empty of faith
- Do what they <u>can</u>
- Seek to be consoled by parents and a parent-like "God"
- Eat what is presented to them—without discrimination
- Practice religion as (and accept medicine and medical advice with) superficial and ego-serving emotionalism
- Full of wanting dependency on the Divine—and on the healer

Adolescent
- *Independent:* wants to be so, but also torn between dependence and independence
- Testy, rebellious, unfeeling, willful, abstract, and self-absorbed
- Do what they <u>want</u>
- Doubt or resist the idea of God or any power greater than themselves
- Eat <u>what</u>ever and <u>when</u>ever they like, as long as they get away with it—to the point of suffering and even death!
- Practice religion (and receive medical advice) in a non-feeling, abstract, willful, and self-absorbed way
- Deny and resist the Divine—and the healer

Adult
- *Interdependent:* realizes the importance of being relational, remaining in relationship to/with everyone/everything
- Strong and balanced; not consoled by secular life; bring love & compassion; positive disillusionment in the world
- Do what they <u>need</u>
- Resort to the Spiritual Divine as a conscious gesture of heart-sacrifice
- Eat whatever brings life and energy to the body-mind—essentially and intelligently by choice
- Practice religion (and the healer's directions) with intelligence in a full-feeling conscious consideration
- Submit whole-bodily to the Divine—and intelligently and accountably to the healer
- Willing to submit to initiating force, understanding the necessity of real growth

Lunch Righteousness

Another side of dieting is what Avatar Adi Da refers to as "Lunch Righteousness." Yes, it takes discipline to do the GLD—which you show by doing it. But, doing the GLD is just basically intelligent. Our demonstration of such discipline in eating pure foods doesn't make us "better" than others. Others may well be where we once were! (And, if we are not careful, we could be back where they are now—and worse!) Have compassion on those who have less discipline. Or those who feel they're hot shit ("better than you") because they're vegan!

By your example, help those around you understand what you've learned—especially if they ask! Do so without berating them for eating as they do, whether you see their diet as superior or inferior. If you're feeling superior, as they say: *"Better to say nothing and let people think you're a fool than to open your mouth and remove all doubt!"* Allow yourself to feel the situation altogether: you are simply like everyone else, trying your best to improve your situation. Relax into it. **Always bring love and good energy to others**—under all circumstances.

The Body is Like a Baby

The gross physical body is like a baby. It requires care. Better care = a healthy baby. Poor care = an unhealthy baby. Best care = an optimally healthy baby (body). You are (or should be) in control of that "baby," the body. What will you do with it? Do you let a baby crawl up onto a table and eat chocolates and get sick?

The body is your responsibility in this lifetime. Will you treat it like a garbage can, dumping whatever you want or like into it? BTW, consider the "context" or Matrix in Which the body (and the world and everything else) appears—the Very Divine. It is real and It is sensitive to what "we" are doing. We honor God, the Divine Person, by eating essentially at Nature' table and otherwise caring for and acknowledging the body as a Gift of the Divine.

Escaping the Tyranny of the "Rich Food" Mind

Since ancient times, the wise among us have always known that our only real "enemy" is…us! Actually, it's the conceptual mind, the ego-mind, an aspect of the brain-mind, that troubles us. The conceptual mind dreams up all manner of difficulty. Everything it doesn't understand is magnified grossly into a "problem." One such "problem" is food, of course. Food obsessions. Exaggerated taste desire. The "problem" of eating the "wrong" foods. The "problem" of not having enuf food. The "problem" of food not being convenient—or sufficiently so. And on and on.

True enuf, excessive intake of cooked and processed foods will harm the gross physical body. This situation is worsened by feelings of guilt and shame. However, we are never separated from the Divine Food Source. We are always being fed our most important "food" by It. Yes, back on the gross level of things, rich foods like cheesecake taste better than raw carrots.

How to rightly handle this? Have some cheesecake *at special occasions* and eat (or drink) the carrots *the rest of the time.* **Appropriate use and intelligent abstinence.** When this principle is understood, and food is rightly used, the "problem" goes away—especially by remembering our Divine Food Source, which is always here. When it is not understood or followed, and we casually indulge our desired craving for the junk, we will pay a price—sooner or later.

The Divine Gourmet Principle

As described by Beloved Avatar Adi Da Samraj, the *"Divine Gourmet Principle"* is the delightful and humorous practice of acting freely and intelligently with food amid a life of great discipline—and when everyone around you is gorging themselves on crap!

Let's say you're at a luncheon with no particular pressure to avoid doing your GLD. However, your personal patterns and tendencies have you experiencing HUGE pressure to taste the cheesecake at the buffet! So, here you are dutifully drinking your liquids while that cheesecake sticks in your mind. Glancing over your shoulder, furtively at first, you remember this principle. You just get up, and with a tiny dish and teaspoon; you take a nip of it!

No, you are not going to burn in hell for that. You are not doing the GLD as punishment for your sins, nor are you doing it to please mom or dad. God will not strike you dead for taking a teaspoonful of your favorite dessert or two wholesome snack crackers with nut butter on them! Or, for that matter, a common soda cracker with bacon and cheese on it. The GLD is merely an intelligent discipline. And the little nip of the Divine Gourmet Principle is a playful and happy way of poking fun at diets altogether.

If your friends think less of you for this act, perhaps they need to enter into a discussion as to why they are so uptight about food. The other side of this consideration is your discipline, your body's needs. And so, in remembrance of this, you easily restrain yourself from taking more than a teaspoonful.

Acting out this principle is not a reward for being good. It is just a humorous gesture, an intelligent and pleasurable display of freedom from the bondage that others suffer on their various "diets!" It also displays your understanding that we are always sustained, Eternally, and Perfectly, by the Very Divine.

Soil Quality and Food Taste

Over the years, we've heard reports of world soil quality diminishing due to such factors as natural post-glacial erosion, rain leaching of minerals, and (more readily understood) mineral and other nutrient depletion from pesticide and chemical fertilizer abuse. Of course, such depletion would necessarily mean a drop in the quality and taste of foods.

Those of us born in the 1940s (including your author) and earlier will remember, e.g., the taste of tomatoes and corn being as sweet and juicy as apples and strawberries. Virtually all other produce was the same. Whereas, most of today's produce by far generally tastes flat by comparison. Why is this so?

Can we attribute this drop in quality and taste to such natural events and human-made practices? If so, what, if anything, can be done to change this, to get better taste—and quality—produce? Apparently, our technology hasn't developed to the point where we can control our planet's weather, guiding rainfall, e.g., to where it's needed most and away from where it's not. And we certainly can't help the fact that we're currently in an interglacial period.

But we can change our practices of farming, moving back to more natural and sustainable means. We can use soil enrichment practices such as crop rotation, companion planting, natural pesticides, and pest control, introduce ground glacial rock, animal waste, and composted kitchen waste fertilizer. Your author has used such methods for many years, and thus produced, via a small garden, far more rich and tasty food than his family could possibly eat—which methods are shared via *GLDLifestyle*.

No point in making an argument for soils contributing to health. That's as obvious as the weather. And just as minerals can leach out of the soil, super-concentrated animal wastes from giant agribusiness farms can and have ruined rivers and aquifers and caused horrible stench for those living downwind. This, of course, is in addition to the far worse damage to the non-humans living in such crowded and unnatural conditions.

We human beings must act responsibly with our fellow Earth-bound creatures. As Avatar Adi Da Says, *"You humans tend to be noisy and to kill everything."* It's high time we stopped abusing animals en mass. If you knew what happens in these "CAFOs" (Concentrated Animal Feeding Operations) and their effect on the environment, you'd be revolted. Now is the time to turn this picture around—with cooperation, tolerance, understanding and love.

The Worst "Sins" of Eating
Rightly done, the taking of food is engaged as sacred activity—as with all the other activities of life. The basic rule is *"Appropriate use and intelligent abstinence."* Using the word "sin" in its original Greek meaning

(hamartia = to miss the mark), there are many ways of sinning, or missing the mark (the "Mark" being the Divine), with food and diet, ranging from mild abuse to extreme insult. Here is a tentative list, including an estimated abuse rating, starting with the worst:

The Worst "Sins" of Eating

- Failing to pray over meals (or otherwise to lovingly and devotionally acknowledge the Divine at mealtime)
- Overeating (which, at the gross level, is likely the worst of all)
- Regular purposeful vomiting of what has just been eaten—as an emotional-reactive strategy (Anorexia)
- Eating while engaging in dangerous activities (eating while driving, operating heavy equipment, etc.)
- Grazing (eating randomly & more or less continuously)
- Starvation dieting (continually and purposefully denying the body's hunger signs and urges)
- Binge eating (Bulimia)
- Speaking while eating
- Strategic eating (eating to become healthy, lose weight, gain weight, or other egoic purposes)
- Eating at inappropriate times (late nite "just for fun" meals, on rising, when upset, <u>when not hungry</u>, etc.)
- Eating in inappropriate environments (noisy, ugly, stressful, dangerous, with bad company people, etc.)
- Inappropriate use of celebratory foods (LQFs; unwholesome, cooked, frozen &/or microwaved foods, etc.)
- Eating while watching TV/movies
- Eating while engaging in other physical activities

No need to be alarmed if you have been doing one or more of these "sins." We egos (or "sinners," if you like) are always finding ways to pleasurize ourselves, since, as egos, our whole MO is self-*fulfillment*—which will never happen, not fully. People are wound so tight these days, stressed out to the max, knowing that any day our so-called "leaders" in government and their Big Corporate bosses could bring the world to ruin at any time.

However, what we <u>can</u> do is handle our personal lives, and maintain at least bodily integrity. We can connect with others at the local level to share our energies and our lives. We can have intelligent and even *wise* friends nearby or on the Net to continually encourage us to higher ways of life, ways that are ego-forgetting, and therefore self-*transcending*—ways that turn us to the Divine. Those are our true friends!

"The food you take into your body and your general environment support a kind of chemical process that produces the etheric dimension. The etheric dimension also derives from the subtle dimension. ...Thus, to treat the physical body wrongly will decrease nerve-force and weaken the etheric envelope, and it will even have some effect on the more subtle dimensions of the being, such as the psychic part of you." —Adi Da Samraj

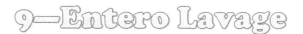

9—Entero Lavage

Paying the Garbage Men Union Scale Wages

Definitions

BMs – Bowel movements

Entero lavage – A French term referring to the perennial, tried-and-true, and even ancient methods of internal bowel washing techniques applied from the outside. In modern times, these can include enema, colema, and colonic irrigation.

Enema – Current use: A thick, flexible rubber "bottle" with rubber hose, plastic clip, and plastic tip, to fill with water or other pure liquid to flush toxic wastes from the bowel and/or otherwise strengthen and/or nourish the bowel.

Colema – A special modern device applied to the toilet onto which one sits, or board onto which one lays, containing a large plastic bucket and hose. Pure water is placed into the elevated bucket; atmospheric pressure on the water causes it to flow strongly into the bowel to obtain greater cleansing than with an ordinary enema.

Colonic irrigation – An electric and hydraulic-powered device that propels pressured water thru purification filters, sometimes with oxygen injection, and into the bowel anally, for excellent cleansing that is capable of reaching to the ileo-cecal area.

Paying the Garbage Men

Regular bowel movements (BMs) are necessary for good health. Dietary fiber occurs in whole raw foods. When less of it enters the bowel, BMs will, over time, necessarily slow down. On the GLD—altho the average BM without stimulation occurs about once every four days—BMs can, with some bowels, slow to as few as once every ten days (see ***LEVEL 1*** in "Applications"). Opportunity knocks!

Therefore, it's good to take advantage of this "quiet" bowel situation to get some special cleansing and purification. This is the perfect time to do an enema (or colema or colonic) to help clean out the residual food sludge now accumulating in the gut—as well as some accumulations that have been developing there for years!

Certain herbs such as Cascara Sagrada (or Cascara Bark) and Senna have traditionally been used to stimulate the muscular walls of the bowel and thereby help bring on a bowel movement. These are the essentially "laxative" herbs. Bulking agents such as psyllium and flaxseed can be placed into smoothies to create enuf material to bring on a BM. Aloe Vera, the greatest of all herbs and SuperFoods, is soothing and healing to the bowel. Your Health Professional will help you decide on which (and if) herbs are appropriate in your case.

The GLD provides an excellent time to use colema or colonic irrigation therapy. *IMPORTANT*: Do NOT go more than four days without a BM! If you haven't had a BM by the end of the 4th day, do an enema or colema, or get a colonic. You really should have a BM at least every four days, natural or via herbs or entero lavage. While this is not critical in most cases, it is important. The "garbage men"—which are the bowel muscles— have to be paid! And they want union-scale wages! Which is also why you need a whole raw salad when you're back on solid foods!

When solid foods are not going into the body on any regular basis, bowel activity slows significantly, eventually stopping—as when fasting and with certain *LEVEL 1* GLD applications. The bowel muscles are stimulated by the bulk and roughage of the natural fibers freely occurring in raw foods. Cooked foods provide little stimulation for the bowel muscles (the "garbage men" of the body) because that fiber is weakened by cooking. Remember: "union-scale wages" or they won't work.

If natural BMs do not occur within 4 days, do an enema or colema or go to a Colon Hydrotherapist and get a colonic. In other words, one can accomplish BMs and waste removal via enema, colema, or colonic irrigation—albeit water-stimulated. PLEASE NOTE: when the water goes up there, the bowel relaxes even more, allowing the water to do the waste removal work. On some *LEVEL 3* applications, there can be natural BMs almost daily. Best is to do an enema or colema twice weekly or get a colonic irrigation once weekly on your 30-day GLD. This is our Rx!

If you are having BMs daily, and long after two weeks on your GLD, you are likely taking sufficient amounts of solids—perhaps snacks and cooked chunky soups—to bring on the BMs. In that case, you will not need entero lavage. However, in that case, you are likely losing weight more slowly or not at all—which, perhaps, is fine. Hopefully, the relative purity of this type of GLD is what you want for your purification.

However, if more and greater purification is desired, (1) get your GLD up above 95% raw, (2) be sure (as always) to get the three basic food groups daily, (3) be certain your liquids are taken as they come from the blender—or even thinned out a bit, and (4) make sure it is all pure liquids. You will receive the full benefits of the GLD when these simple rules are followed. BMs will slow down accordingly.

BM Expectations on the Levels of Application

LEVEL 1 – Entero lavage will be needed every 3 days

LEVEL 2 – Natural BMs may average every 3 to 4 days. No entero lavage would be strictly needed in that case, but is recommended, anyway, after the first week, for the sake of assisted bowel toxin elimination.

LEVEL 3 – BMs will depend on your GLD application—mainly, liquid viscosity and use of snacks. We suggest doing the entero lavage as a preventive measure for continued bowel maintenance and function.

Hot Water as an Aid to BMs

One of the easiest ways to prompt a BM is via hot water. No need to use pure water, because in this case, the water is for outside the body. Common tap water is fine. If BMs seem a bit stubborn in coming, or if you otherwise feel the need for a BM, simply pour or pat some hot water directly onto the anal area. If the water is too hot for your hands, it's too hot for your backside. Somehow, anal tissues can handle rather hot water—and they seem to like it!

For whatever reason, the hot water strongly encourages the lower bowel to release its contents. A quart-size plastic bottle with a large mouth is usually best for this practice. We recommend pouring with the right hand (while sitting on the toilet seat) and patting the water into place (against the anus) with the left hand.

With practice, after the BM and with using the remainder of the water, the anus and surrounding tissue will be clean at the end of this process. Then, pat your backside dry with a hemp towel. ***IMPORTANT***: For the sake of hygiene, finish by washing your hands. Notice another positive quality in this process: no toilet tissue is needed!

Of course, **if you have a bidet**, you have the better way to cleanse the anus after a bowel movement and to stimulate one. **The bidet is the superior method of anal hygiene**. A bidet with seat-warming, water-heating, deodorization, and warm-air blow-drying capability is most desired—but at least the seat-warming and water-heating. These bidets offer the user advantages and pleasures not afforded those who are reduced to participating in the destruction of forests for toilet tissue to smear feces over their backsides!

Google "bidet" and see what you get. In some countries (Japan, e.g.), they're SOP—standard operating procedure. Almost everyone has one. Very popular in Europe, too. Costco sometimes carries them. Check out the *Toto*

Washlet. Once you've used a sanitary and hygienic bidet, with water-stimulated BMs, warm toilet seat, water washing, air drying, and odor-erasing, you'll never go back to the old toilet tissue routine. Toto© Washlet bidet models start at about $200USD and go up to about $650 or so. Completely worth the money.

Performing an Enema

Enemas are easily done. Purchase a strong thick rubber enema bag, e.g., Faultless®, about $20USD with its accessories, from any USA drug store or large department store (e.g., Wal-Mart). Also see www.enemasupply.com and www.optimalhealthnetwork.com and www.enemabag.com. Do not purchase a "fleet enema" bag, as these are flimsy and will not do the job for the kind of use you will be putting the bag to.

Wash out the bag with hot soapy water before each use to remove any possible harmful bacteria. *Use only pure water in the enema*—altho "nourishing" enemas (Vitamin C, e.g.) and "parasite-destroying" enemas (adding blended raw garlic, etc.) are possible (see below). Warm the water a bit before placing it into the enema bag. Best is room temperature or warmer.

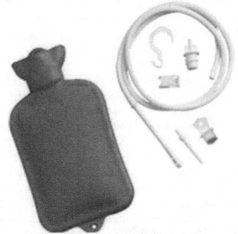

The enema kit you want comes with a plastic hanger for hanging the bag on any fixture above the body (like a soap dish in the shower stall or bathtub). Atmospheric pressure on the water inside the bag will cause it to easily flow down thru the included hose and into the anus. It's good to blend a chunk of fresh garlic into the enema water (be sure to blend well to avoid large particles left). Other items that can be blended into the enema water include crystal vitamin C, plain yogurt, and powdered antiparasitic herbs (Wormwood, etc.—check with your healer).

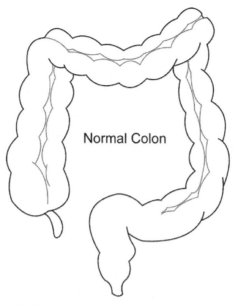

Normal Colon

When ready for your enema, place the stopper clip about 6 inches from the nozzle tip so you can open and close it easily. Fill the enema bag with the pure warm water and any other addition (garlic, etc.). Hang the bag in the tub or shower enclosure as high as possible. Strip naked and lie on your back. Place a few drops of coconut oil onto the tip of the enema nozzle (at the end of the hose) and on your anus. Gently push the nozzle well into your anus.

Reach back and open the clip, allowing the liquid in the enema bottle to flow into your rectum and sigmoid colon. When the bag has emptied, get up and sit on the toilet, allowing the water to flow out with the residual accumulated waste materials. When finished, carefully rinse out the enema bottle and wash the tip with hot soapy water. You're finished.

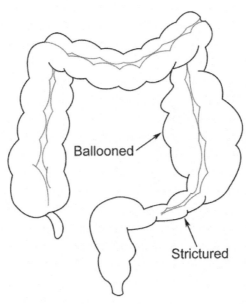

At first, you may not get thru the whole quart of water in the enema bottle before you feel a powerful urge to eliminate. Over time, you will be able to retain the whole bottle before releasing it. This is especially useful if you are doing a therapeutic enema, which includes the use of various bowel stimulating and anti-parasitic herbs, garlic, plain yogurt, and vitamins.

And, don't be surprised at what comes out! Often this can include worms, thick mucus, strange-looking formations, and rubbery shapes that appear to conform to that of the inside of your bowel. Better out than in!

Here is an example of a problem bowel and one that is of normal shape. We can, via the GLD, start to feel better long before the bowel gets near the normal shape, but some change has to take place first. Your right use of the GLD will accomplish this.

Remember, once you've started doing enemas on your GLD, your bowel will relax and let the water do the cleansing. So, don't wait for a natural BM after that. It's less likely to occur after an enema. Just do a series of enemas, colemas, or colonic irrigations to allow the important extra entero lavage, the added purification.

Reintroducing Beneficial Bacteria via Rectal Syringe

Besides adding some plain yogurt to your enema (nourishing enema), another even quicker way is via the use of the bulb rectal syringe (see image). This can be done in the bathtub or shower enclosure or even on the toilet. The syringe is about fist size and holds 8 oz. of water or other liquid. In this case, watery plain yogurt. In a bowl, mix two heaping Tbsp. of plain yogurt with 4 oz. pure water. Thoroly rinse out the bulb and squeeze it empty.

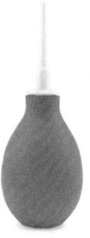

Allow the bulb to suck up the watery yogurt mix. Place a little coconut oil on the tip so it will slide into your anus easily. Holding the bulb upright (tip up), squeeze out any air until the watery liquid is at the tip. Then, slowly and gently insert it upward into the anus—preferably all the way to the bulb.

Squeeze the bulb until it is closed (until you've made a fist squeezing it). Gently pull out the bulb. Hold the liquid in as long as you can before releasing the contents into the toilet.

While some of the watery yogurt will come out into the toilet, some will remain in your bowel—along with a now-proliferating friendly batch of bacteria—which is the whole point of this little operation. You can do this three more times in order to get a good positive inoculation of friendlies into that gut. Good job!

How Long will it Take for me to Get Well?
We address this question in another part of this book. Several factors are involved. Here, the bowel comes in for special consideration. The bowel is not often discussed by medical professionals when considering most diseases. But its functioning is crucial to our well-being. A major factor in the time it takes for us to get well from mild to chronic diseases is the shape and condition of our bowel. If it's all twisted, contorted, strictured and bulging here and there, we've got a way to go before we can expect to feel well.

10—Signs and Symptoms

Disease and Healing on the GLD

Various signs necessarily appear during the course of your GLD. Some signs are negative and unnecessary. Some are welcome signs of cleansing and purification—the signs we want to see. These are not always pleasant, but they are important, and should be welcomed by you and your healer. Their various accompanying symptoms will tell whether you are engaging the GLD correctly or not. They show you your body is eliminating unwanted materials.

There are basically two kinds of symptoms: (1) disease symptoms, and (2) cleansing and healing symptoms. Disease symptoms occur most often as a result of diet and lifestyle abuse, or (less often) as a result of accident or injury. Disease symptoms can, and often do, last far longer than do most cleansing/healing ones. Cleansing symptoms occur only when the body is getting what it needs: pure diet and life-positive lifestyle. *Only cleansing and healing signs will appear on the rightly-done GLD*.

As you progress during the first few days and weeks on your GLD, you should notice certain changes in the way your body feels. The first signs occur in the first few hours—hunger! You will feel hungrier than usual because your body has been used to getting solid foods, and (for most people) mostly cooked foods—on a fairly regular (or perhaps very regular) basis and probably more in amount than you need for good health. Now, on your GLD, you're taking these liquids, which are thinner and more nutrient-dense than solid foods.

This change can therefore produce signs resembling hypoglycemia. You may feel a bit light-headed, or even slightly dizzy. Take some juice, blended soup, or a smoothie. In your bodily activities, relax; slow down a bit, put out a little less energy. This will pass. Your body will adjust to this new regime, usually in only a few days. Or, such symptoms may persist over several days, but they will eventually end—even for those with major sugar and carbohydrate metabolism problems (so-called "diabetes").

Next, you will notice that your body feels better. There are fewer or otherwise diminished aches and pains if these were among your disease symptoms. Your weight will come down. These signs usually occur within the first few days—if you are doing your GLD correctly. If, on the other hand, you are indulging in more cooked liquids than raw, and sneaking whole handfuls of snack crackers and cookies and such, you will only postpone these signs of purification, perhaps even indefinitely.

Your weight loss and improved health will occur to the degree that you follow the GLD more precisely, gradually increasing the percentages of raw liquids above the basic starting point of a minimum of 75%—and avoiding the LQFs. Those with entrenched or chronic thyroid problems will tend not to lose weight as much as otherwise unless they're on whole porcine or bovine thyroid and kelp (talk with your healer about this).

You may, on your GLD, experience occasional sleeplessness, fluctuating energy levels, sudden surges in energy, and sudden clarity of the senses (especially eyesight). On average, you'll need 20% less sleep on the GLD compared to when on solids (30% less while fasting). It is fairly common to experience improved visual acuity, increased hearing sensitivity, and a better sense of smell. "Gas," or "wind," or flatulence, is virtually eliminated.

Stomach and bowel rumblings are quite common, can occur daily, or several times per day, and can last for weeks. The body—especially the gastro-intestinal system organs, including the stomach, small intestine, and large bowel—is simply making many adjustments within, and adapting to the new dietary regime of cleansing and purification. All of this is normal. Stay with the program, varying the drinks and liquids from time to time, even perhaps daily, to maintain variety and interest.

Signs of Cleansing

- Light-headedness
- Brief fever and chills
- Stomach and Bowel rumblings
- Body Temperature Fluctuations
- Increased energy/energy fluctuations
- Uneven sleep; occasional sleeplessness
- Energy surges, sudden energy increases
- Yellow or green discharge from the eyes
- Excessive sinus drainage and throat phlegm discharge
- Coated tongue (eventually clarifies on rightly done GLD)
- Brief recurrence of past disease symptoms (cold, flu, etc.)
- Gradual elimination of all symptoms (on correctly done GLD)
- Increased sensitivity and clarity of the senses—especially the etheric

---

Your Body will Smell Better—and Be Better!

Another cleansing sign is your breath. The deposition on the tongue of waste matter from the body (which especially happens overnite and right from the start) is a long-recognized sign of cleansing. A tongue scraper (available in drug stores) can help this situation, after which you can brush your teeth—and your tongue. Eventually, over time, this deposit will disappear, showing that your body is achieving a new level of cleanliness.

Body odor is another such sign of cleansing. The body takes on the aroma—or stench!—of whatever is put into it. Smoke cigarettes and smell like a burned-out corpse! Eat junk food and smell like a garbage heap. Eat raw foods and your underarms and other body parts will eventually actually smell a bit musky but good. Even your feces will no longer have a foul odor. Don't believe it? Try it!

Other Signs and Symptoms of Purification
The sinuses may suddenly, one night, begin discharging large amounts of mucus, accompanied by throat mucus discharge, both of which may go on for 1-3 hours. This commonly results from dairy abuse and/or excessive use of pharma drug sinus inhalers used to temporarily shrink sinus membrane passages for more easeful breathing. Eliminate the need for such inhalers by right use or elimination of animal dairy products.

Yellow, greenish, orange, or other odd-colored discharges may emit from the eyes or nose as a result of having taken certain pharma drugs thru the mouth, eyes, or nose over periods of time. The body is always looking for a chance to eliminate these foreign substances. It will often store excesses that it cannot easily and quickly eliminate, sometimes as tumors. The GLD provides the right cleansing opportunity.

You may suddenly experience symptoms of bronchitis. It has been years since you suffered that malady, so you are now wondering why the recurring signs. When drugs suppress such disorders, symptoms often return on efficient cleansing programs such as the GLD.

Stronger strains of the organism, desperate to avoid the drug and your weakened immune system, build a spore around themselves as protection, hiding out until the body is sufficiently weak. This is what these guys do! And why drugs are rarely helpful in the long run. They *suppress*, not *cure*!

However, on effective cleansing and purification regimes such as (and including) the GLD, the body, with its renewed strength, breaks open long-suppressed tissue areas of embedded disease organisms, parasites, and toxins. Your immune system, strengthened by dietary purity, SuperFoods, life-positive lifestyle, positive visualization, and attention to the Divine, is far too powerful for mere parasites and embedded toxins. Victory is at hand!

The GLD is your opportunity, and that of your healer, to witness this aspect of the disease process. It is an important one that is not yet taught in medical schools—and yet known for millennia by the Traditional Naturopaths and experienced old-school healers.   Adi Da: *"Life is a school, and class is always in session!"*

Estimated <u>Relative Potential</u> Rapid & Thorough Cleansing Effects
of Fasting & Various Diets over the Same Period of Time

- Juice Fast, 100% natural...100%
- GLD *Level 1*..97%
- 100% raw all-natural strict Vegan diet w/no use of LQFs........95%
- GLD *Level 2*..94%
- GLD *Level 3*..91%
- 100% raw mostly-natural Vegan (no animal) diet w/rare use of LQFs...93%
- 66% GLD (1 hi-raw natural solid food meal, few LQFs)...84%
- 100% raw mostly-natural Vegetarian diet w/rare use of LQFs...83%
- 33% GLD (2 hi-raw natural solid food meals daily, occasional LQFs)...72%
- 75% raw partially-natural solid food diet w/some LQFs...72%
- 50% raw partially-natural solid food diet w/some LQFs...60%
- Strict 75% raw Vegetarian Diet w/occasional LQFs...59%
- Average Blood Type© Diet.......................................36%
- Average Jenny Craig© Diet.......................................34%
- Average Weight Watcher's© Diet.............................30%
- Average Atkins© Diet..26%
- Standard American Diet (SAD)...............................9%

Notes: Gross level cleanse effects are expressed here in terms of percentage of overall tissue purification accomplished in the shortest period of time. There are, of course, many factors to take into account here, including the person's age and relative vitality, the quality of the water used, machines utilized, natural vs. non-natural nutrition sources, and more. The fact that the SAD diet can allow any cleansing at all is a testament to the power of the average human body to cleanse itself under challenging conditions. The above SAD diet inclusion represents where the person might be a little more conscientious than average.

More on the Return of Symptoms

Following your GLD over time, you may or may not experience a repeat of the symptoms of disorders you've had in the past, beginning with the most recent and then the one before that, the one before that, etc. This happens about 30% of the time. These may seem like the same diseases coming back to haunt you. Once again, they are merely the body's way of finally eliminating a problem that was suppressed by drugs or other means and otherwise never allowed to finish their full natural course.

This process may continue over months, or it may not occur at all. The intervals between such cleansing events are often three months. The actual cleansing events are usually far briefer than the original disease condition, lasting an average of 5 days. At these times, be sure to remain calm and steady on your GLD. E.g., an average "cold" or "flu" (*disease* process) comes on gradually over a few days, lasts around 2 weeks, and then gradually disappears as the immune system gains strength in the body.

With a *cleansing* process, on the other hand, symptoms come on within hours, last 3-5 days (depending on several factors), then leave within 24-36 hours. Big difference! These purifying events, or return-of-symptoms cleanse events, tend to occur more often *10 days to two weeks AFTER a fast or GLD.*

Gone—and Good Riddance!

As you continue over days and weeks, your disease(s) will continue to decrease in intensity. In most cases (unless they were already too advanced when you began), they will eventually leave altogether. *With chronic degenerative disease processes, the patient must be monitored thru the earlier stages of purification until all medications are eliminated and all symptoms are either diminished to the point of insignificance or themselves wholly gone.*

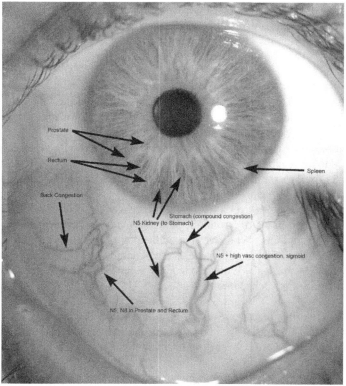

If symptoms are greatly diminished, simple and temporary or even long-term self-applied remedies may be employed. The now self-guided patient may then continue on the GLD, some modified form of it, or a hi-raw (80% +) or all-raw solid food veggy diet. For most of us, by far, (97% of us), only fresh raw untainted natural food will both get and keep us symptom-free. And liquefying these foods makes things that much easier on the body.

Mystery Disorders

Take note, too, that some chronic diseases appearing lately have no names. There are so many chemicals already in our environments, and more being added every day, that it is no wonder these strange symptoms continue to appear—including some that in certain ways mimic known disorders. Some of these can take a great deal of time to resolve. Added to that, many people have multiple disease processes going at once and are aware of perhaps only one. At Grand Medicine, we have seen this numerous times—in fact, this is the case more often than not.

We are also fortunate to know the Eyology sciences, where we can take images of the irises and scleras and compare eye markings with the patient's signs and symptoms. We can integrate other data from health practitioners, as well as from the patient, to aide in our assessment. The eyes do not have names of diseases written on them, but describe congestion in generic terms that are understandable—and universal! Thus, we can see disorders developing up to three years in advance of their presentation as symptoms. This is all a great advantage to the healer.

Drugs vs. Herbs
As we've stated, each healing modality has its unique place. There are many such modalities: Acupuncture, Allopathic, Naturopathic, Massage, Acupressure, Reflexology, Radionics, Chiropractic, and many more. Allopathic dominates in medicine now only because the Rockefeller family decided to make it big selling drugs. And they did. So, MDs get exaggeratedly high pay for the same work effort as others—in healing and in other fields.

At Grand Medicine, over more than four decades of clinical experience, we've seen and heard of (from our patients) many instances of the abuse of pharma prescriptions. When we studied the purported reasons for these drugs and the damages they could cause, we wondered how they could ever have cleared FDA approval. We don't wonder anymore. The profits are so high that fast-tracking has become SOP.

Still, a few drugs are useful, albeit on a temporary basis, especially certain pain-killers. Some others can be said to be moderately useful, while most, by far, we contend, should never have been approved.

Once, on a trip to a foreign country, I returned with an infection in a finger that just wouldn't go away. It spread to other fingers on that hand, and then to the thumb. It looked awful, like the skin was rotting away. I tried any number of herbs and combinations thereof, but nothing was working. This was, of course, quite frustrating. I wanted a natural remedy, but was there one? In this case, I thot, maybe not.

Consulting with a friendly MD, I was given a prescription for a cortisone gel. At the pharmacy, I was shocked to learn that the 1.5 oz. tube cost me $62USD. It probably cost the company 75¢ to make, tube and all. I applied it and, wow! it worked in 2 days! But two days later, the infection came back. Like a good patient, I re-applied it. Once again, it was gone. And once again, it returned! Damn! What's going on here? One more time. Same result.

So, I finally listened to my intuition, which told me there was a natural remedy that I had to apply and stay with. I dipped some gauze in coconut oil, wrapped the infected fingers in it, and covered the bandages with plastic wrap. I changed this soaking and bandaging process nightly for 10 days. By the 10th day, the infection was gone—and it has never returned.

On the other hand, I've had street people come into my office who were massively infected. I knew very well their only hope of eliminating that infection quickly and effectively was thru antibiotics. The only trick in those cases was to get them to the hospital—and admitted. But then, many of the bugs that used to respond to antibiotics have adapted, so ever newer drugs need to be invented. But take note: bugs will never adapt beyond the ability of natural remedies to manage them. And there's a natural remedy for every disease—as long as it's known and rightly applied.

A Difference in Approach
All types of medicine have a place of propriety and effectiveness. **Rockefeller-Big Pharma Medicine**, which is something over 100 years old, is essentially about treating symptoms. It can be excellent at diagnosing, altho many such procedures are invasive and some downright harmful. It excels at dealing with emergencies. But with chronic degenerative diseases, its procedures are *palliative* at best—and *lethal* at worst. From medical error alone, it causes over 400,000 deaths per year in the USA.

Natural Medicine has many forms, ancient, traditional, and modern. Naturopathy is our oldest medicine. BTW, it is where surgery (called trepanning) began. Anthropologists currently estimate surgery as being about 60,000 years old. Naturopathy looks to find the cause or root of the disorder. As such, it asks many questions of the patient and treats the cause. At best, it works to empower the patient toward health self-responsibility. With perhaps only a few deaths per year from error, its acceptance by the public is legendary.

Pharma Medicine, seeking to protect its power and profits, has a long and sordid history of suppression and persecution of virtually all other forms of medicine. Obviously, it is to the advantage of everyone to allow and promote all forms of medicine that prove to be beneficial. The only way this will happen is with open-mindedness and fair and open testing of each modality.

Healing the Part vs. the Whole
Both Allopathic and Naturopathic and even Ancient healers very often make the mistake of simply *treating symptoms* in an effort to bring about a cure. This is entirely understandable under the current regime of Pharma Medicine—as well as from the standpoint of our compassion for the patient— just wanting them to be well and not have to suffer. However…there is a much bigger and more important principle here they are missing.

"If you are busy diagnosing the system and then coming up with a remedy to attack a 'problem,' you are not taking into account the whole system. You are just using your analysis, which is detached from the whole. You should take all of the data as a means of understanding what is going on systematically in the individual case, and then you should address the entire system.

"You must address the whole body, which is a system of many organs in relation to one another, and so forth. Healing is about the entire system and what it is going to do itself. It will self-organize. It will self-purify. It will self-correct. You simply must help the system to work. This is whole-body thinking, non-seeking thinking."
—Adi Da Samraj

Rather than try to bring about a cure based on seeking, it's far more prudent to simply "searchlessly" work with the whole body, allowing the body its wisdom. As Adi Da points out in the book, <u>*Conductivity Healing*</u>, the body is self-organizing, self-correcting, and self-rightening. Rather than focus on treating a rash on the skin, we are far better considering the whole person and allowing the body to correct itself—which does not obviate treatment.

What we typically do as healers is focus on "the problem." A problem needs a solution. Taking the Radical Healing approach suggested by Adi Da means a systems approach to healing. Consider everything, all the available data, making appropriate recommendations, starting with diet (since the gross body is a FOOD body), and making sure the patient is doing **The BIG 7** to the best of their ability, but then allowing the body to do its work.

The "cure" is not the goal, then. There is no search, no goal. Make sure everything is in place for the body to do its purifying, balancing, correcting, and rightening. Give the body what it needs to do this. *Make sure the patient is doing their part* in this responsibility for bodily health. As long as there is no need to intervene in life-threatening signs, this eclectic, systems, non-seeking, or Radical Healing approach is the best one.

"It does not make any difference what the so-called 'problem' is. You should always serve systems, not 'problems.' The system is a whole. And it is intrinsically self-correcting if permitted to do so. Always assume the whole-body approach. That approach is about how to balance the whole body and how to 'consider' the range of substances that will serve the self-correcting process of the body. ...[This] is about how you manage health in a searchless manner, trusting the system to work."
—Avatar Adi Da Samraj

At Grand Medicine, what we have seen clinically, and experienced in a life now approaching 80 years, is that there is always some damn thing wrong with the body. An infection here, a sore back there—it's always something. Bodily health is not about perfection. The body is always a work in progress—even to its end. This in no way suggests we should not keep engaging right life practices. No way, Jose! These practices are merely appropriate.

In another place in the book, <u>*Conductivity Healing*</u>, Avatar Adi Da mentions our tendency to be obsessed with perfect health. He says, *"You have to be willing to practice no matter what is happening in your life. ...good health is not an absolute... People become unhealthy for all kinds of reasons and at various times. For some people, conditions persist regardless of their practice of healthful disciplines. One should merely continue life-positive health practices which are counter-egoic...whether or not it produces perfect health."*

And later, *"The practice of health is rightly about counter-egoic self-discipline in devotional turning to [The Divine Reality]. It's not about improving or developing the individual 'self.' Prior Perfection is always already the case, so perfection of any [bodily] condition is both impossible and unnecessary."*

In the below Left Lateral Quadrant sclera photos, the patient presented at our clinic on the 15th day of a combined 30-day GLD and juice fast. The top image was taken on the 15th day, the bottom one on the last (30th) day of the GLD/fast. The same camera and lighting were used in each photo. The improvement in his health is clearly reflected in the sclera line changes.

The thinning and fading of the sclera lines indicate the purification, cleansing, and healing that has taken place. He lost about 24 lbs. on this regime. He looked to be in excellent health, symptom-free, slim and trim at age 63, and claimed he felt better than he had in years. He plans to do the same 30-day GLD each year for the rest of his life.

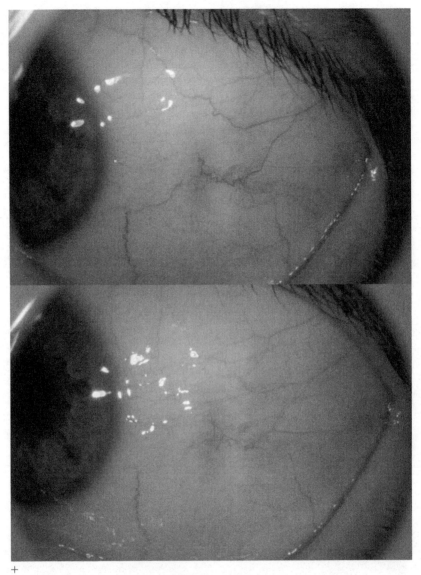

+

Of course, this is just one of the many, many ways the benefits of the GLD can be clearly seen in those who rightly participate.

11—Weight Control

How the GLD can Do It Better—and Why

How much weight will I lose? Could I lose too much weight?

It has long been known that rapid weight loss programs are generally not as successful as those in which the weight comes off more gradually. However, the more crucial factor, in most cases of overweight, is the understanding of the person who suffers the weight problem. In fact, in many cases, there is no overweight "problem" to begin with! The "problem," in many cases, is the *culture of sameness*, where we are told we all must look a certain way.

Frame Size and Metabolism

Some bodies were never meant to be "runway model slim." Some of us are large-boned (or large framed). To find out, place one hand on the lateral side (away from you) of your other wrist. If you cannot easily (without squeezing) touch the middle finger to your thumb at the wrist line, you're large-boned. If you can, with little room to spare, you're medium boned. If you can touch your index finger to your thumb, you're small-boned. Other ways of determining frame size are found on the Net.

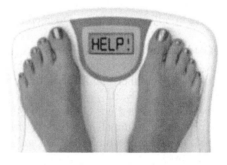

Metabolism is another factor in weight control. Inactive people can develop slower metabolic rates. Age and other factors can contribute to this— which is where pure diet and life-positive lifestyle come into the picture. A slower metabolism means more gradual weight loss. But, it doesn't mean NO weight loss. The GLD eventually tackles all weight control situations. Meanwhile, rather than have someone tell you you're overweight, why not ask yourself? What was your weight when you felt functional, comfortable, flexible, and generally easeful in the body?

On the GLD, if you feel or are overweight, your excess weight will more than likely gradually, effectively, and safely diminish. Weight loss, however, could be slowed significantly by low thyroid (hypothyroid) conditions. A home self-test for thyroid function is provided to *GLDLifestyle* members. For help with thyroid testing &/or thyroid function, ask your Natural Health Practitioner. You may need Armour thyroid and kelp.

Eventually, if you remain on the GLD long enuf, and if your GLD is sufficiently high in raw juices and green smoothies—in other words, if you're doing your GLD correctly—your body will take the shape it was meant to have by Nature all along.

Maintaining or Gaining Weight on The GLD

If you're **a thin-body type**, you may be able to keep your weight by strategically using rich nut-seed smoothies and other hi-calorie drinks. The avocado-coconut smoothie (see Appendix A) is an example: rich, thick, delicious, and high in the good fats. If you're an *extremely* thin-body type (only about 1.3% of the population), talk with your Natural Health professional about how to apply the GLD in your case, and whether a few days of a mono diet might be a good place for you to start.

In other words, most thin-body types—those who generally have trouble keeping weight on—are not in this very small percentage, and therefore they can do the GLD with minimal consultation. In their case, their weight may initially come down to a certain level and stay there, just like with the "average" and heavy-body types. Again, please take into account exercise, drink viscosity, and other liquid and lifestyle activity factors regarding weight control. Burn a lot of calories with hi exercise and you're going to lose weight. Exercise lightly and you'll tend to keep it.

GOOD Fats and BAD Fats

The body needs fats to be healthy. There are fats (and oils) that are healthy for us and there are fats (and oils) that are not so healthy—some, even harmful. Essentially, the "good" fats (and oils) come from natural, living nut and seed sources and are either totally un-processed (non-processed, eaten raw) or at least minimally processed. Minimally processed raw, expeller-pressed) oils from natural "live" nuts and seeds can be considered "good", or healthy for us.

The good fats are naturally found in living foods such as coconuts (a nut), almonds and most other nuts, and sunflower seeds, pumpkin seeds and other seeds, and avocados (botanically considered a berry). Many natural foods have small amounts of fats in them, but, basically, raw nuts and seeds are highest in these "good", healthy fats. At the top of our "good" list are coconuts—a true SuperFood (see Appendix C)—and almonds, queen of the nuts.

For other good fats and fatty oils, we can go to the minimally-processed raw butters such as almond butter, coconut butter, and other nut butters (altho peanut butter—peanuts are a legume—is not particularly recommended). If you must have animal butters, ghee butter is most acceptable. Cacao (cocoa) butter can also be included here. As for oils, stick with the MCT oils, including (especially) raw natural expeller-pressed coconut oil but also the other natural and minimally-processed nut and seed oils. Tip: get into making your own nut and seed butters!

On the "bad guy" side, we have the processed vegetable oils, even olive oil (!), lard, essentially most animal-based oils, common animal-based mayonnaise, all processed foods, common salad dressings, cereals (grain-based), pastries, canola oil, corn oil, commercial snack foods and other such packaged foods, most condiments, fast foods (of course!), candy bars and most nutrition bars, and most commercial desserts (pies, cakes, etc.).

Snacks can and should be taken by thin-body types who wish to either maintain their current weight or even gain weight on the GLD. The emphasis will be on nuts and nut butters, seeds, and seed butters—preferably but not absolutely necessarily homemade. Several quite delicious raw nut and seed butters are currently commercially available. Several beg Tbsp. of any combination of these can be taken throughout the day.

Chips and dip, hummus, salsas, guacamole, mixed sauces—these are all fair game for the thin folks. The very items those of us who only wish we could be eating are allowed, and in some cases even encouraged for the skinny people. HOWEVER, snacks must be (1) pure and wholesome as possible, and (2) used intelligently—not indulged exclusively while avoiding your smoothies. Pure juices may be bypassed, but remember, this is a liquid diet!

Meaning that while purification will continue for most thin body types even while taking appropriate amounts of nut and seed butters, veggy dips, and guacamole, the green smoothies and other liquids have to be there for right purification to occur. The amounts of these dietary items will depend on several factors, such as your current height and weight, your health condition overall, disease processes, age, etc. If, as a thin-body type, you are continuing to lose weight, your experienced health professional will help you make the needed adjustments.

What Did You Call Me? Chubby? Tubby?

Of course, *the thinner the liquids the greater the purification*—and (in general, all other things being equal) the swifter the weight will come off. However, remember that first and foremost on your GLD are **purification** and **equanimity**. Weight loss and improved health are secondary to them. And emotional issues are often the biggest consideration!

Some gain weight and keep it on to spite a parent or parents who were strict disciplinarians. This is called an "Oedipal" reason, referring to the early life relationships between us and our parents. Then, there are those who gain weight to protect themselves from rape or other physical abuse. Of course, there are many more reasons for weight gain. In any case, your GLD allows you to confront these issues and more beyond them.

You will necessarily face these while on your GLD. You will be tested by this whole GLD process regarding your restraint and will power. No worries, tho: you are not in competition with anyone while on your GLD—not even yourself! Doing the GLD rightly, there will be times when your weight will remain the same—or perhaps even go up a bit! Possibilities include one or more of the following:

(1) your body (thyroid, pituitary, hypothalamus) is going thru certain special metabolic adjustments
(2) you need to apply the GLD differently, taking more raw juices, herb teas and thinner smoothies
(3) your exercise regimen needs adjusting
(4) all of the above

Once again, regardless of adjustments, never miss your green smoothie!

Be very wary of any tendency to opt for taste. Food desire is so easy to abuse—and with potentially deadly results—at least! The whole thing about diet isn't essentially about taste, anyway—it's about purification, health, balance, purity, equanimity, what's appropriate for the body, what brings life to the body, what foods are easily assimilated and in modes that allow wastes to be easily eliminated. So, be encouraged. Avoid the "easy way out" (taste). Choose among healthy alternatives. Always do your best to maintain diet purity while on your GLD.

Example: I'm overweight and on a modified GLD (one solid food meal daily). It's late in the day, I'm not really hungry, and have a green smoothie in front of me. Another big glass of green smoothie is in the frig. I'm thinking about my salad, a half piece of toasted sourdough bread, and a hot chocolate. Which way to go? I opt for taste—the salad and hot chocolate. Next day, I've gained two pounds! Ouch! Lesson learned! Thank You, Lord!

Remember what you used to look like as a child? What have you always wanted to look and feel like—whole, trim, strong and well—regardless of body frame. **Keep this vision in mind**, because *it is going to happen* when you rightly apply your GLD! It is just flat going to happen! Visualize it. Keep a picture of it *clearly in mind*, this vision of the new you. Think of it often, like many times a day.

Radiant health is your birthright. You're supposed to have it. You deserve it simply by virtue of having been born into a human body. It's natural to feel and look this way in youth. But, after age 25 <u>you have to earn it</u>! You must act intelligently with diet and lifestyle after age 25. Certain metabolic changes occur after age 25. Yes, there are herbs, breathing, and other lifestyle practices that can mitigate this process (join us at **GLDLifestyle**). Meanwhile, your GLD is the best way we know of to keep this youthful vision going.

One of the many advantages of the GLD is that your "bioFOODback" is much quicker than on other diets. Healthy results—and personal lessons—come faster than on anything but true fasts—and you cannot do a fast nearly as long as the GLD...or as often! So, go for it!

Keep your spirits up by reading this book over and over, and by talking with others who are also on the GLD. Form a GLD Group and do your yearly 30-Day GLD together. This is how we inspire each other, encourage each other, and hold each other responsible and accountable for increased health, detox, purification, weight loss and maintenance, and real human growth.

Avoid those who disparage what you are doing. If you're afraid they will disapprove, don't tell them you're doing the GLD. Keep the good company of those who are life-positive and open-minded. Your continually improving health and bodily feeling will prove you right—and your bathroom scale and any blood tests and other physical exams will back it up!

Eventually, everyone will notice your new appearance and health improvements. Remember this when your past body habits tell you to quit and get a Big Mac! (A green smoothie may not taste as good as a Whopper, but a green smoothie won't kill you, either! Just the opposite.)

Right Weight Loss and *Wrong* Weight Loss

You see them on TV, on Weight Watchers®, on the plastic surgery medical shows, and on the street. They've "lost weight." Somehow, they look better—but still unwholesome. There's loose fat dangling from their arms, legs, and abdomen. They look chunky, lumpy and bumpy. They look unhealthy. Because they *are* unhealthy! You can lose weight the "wrong" way. You can eat only beefsteak for days and weeks at a time and lose weight—and junk up your body full of uric acids, ammonia, and purines.

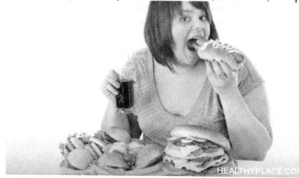

You can eat "low calorie foods"—simple carbohydrates, processed foods—and lose weight—and be sick! You can even "go on liquids"—coffee, beer, black (caffeine) tea, whiskey, sodas, and dairy milk—and lose weight. You can exercise like crazy and eat crap food "as a reward." You'll lose weight by these means. But you won't be healthy.

So, how do you correct these situations? Simple! It's the *quality* of the food, solid or liquid, that makes the difference. And, we're not talking about superior quality beer! We're talking about substances the body recognizes as food. The only way you will ever learn what your body was supposed to look like by nature is by eating raw food for a period of time. What period of time? Unless you're grossly overweight (which will take longer), we're talking ninety days minimum on solids—less on pure liquids.

On average, 90 days is the amount of time it takes *for the average human adult* to get cleaned out and balanced via solid raw fruits, veggies, nuts, and seeds. Variously longer for those with chronic degenerative diseases. You can do this quicker and easier—60 days, on average—on raw liquids. The GLD! The people with the saggy skin need to get into pure diet and life-positive lifestyle, not spend tons of money going back repeatedly to plastic surgeons. They'll never really achieve the health and beauty they want via surgery. That kind of surgery is just a temporary fix.

Not that surgery in and of itself is bad for you. Even plastic surgery can be a great aide to those truly in need, especially those injured or otherwise disfigured where such treatment would clearly help both physiologically and socially. Even those suffering severe emotional complexes re physical appearance. Meanwhile, what will Nature do in even these circumstances via dietary purity and life-positive lifestyle? So, do the surgery when necessary. Avoid it otherwise, choosing in all cases the Way of Nature. This is only smart and basically intelligent.

How—and How Much—We Eat

An old Hindu saying says: "*Fill your stomach half full of food, 1/4th full of water, and 1/4th full of love of God!*" In Western Countries, we typically have the ability to purchase whatever kinds of food we want and in whatever quantity. But, we're typically not as careful about the quality of the food we eat. And we are not very careful about how much we eat, either. And it shows.

Country by country (in 2018), Americans were the 12th most obese people in the world—and the most obese in North America. Some 38% of the population had a BMI of over 30. Some 80 million adults and 14 million children were overweight, with the adults 26 pounds heavier than they were in the 1950s. Why? (1) Stress—we overeat to deal with it. (2) Fast foods are cheaper than quality foods. (3) We depend on grocery stores and big box stores for much of our food—which get much of their (chemical compromised) food from Big Agriculture. (4) Not enuf of us are growing, sharing, and eating our own.

Re gross food, ***one of the worst "sins" is overeating***. We are usually so busy enjoying our food that we don't pay attention to how <u>much</u> we're eating. In fact, while eating, we are often too busy talking, watching TV, excessively thinking, worrying, or engaging in some other activity, to even notice how much we ate or even how the food tasted! We are typically so stressed out, we tend to choose taste over quality. And when it's cooked food we're talking about—which it <u>is</u>, most of the time—we're going to put on the pounds!

BioFoodBack Instinct

We actually need far less food than we typically eat. Cooked food has no feedback mechanism to the brain associated with it. Raw food does. If our diet is all raw food, we won't be fat. It is quite difficult to be overweight on all raw food. But, not to worry: the GLD isn't necessarily about eating all raw food (altho it certainly can be).

We know instinctively when to stop eating any <u>raw</u> food—because even fresh, raw, ripe fruits and veggies simply don't <u>taste</u> good anymore when the body has had enuf of it! CAREFULLY NOTICE THIS! However, we can eat <u>cooked</u> food until we feel stuffed, with our stomach painfully full. And even after that, cooked food <u>still</u> tastes good! **Because there is no instinct for cooked food**! The GLD allows us to see this mechanism in action.

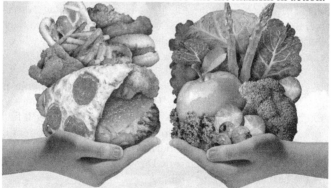

The GLD involves more raw food than cooked—by far. Even **all** raw food. We notice, especially as the days and weeks pass on the GLD, that we are developing a taste for purity. We develop a different kind of hunger, too, one that is satisfied by far less food than when on solid foods—especially solid *cooked* foods. What is this saying to us? It is pointing us to our true diet. You have to experience it to "know" at that level.

With this kind of "knowing," you'll never be fooled again: we need far less food than we typically eat. This is very clearly discovered on an all-raw diet. So, we need to eat more of our diet as <u>raw</u> to find this out! Eating mostly cooked food, the body is being starved for the pure nutrients it gets untainted from the trees and fields.

Eating on Cue

Another reason we Westerners (and newly-enfranchised Easterners) get fat is that we tend to eat "at the right time." It's Breakfast time, so we eat. It's lunchtime, so we eat. It's dinnertime, so we eat. No matter if we're hungry or not. We eat! Most of us don't even get hungry until noon, anyway, but everybody knows you're supposed to eat breakfast, right? A no-brainer, right? So, let's eat. What? Not hungry? Something wrong with you? Are you sick? Don't like the food? Eat something else! Eat, eat, eat! Breakfast is the most important meal of the day, right? Wrong!

It's Billy's birthday, so we eat. It's Mary's graduation, so we eat. Hey, our team won, so let's party! Which means food! Granma died, and that's depressing. Let's order out for pizza. That'll bring our spirits up. Don't leave any food behind. Our host will be insulted. Take an extra helping. Someone left some food on my desk. Better eat it before it gets stale. It's just sitting there, tempting me. Better eat it. There are so many reasons to eat—except for the best one: being hungry!

Ever get so hungry you thot you could eat a chair? Ever miss a meal, only to find out within a few minutes there was no problem waiting 'til the next one? Hunger—genuine hunger—is a good thing, especially for Westerners. Most people who can afford to buy whatever food they like, and whenever they want it, have this problem. We eat whatever we like whenever we like, ***not waiting until we're truly hungry***.

On the GLD, you'll know hunger. Not the extreme hunger of starving people in certain countries. Hunger happens when you switch from solids to liquids. And you'll see how hunger serves you. You'll finally get to the point of not being desperate for food anymore. The wisdom of this whole process of eating and being truly nourished whole-bodily is described in the book, <u>*Green Gorilla*</u>, by Avatar Adi Da, which is our favorite, the one we consider the best ever written on diet.

Why We Are so Desperate for Food

We feel disconnected from the real and true Source of our food—and from Real Food Itself. It's like what happens when we're born into the world. We are suddenly broken away from the mother, our safety blanket, our soft, comfortable, and warmly secure womb world—where everything is provided and with which we're totally identified as a unity. While we were in there, we had complete faith in our environment, with which we felt utterly "at-one."

110

Then, boom! We're burst into the world, often crying from that slap by the delivering doctor.

From then on, we identify with the body. We feel this separation, this separateness, this separativeness. And we try every conceivable way to get back to that sense of peace, security, and unity. This is the ego, the separate one—which, paradoxically, is never "separate" from anyone or anything! This sense of disconnection is why we're so craven. For food and everything else. In a true Wisdom Culture (see Appendix G, and www.eyology.com, and also the book, *The First Three Stages of Life*), this process is handled lovingly and carefully all thru infancy and childhood.

This is where the Divine comes in: to Teach us out of our sense of separateness, to show us the way of Real Happiness, where we are always already connected to and feeding from the True Food Source, always already in Eternal unity with everything and everyone. For those who have tasted this Source, no further explanation is necessary. For those who haven't, none is possible.

Slow and Fast Metabolizers

We have mentioned how some of us have slow metabolisms, and some have fast. Metabolism involves vital chemical reactions in the body that convert food to energy, change foods to proteins, fats, etc., and eliminate nitrogen wastes. Fast metabolizers can eat the same meals as slow metabolizers and not gain any weight—even lose weight.

Those of us with bodies that have slow metabolic rates wish we could speed things up a bit so our bodies wouldn't hold onto weight so much and so easily. We seem to gain weight simply by thinking about food. One little foray into pizza-land and, Pow!, 6 pounds. It's not fair! Food appears at once to be our dream-come-true pleasure-palace and at the same time, our mortal enemy. But metabolism can change—at least temporarily.

Various substances have been used to **speed up metabolism**. Perhaps chief among those is caffeine. Then, to a lesser extent, there are Theobromine, Theophylline, and Chlorogenic Acid, all found in cocoa and coffee. Increasing muscle mass, drinking extra water, and taking in more protein are other tricks. They are all temporary means. When we fast, metabolism is not sped up—unless we exercise. Energy is burned just by sitting. Not much, but some. Coffee works for the short term—until your body adapts to it.

Certain stimulating foods can increase metabolism, such as cayenne, jalapenos, and habaneros, for example. Add broccoli to this list. All of the SuperFoods do the same (see Appendix C). Green tea and Oolong tea can help. The medium-chain fats in pure coconut oil are known to increase metabolism, whether taken directly (in smoothies, e.g.) or in cooking. High-intensity exercise workouts are almost always mentioned by "the experts" as increasing metabolism.

We want our food to entertain as well as nourish us, and yet, for some of us, whenever we eat it, we put on the pounds. It almost seems like it doesn't matter what we eat—we put on pounds. What's fair about that? OK, it's flat the fact with some of these bodies, but that's not consoling. On the GLD, this is handled so nicely. Drinking pure liquids, we don't gain weight. First, because it's mostly or all raw foods. Secondly, because the foods we typically eat (often crap!) are just not on the GLD in the first place. The GLD is the perfect diet for slow metabolizers.

Mainly, **the way the GLD helps us** is by showing us what works and what doesn't. We have a full 30 days to learn—and learn we will! The GLD is an adventure, a challenge, a full-on learning experience. Some certain foods and behaviors serve health, weight management and purification and there are those that do not. It's in varying degrees different for each person. Each learns at his and her own speed. Do your GLD, and this learning, this growth, is assured.

Snacks for the Stout

OK, large bone structure and slow metabolism. Now what? We've struggled all our life with this situation. Nothing has worked to keep it handled. Enter the GLD. Now, it suddenly happens! And, best of all worlds, you can have snacks! You can enjoy Holiday food! You may even take little nibbles daily without punishment—meaning, without gaining weight. How does that work? It's called *confronting the pattern*—fearlessly!

Here's the trick: Let's say you like snack crackers with smoked salmon spread. You can do it! Take two of the suckers and savor them, eating very slowly. Wow! Raw pleasure! Maybe even a teaspoonful of some cooked mixed veggies your spouse is having for dinner: *The Divine Gourmet Principle*. No biggie!

The rest of your diet that day is pure raw nourishing liquids. You are always sure to do your morning Power Walk or calisthenics routine. That's a given. And, you're so busy with work that you don't bother with food, anyway, until you're genuinely hungry. This is how it's done. You're going to lose weight. It's gonna happen. Don't believe it? Watch the scale.

Obesity vs. Overweight

There is a difference between overweight and obesity. Clinically, we've met the exception to the fat person rule that overweight people are often obese. *Overweight* means the weight of the body is more than the body was designed by Nature (genetically) to handle efficiently. ***Obesity*** means increased weight from excessive fat. So, we can be thin *in appearance* but obese in fact, in body fat. However, except in cases of genetic extremes, both are diseases and are curable via the GLD.

Motivation

Your author confesses a lifelong struggle with overweight—until age 66. Some of us are just large-boned, with a slow metabolism, and not meant to be thin like those models in magazines, on TV, and on the Net. I would fast and lose weight, and then gain it rite back. I was "big." I hid it from friends and family. It was painful to look at all that fat in the mirror. The body was not supposed to look like that, and I knew it. Only when I got onto the GLD and exercise did the problem get finally handled. The **tendency** to overeat and avoid exercise is still there.

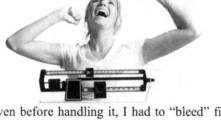

But, even before handling it, I had to "bleed" first: I had to suffer overweight long enuf, feel the pain of it for a sufficient period of time, and get **so fed up** that I was genuinely ready to make a change. Then, I visualized what this body was supposed to look like by Nature. I saw it clearly in mind— and kept it in mind while I did my liquids and my exercise—regularly. And now, it stays that way. I know what to do—and I do it. Oh, thank You, God!

We all can make this gesture. Some will, some won't. Some will do it this much and some that much. That's fine. The visualization helps. Seeing the pounds actually melt off when watching the scale helps even more. Nothing succeeds like success. The GLD makes success easy. And if you mess up, and you probably will, you can always get back on—and get stronger as you go. There's nothing that says you can't do TWO GLDs in one year! I have. The more you do it, the more you learn.

The GLD is always there to help get you back on track. And remember: the exercise is crucial. However, if you're bed-ridden or otherwise incapacitated, it'll still work with just the GLD. It'll just take a while longer. Keep looking in the mirror and having that vision before you. It works! There's no time limit. It may have taken years, even decades, to achieve your body's level of toxicity and disease. Thru the GLD, Mother Nature will do her work. She may seem slow, but it won't be anywhere near as long as it took to get that body junked up.

"When one presumes that the body is a 'problem' to be 'solved,' rather than a system to be lawfully managed, then exaggerated and systematic efforts to 'cure' the body only interfere with the body's self-healing ability... Rather, you have an obligation for health, and not a 'problem' to be corrected. When the body's functioning is limited in any way, yield the body to the lawful situation in which the condition may be set right, rather than presuming a 'problem' and seeking a solution."
—Avatar Adi Da Samraj

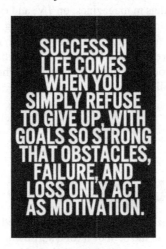

Food Addiction and the Eating Gorilla

Until we finally understand the true Source of our sustenance, we are (as Avatar Adi Da Describes) like the gorilla in the desert. We are obsessed, craven, desperate to get and have our food, to always have it with us, to never be separated from it, and fearful of losing it. All the while, the Source is with us: the Very Divine. Fortunately, we can't escape It! We're living in Its Wonderful Energy!

Our Perfect Food Source is the Matrix in which we appear, the Sustainer of everything and everyone, the Energy and Consciousness of us. We humans tend not to notice this, to not be aware of it at all. We are fearful and craven. Whereas, the gorilla <u>in the forest</u> is happy. He knows that his food is all around him. He sees you. You are eating food. He doesn't feel threatened by you. So he sits down and happily munches on his cabbage!

Until we understand this principle, we are like the gorilla <u>in the desert</u>. We are obsessed with food. We go out with friends to a buffet. Terror! And delight! You mean...I can eat anything I want? As much as I want? Wow! So, we get as much as we can fit on our plate, when <u>we're</u> finished we'll go back for more...and more...and more. Look at those desserts! Gotta get some of that.

At restaurant buffets, we don't want to miss this opportunity to taste and enjoy as much as we can. We feel we've gotta taste everything. Pie—with ice cream on top. And whipped cream on top of the ice cream! Yahoo! No restraint. No control. No discipline. We unbuckle our belt to its last notch. We leave the restaurant embarrassed, ashamed of ourselves. Damn! I did it again! And then, the next day (or even that nite), the pain. The bodily irritation. A few days of suffering. The scale—our worst enemy! Undisciplined, self-indulgent—you always pay a price.

Without this understanding, it's a losing battle. We only have to see what we're up to, our patterns regarding food. We have to feel the pain of them to the point of understanding. Then, we're free. Then, we have the chance to sense that we are always already perfectly sustained. The True Food is literally everywhere. We breathe it in. Until we've breathed enuf of it, tho, we're going to be craven like this, always worried about our life, always looking at the clock to see if it's time to eat, always looking at food as our sole source of pleasure, to see if there's still enuf left for us, desperate, as tho it soon might not be there.

Connecting or communing with the Divine, God, in the Person of the Spiritual Master (e.g., Adi Da Samraj), we forget our usual problem consciousness. Gradually, we take on the disciplines He Gives us thru His Teachings. The body-mind comes slowly and surely into balance. The Divine Showers His Wisdom and Grace on us. We feel It. We taste It. We want more! There *is* more! We're satisfied at ever-deeper levels. We feel happy. We're home!

Everything in life is a lesson, a blessing, or a test—or some combination thereof.

So, we're back at the buffet. It's test time. What will I do this time? I've been gradually taking higher percentages of raw food in the diet. I switched to a yearly 30-day GLD—starting early January. The whole concept of eating and what it means altogether—sustaining the body, what kinds of food bring this balance and good feeling, the pain of being silly with food, of overeating, the knowledge of my tendencies—this all comes into consciousness.

OK, here's the food. It's all right in front of me—including that great looking, great smelling, and (yes) that great tasting cooked and processed food! I'm here with friends, so it's all very conscious this time. Smaller portions this time. Little bites of this and that. Dessert, too. The meal ends.

It was pure enjoyment. But, it was much more conscious. I'm still a little hungry—for **life**. Best time to quit! Lesson learned. Positive ending!

Discipline

There's that word again—that hated word. Why can't I just eat whatever the hell I want and stay looking like I did when I was 17—or at least the way I always wanted to look? Some of us are not supposed to be thin (or what we tend to think of as "thin" or "slim"). BUT...there is "stout-healthy" and there is fat, overweight, obese, unhealthily so. This means facing it and being intelligent about facts—meaning strapping on our "adult."

Discipline—according to Adi Da—"...*is the hallmark of an adult human being.*" The infant, child, or adolescent in us wants mommy or daddy to do it for us. The adolescent in us wants to think of itself as being disciplined—or "*I'm going to do it.*" But while it may happen, it is only in fits and starts. The adult in us takes it on—seriously. Not <u>grinding</u> seriously, but <u>Happy</u>-seriously, as part of the understanding of what it is to be an adult.

The adult in us honors the bodily Gift we've been Given. We allow ourselves to feel this Gift. We see how so many trash the body in their desperate search for self-fulfillment. At some point, we see that we can't let that happen to us. We won't. As an adult, we embrace what we've been Given and treat it intelligently. It's hard! It's very difficult—sometimes it seems impossible. But, we have The Very Divine Help! That is our high card! USE IT!

In that most difficult time, when you're reaching for that sandwich, that glass of wine, that bag of chips or candy, look at the murti image, the foto or drawing of the Spiritual Master. Ask for Divine Help in that moment—and in any and every moment of need or difficulty. The Divine Reality <u>is here</u>— Always. It wants to be used. It can't Help us unless we ask, unless we submit, turn to It, The Happy Truth. <u>Turn—and you will get that Perfect Help</u>!

116

12—The LQFs

How the Low Quality Foods (LQFs) can be used Appropriately

An ancient expression says, *"The body is the temple of God."* Is it, really? Or is it a dumpster? To answer this question, look at the way we eat? If, in order to make the body a *"Temple of God,"* in other words, to honor it as a sacred vehicle that was Given to us as a Blessing, we must eat *"the fruits of the fields and of the trees"* (Genesis 1:28). We seem to have somehow strayed a little from that admonition!

Witness: Twinkies® and Ding-Dongs®, TV dinners, powdered chemicalized coffee creamers, donuts, hamburgers (that literally last indefinitely on a shelf), and commercial soft drinks—you know the list. It's long—very, very long. It's what we eat. It's what Big Corporate sells to us as "food." Some of it no animal would ever touch. It makes us fat. It makes us sick. It makes big Corporate rich. It makes Big Pharma rich. They love it! And they want us to love it—which is why they pay big money to keep this crap food racket going.

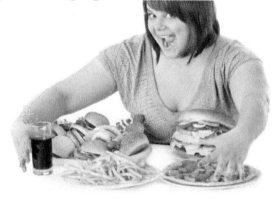

Crap food on shelf after shelf in all the supermarkets of the world. Then, tucked toward the back, there's the produce section. And, in the big-box stores, even the produce has been tampered with. These days, to protect our health and that of our loved ones, we have to find local sources of natural produce—or grow our own. So, it's our choice—once we know better. Once we value our health.

We've been raised to "like" all manner of refined and processed foods—and, at the gross level, this is exactly why we are in such trouble with health. We eat what we like instead of what we know is good for us. Time for a change of meals! The good part is that after you've been on raw liquids for a while, you tend to choose purity. The body brightens up, smartens up, gets clarified, detoxified and purified—and starts insisting on the good stuff.

Don't expect to be encouraged toward pure foods on the Big Corporate-owned mainstream media (MSM). Food, Inc., owns the factory farms that do major polluting. And 70% of TV advertising comes from Big Pharma, the nice folks who push the drugs that you have to take after getting sick from eating all that crap food. These wonderful folks want you to get and stay sick—or just well enuf to have to continue to take their poisons—for life!

While on your GLD, you will generally avoid solid foods of all kinds, except perhaps (altho not necessarily) for some occasional naturally relatively wholesome crackers, and possibly other items (nut butters, etc.) as described elsewhere in this book and as appropriate to your specific health circumstance. Even more important, tho, is dropping all use of the Low Quality Foods (LQFs), as listed below.

These are usually the substances that got us into the diseases we've suffered and may now be suffering. We must learn how to use them in ways that they will not hurt us—or ignore them altogether—which is even better. However, as we've suggested, it is not necessary to utterly avoid them forever and ever. It's just a matter of "*intelligent use and appropriate abstinence.*" When we "just have to have them" is where the Divine Gourmet Principle comes in.

AVOID THESE — the Low Quality Foods and Substances (LQF's)

- Caffeine products
- Chemicalized foods
- Microwaved foods
- Alcoholic beverages
- Cesium-irradiated foods
- Gluten-containing products
- Refined and processed foods
- **GMOs**, or genetically modified foods
- Smoke (cigarettes, cigars, vaping, etc.)
- Fried & fired foods, super-heated fats and oils
- Animal products (red meat, fowl, fish, dairy, etc.)
- Commercial soft drinks (Pepsi, Coca Cola, Dr Pepper, etc.)
- Street, OTC and all but emergency / temporary prescription pharma <u>drugs</u>
- **Refined sugar**, its many analogues, and all products containing it (see Appendix D)
- Foods exposed to pesticides, herbicides, fungicides &/or grown with chemical fertilizers

The LQFs—a Closer Look, and One at a Time

Alcohol

Alcoholic beverages have been around for thousands of years and will likely continue indefinitely. They're to be considered celebratory substances only. We've had patients ask, "*Ah, c'mon now, Dr. Leonard. You're not gonna ask me to drop my two beers a nite, are ya?*" It's as tho I'm removing his only pleasure in life. He's <u>indulging</u> himself, pure and simple. There's a time for alcohol—IF you're going to use it, and a time to avoid it—which is most of the time. Alcohol has no substantial food value, and when taken regularly, it tends to be addictive.

Some of us are far more vulnerable to alcohol's addictive nature than are others. As such, lives have been weakened, harmed, and even destroyed by it. If and when you do take it (on these very special occasions), <u>be sure others see you</u>. This is the **adult** way to use these addictive substances. Drink only in the presence of others. Why? So you will be <u>seen</u>, so you can be

<u>responsible to others</u> for your actions, so you won't be "hiding out" like a teenager, like an adolescent **with his secret life**.

Some wish to reduce the risk even more by drinking certain wines and beers ("near-beer") containing extremely low amounts of alcohol. This strategy is acceptable at these celebratory occasions, but even in their case not recommended for regular consumption. Those with certain tendencies to alcohol addiction must, of course, avoid these low alcohol content drinks altogether. (And your author describes this "right use" principle in some sense *painfully*, as he dearly enjoys his liqueurs!)

"Some of us have to bleed before we make a change."

Twice, to get a sense of what patients and even relatives go thru with alcoholism and its recovery, I ventured into local AA (Alcoholics Anonymous) meetings. (As it turns out, anyone can attend.) I was in tears both times. I listened while person after person came up in front of the group, and, after introducing themselves by their first name only, and confessing alcoholism, described how their addiction variously ruined their health and/or their life. This, of course, was heart-breaking—person after person! Very instructive! You don't want to get to that place.

Live long enuf, and in certain parts of town, and you'll see the man or woman in wrinkled clothes lying asleep or otherwise unconscious in a gutter, sometimes having urinated in their pants, clutching a bottle-shaped paper bag. You don't want to get to that place.

God Knows we are all under stress, all suffering sometimes enormous frustrations. Our freedoms are being taken away from us by the powerful elites, the super-rich and their dark minions, their lackeys in Big Corporate and government at all levels. In these Dark Times, money and power reign supreme. With this stress and frustration, no one can be blamed for taking an easy way out, indulging in drink, smoke, sex, or something at least tasty to eat. Few have the strength to resist at least some self-indulgence. We are each just where we are—no praise, no blame.

> Re our attitude toward the ego-madness of our current world…
> *Jesus* reputedly said, *"Be as wise as serpents and as harmless as doves."*
> *Adi Da Samraj* said, *"Positive Disillusionment—remain positive and loving, and have no illusions."*

However, when we make that crucial connection with Wisdom, and learn the Law of Love—which is associated with breathing, the etheric, and feeling—and that human responsibility for reactivity amid the events of life involves this Law, then we have a chance. We can conduct the universal life force (the etheric, the breath) in the circle of the body, remaining feeling-radiating as love in this midst (*__Conductivity Healing__*, pp94-95).

What is not told in our crazy random culture is what Adi Da Samraj has said about *"**The Addiction Affliction**"* (a brilliant audio talk: www.adidam.org). Both our pleasures and our pains potentially aberrate us. Sex, e.g., feels so good, we just want to do it all the time. We want that hit. It's the orgasm. We think, *"Why can't we feel the orgasm constantly, continuously?"* We tend to think that must be what Heaven's like! But it ain't. It's better than that.

So, our pleasures can cause us just as much suffering as our pains. Just as much. We tend not to think so, but it's absolutely so. In one sense, this points to the "life of moderation" mentioned by the ancients. Altho moderation is not a *higher* way of life, it is undoubtedly a *better* way—than most people suffer.

Life in this Earth realm isn't like our mental concept of "heaven." It's about opposites: up and down, good and bad, pleasure and pain. It's all of that—until Divine Realization. If you have a body, you're gonna suffer. Sooner or later, living life in this realm, you realize that life here is essentially suffering. This is your motivation to, and the sign of your readiness for, Divine Life. Until then, you're just wandering the realms of possibility.

"You are locked into your suffering, and your pleasures are the seal." —Leonard Cohen

These days, watching TV or Net movies, you can get the impression that "drinking", meaning consuming alcoholic beverages, is a completely natural and normal activity that we all do regularly—especially "after the game", to celebrate a victory of some kind, to unwind after a tuff day, and on so many other occasions. Drinking has become institutionalized as an activity. But, none of that makes it healthy—or necessarily intelligent.

In saying this, I am not in any way saying you should give up your nightly glass of dinner wine, or your beer at the game, or whatever your favorite drink is, and for whatever reason you take it. I only offer this for your consideration. Not to spoil your fun or enjoyment. In and of itself, alcoholic beverages have little or no real *nutritional* value. They can, at times, have *emotional* value. Finally, you have to be the judge of your use.

So, why do we use alcoholic beverages? What does "the sauce" do for us, anyway? It "takes the edge off," right? It dulls the senses to one or another degree, so we feel relaxed—but against what? Why do we feel we need the senses dulled? Because of the goddam stress and frustration of everyday life, that's what. Anyone with half a brain knows we're being screwed by the elite, our "controllers" and their henchmen. And we can't think of anything effective we can do about it—other than somehow escape it, which means the bottle, liquor, "spirits."

And it works! But it's just a temporary fix. Worse, it's addictive and can hurt us—when we don't use it rightly, which wrong use is called "substance abuse." But, above realizing yourself as an addictive personality is realizing you are identified with this body-mind as your "self," somehow a separate, separative, and separating entity (that doesn't really exist as such). As such, you are struggling for fulfillment—"self" fulfillment, which is why you take the sauce, why you do everything in life as this "ego", the (actually non-existent) "separate" one.

This *alcohol cure* approach to life, like all self-fulfillment or self-escape approaches, high or low, is a dead end. It never fulfills the heart. It just leads to more frustration, until you get so tired of it, so exhausted from it, you either want to end it all (which is a total waste of the life Opportunity) or you're ready for a more life-positive alternative—something heart-deep capital "F" Fulfilling—which is discussed in Chapter 15.

Irradiated Foods
In recent years, there has been a movement by the food processing industry to place certain easily spoiled foods such as fruits near spent objects of plutonium, waste products of the fissionable materials industry. It was found that by doing so, the food would last far longer than by other methods, and with far less cost. Only trouble with this: the food is now contaminated with nuclear radiation. Tests done by the industry claim no appreciable or otherwise dangerous radiation involved with the food. **Question**: Do you want to take that chance?

Chemical Pesticide-Laden Foods

There are *chemical* pesticides and there are *natural* pesticides. Yes, certain chemical pesticides have been effective and efficient in destroying bugs and preventing their predation—*in the short run*. However, now that we've seen their effects *in the long run*, namely the awful and damaging effects are they having on the body and on our natural environment, what will we do?

DDT has been proven to cause much damage to many creatures—including humans! Many other such pesticides are highly suspect and should be observed quite closely in small experimental areas by trusted, valid, 3rd-party studies, before being released for sale and use on farms and by the public. However, the blatant irresponsibility of Big Chemical is shown by the fact that it is only long after their introduction into use by everyone, that their terrible damage is being seen and felt as ruinous to EarthLife. Even then, they try to shirk responsibility.

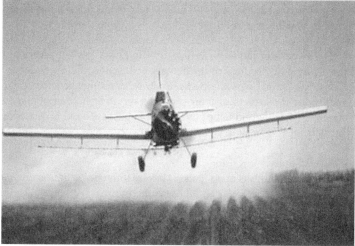

Meanwhile, natural pesticides such as rotenone, marigolds, ladybugs, and praying mantises have been used successfully for many years in many cultures. Strong, well-prepared soils don't need pesticides, as many natural farmers well know. Moreover, while bugs can and will adapt to human-made chemical poisons, they somehow never adapt to natural ones. Mantises and lady bugs are great garden protectors, but chemical pesticides kill them.

Natural compost is the best food for almost every plant. It can be prepared in as few as eight days via the strategic use of chipper-shredders. It's about mixing equal amounts of fresh organic wastes with manure and dry wastes (leaves, sawdust, etc.). Add some ground glacial rock dust, and you have the formula for good soil. Avoid foods grown in chemical pesticide soils. *GLDLifestyle* describes this process in detail.

Clearly, we need to get back to small organic farms and to encouraging home and community gardening. We need cooperative communities (CoOpComs) of 16-25 persons. Both can produce all the food needed by humanity—safely, efficiently, and in harmony with Nature. In CoOpComs, we have always had our own build-in community of like-minded people to care for and who will care for us—birth-to-death, cradle to grave. With a climate-controlled GardenDome, we can have all types of organic produce year-round (see Appendix G).

Chemical Sweeteners or Sugar Substitutes

There is a whole literature around the human suffering caused by chemicalized, or human-made, refined sweeteners, "fake" sugars or sugar analogs. We at GranMed have seen clinically that chemical sugars ("Sweet-n-Low®," "Equal®," "NutraSweet®," "Spoonful®," etc.) do much harm. Among the worst of the ingredients therein is aspartame, which has been implicated in cases of multiple sclerosis, lupus, and many other disorders. Along with ordinary refined sugar, which is terrible as a food and is actually a poison, they should be carefully avoided.

The sweetener industry, as part of "Big Food," or "Big Agriculture," is in it for the money, heedless of the damages caused by their products. Most of Big Corporate is run by psychopaths, anyway, corporate heads that have no real empathy for the effects of their products on other human beings or the environment. A fairly good list of these junk sugars is found in Appendix D. Read your labels! These junk sweeteners are everywhere.

Chemicalized Foods

Ah, the ubiquitous chemicals! They're universal. *"Better living thru chemistry!"* Since the late 1930s, that was the motto. We were all going to be moving into the future thru modern chemistry. What has actually happened has been more like moving toward death! Until the early part of the 1900s, one couldn't even find chemicals in foods. Everything was "natural"—altho not called as such.

When the food processing industry was in its infancy, it had nothing like the technological sophistication it has today. Now, they can "doctor up" foods with all manner of chemical processes. And doctor them up they have! And our idiotic government has made matters worse. Mainly, government subsidies incentivized them to turn farming into a huge financial profit industry, which forced small organic farms almost into oblivion.

It's a chemical feast out there. Everything's got chemicals in it these days (2019). Surfactants, coloring agents, anti-caking agents, fillers, thickening agents, thinning agents, artificial flavoring agents, preserving agents, conditioning agents—the list goes on and on, anything to make the product look better, smell better, taste better, and last longer on the shelf!

Speaking of shelf life, McDonald's© hamburgers have been left, forgotten on shelves in peoples' kitchens, for 15 years and more, and appeared virtually unchanged from when they were left there! How did this happen? What on Earth is in them that preserves them without mold or bacterial action destroying them? These products are miracles of modern chemistry and processed foods—in the unhealthy and otherwise negative sense. What will they do in your body? What effects are they having on your health? What diseases are they causing?

When is the last time you picked a *butylated hydroxyanisole* from a tree and ate it? That's "BHA," a common chemical added to packaging to keep its contents fresh. Can the liver—which organ is mainly responsible for detoxifying these substances—effectively contend with BHA and continue its role in helping the body remain healthy when many more chemicals than BHA are constantly coming in? Just how much punishment can the liver (and the rest of the body) take in this chemical onslaught? Do you really want to find out? Or, have you already? It is unlikely your doctor will name chemicals as having caused your disorder.

How much are these modern food processing chemicals contributing to our sickness and disease? Will we ever know—without taking a step back (or at least to one side) and attempting to assess the situation. It may well mean stopping their use almost entirely. "Almost," because there may be a few that are "fairly" safe. But, with certain technology—including climate-controlled greenhouses—we actually can live without any of them.

Meanwhile, on a typical trip to the grocery store or supermarket, we see row upon row of "foods" in bottles, cans, and boxes—or otherwise packaged. With the advent of agribusiness—or industrial farming and CAFOs—chemical fertilizers, inhumane animal treatment, antibiotics and other drugs fed to or injected into animals, genetically modified food (GMO's), and irradiated food, purchasing foods in packages (or even whole) these days is almost in itself hazardous to one's health. There is so little trust in the modern marketplace today that in order to be healthy we almost have to grow all of our own food ourselves!

To be on the safer side, we're much better off at least heading directly for the produce section and doing our food shopping for organics there. Except that most of that food is sprayed with chemicals! So, we're at risk nearly everywhere, unless we're in one of the newer Natural Food Markets, where at least most of it is *at least labeled* natural and unsprayed and grown in non-chemical-fertilized soil.

As we've said, the best scenario is raw, ripe, un-sprayed, natural in-season food that has been grown locally (which means that it has the local energies in it). Of course, the safest food of all is almost always natural organic home-grown. This is reminiscent of the home "Victory Gardens" of WWII. During that time, Americans were urged by the federal government to plant their own gardens in their yards at home in order to take the stress off farms—whose young men were off at war. People got healthier as a result.

Home-grown is optimum, and it's easier when living in a cooperative community (see Appendix G). In a CoopCom, others help—because they want to, they care. They do so voluntarily or otherwise by agreement. Bottom line: The food we eat turns into the flesh, bones, and blood of our own body. Pay whatever price you need to pay, but get the best. This is your best chance of being healthy in the body at the gross food level.

The Price of Good Health

We pay a price for whatever we do in life—including whatever we eat. We pay more, or we pay less. Quality usually costs more in dollars, in energy, but we're usually willing to pay more for better goods. Good car, good performance. Junker, always in the shop. How about when it comes to health—especially food? Natural raw produce usually costs more at the grocery. Pay whatever price for purity. Result: a healthier body.

When fasting, if you take a little hit of this or that solid food, you won't lose as much weight or get the level of desired purification. You pay the price for not being strait. What price are you willing to pay? What are you willing—or not willing—to suffer? This is not about strictness to the point of pain, or some silly, lunch-righteous attitude that irritates everyone. The rule is *intelligent use and appropriate abstinence*, a balance that comes with self-understanding. Self-understanding comes from love of the Divine, which is worth whatever price we pay.

Coffee and Other Caffeinated Beverages

No way is coffee going to suddenly go out of favor. It's been around for nearly two millennia, apparently starting with Arabia in 675AD. The caffeine in coffee and other beverages is classified as a mild stimulant. It's this stimulating effect that wakes us up in the morning. However, consider this: *the body should not have to be stimulated into wakefulness*—unless in an emergency. We should be counting on natural bodily energy from the time we arise 'til we go to bed. And we can, from our diet and lifestyle.

So, what happens with this caffeine stimulation? The nervous system takes the first hit. Then, the liver has to detoxify the caffeine and any other life-negative substance therein. Lastly, certain friendly bowel flora is destroyed with each cup. Some evidence suggests that coffee encourages breast cysts in women. OK, we all like the taste of coffee. And there are certain nourishing factors in it. But, does that merit taking it on any regular basis?

And, it's not just coffee. Caffeine is found in higher amounts in black tea, orange pekoe, and other forms of tea—and other products, as well. Caffeine is habit-forming. We get addicted. It usually takes 3 days of headaches to quit the coffee habit. One healthier alternative is organic free-trade decaf. Tastes like coffee but without the kick.

Our Rx: keep some coffee around for when you have to stay up late to finish a report, or pick up Aunt Mary at the airport at 2 AM, or attend someone at hospital. Emergencies. You're driving home late from the Mountain of Attention Sanctuary to San Diego and falling asleep at the wheel. Pull off the freeway and into Mickey Dee's for a hot cup of java. Arrive alive. The rest of the time, stay the hell away from the stuff!

Commercial Soft Drinks

Immense evidence clearly shows that commercial soft drinks, including Pepsi® and Coca Cola®, are dangerous to our health. Hot chocolate, tea, and coffee are not considered soft drinks. "Soft drinks" are usually carbonated, the cola-type drinks—as opposed to alcoholic drinks, which are "hard drinks." We at GranMed predict that at some point in the foreseeable future, there will be cola bashing like cigarettes were in the past. Similarly, these products are life-negative and should not be manufactured for public sale in the first place.

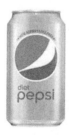

However, it's not necessary to make laws against their production. (We have too many laws as it is.) When we understand, as a culture, the suffering the body has to endure by their use, their production will automatically diminish. The book, ***Excitotoxins: The Taste That Kills***, by Dr. Russell Blaylock (Health Press 1-800-643-2665), provides the gruesome details on taking these commercial cola drinks on any regular basis. One reason is aspartame. Multiple Sclerosis, birth defects, and many other degenerative conditions are associated with their regular use. You'll see them in peoples' grocery baskets at market.

One of the physically most beautiful women I ever saw at Grand Medicine came into our office in San Diego, presenting with bowel cancer. She was only 26 years of age. She'd begun on a cup of Pepsi at age four, gradually increasing her "dose" over the years until she was drinking upwards of a case per week! She was too far gone for us to help her. She died within a few months of her visit. We could provide more stories, but you get the picture.

One could make lube grease taste good, but does that mean we should eat it? Read the label: besides the sugars and acids, other soft drink ingredients of concern often include <u>caffeine</u>, which, besides being a mildly addictive stimulant drug, also increases the excretion of calcium; then, there are artificial colorings, especially <u>Yellow #5</u>, which promotes various diseases in children, including hives, asthma, and other allergic reactions.

Other common soft drink ingredients can include *acesulfame potassium, high fructose corn syrup (HFCS), aspartame, sucralose, bisphenol-A (BPA), saccharin; sodium benzoate, sucrose, citric acid, sodium benzoate, modified food starch, artificial flavors, sucrose acetate isobutyrate, sodium polyphosphates, brominated vegetable oil, caramel color, artificial dyes like Red #40, dioctyl sodium sulfosuccinate, phosphoric acid*, and *MSG*.

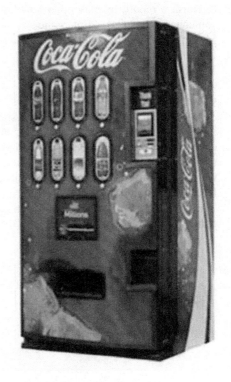

A Harvard University study showed that soft drinks may be responsible for the doubling of obesity in children over the last 15 years (probably by stimulating appetite)—and that those taking soft drinks are more likely to develop diabetes in later years. The phosphoric acid in Coca Cola is reputed to be excellent for removing rust stains. It is also reported that Coke® and/or Pepsi® are used by police to remove blood from the highway! Also excellent for cleaning toilets!

It gets worse. These junk food companies pay junk wages to (and horribly mistreat) workers in their bottling plants in foreign countries—especially in Central America. These activities and other practices of these "beverage companies" are criminal. At some point, these purveyors of pain and suffering will pay a terrible price. Meanwhile, just don't drink the stuff!

One last note: Taking advantage of America's position as the most dominant and militarily powerful nation in the world, soft drink companies have insinuated their way into various countries to produce their awful product less expensively. In many ways, this has had disastrous results for locals in these countries—and not just in health terms.

In the USA, these poisonous commercial soft drinks have gotten into our schools via vending machines. Vulnerable school children are their easy prey. Teenagers and adults see sexy and fake humanitarian ads on TV extolling the "virtues" of this junk. *"We'd like to teach the world to sing (bring the world together) in perfect harmony."* This is blatantly immoral and criminal behavior, reminiscent of the old cigarette ads and the continuing horrendous drug company abuses. It only persists via money, power, and corrupt political influence.

Dairy products

Milk and other dairy products are not generally the best foods for human beings. Dairy milk is best for calves. It is high in fat, designed to make calves grow very big, very fast. For human infants, as well as for human adults, it is not nearly as digestible as human milk. Moreover, it causes problems in the human digestive tract. A certain percentage of human adults develop allergies as a result of taking dairy products.

Yogurt is curdled milk that has been exposed to lactobacillus acidophilus, Bifidus, and other bowel-friendly bacteria. Yogurt can be useful in a variety of bowel situations, including those overdosed by antibiotics and/or refined sugar. Some people seem to do well with a little occasional plain yogurt and/or kefir. Especially blue-eyed persons should avoid dairy, which causes excessive mucus production in those with that genetic eye color.

Unsalted raw butter and/or ghee (clarified butter) can be useful in certain dietary circumstances involving the health of teeth. Most persons, however, don't need butter for regular good health. The same goes for cheese and the other dairy products—delicious as they can be. They are fattening and mucus-producing and better generally avoided—except, perhaps, on special celebratory occasions.

At Grand Medicine, we have known many patients suffering arthritis and cardiovascular diseases attributable directly to animal products in general and dairy in particular. The breakdown in the body of these products produces only acidic results, effectively (over time) pulling minerals out of bones and forcing them to harden on bony ends, unable to re-enter their places of origin—inside the bones. This fiery situation burns the life out of the body.

Drugs

It has become common for teenagers to experiment with various "drugs" to "get hi," change consciousness, or feel connected to or accepted by certain others in their chosen group or whomever they wish to impress. But, of course, some "drugs" have their dangers and are not healthful. Altho some so-called hallucinogenic "drugs" (LSD, Ayahuasca, e.g.) can be useful under certain circumstances, others are potentially deadly.

Some items labelled "drugs" by our wonderful idiots in government have been used by the people for millennia for healing, sacred ceremonies, textiles, and more. Cannabis, e.g., better known as marijuana, was classified as a "Schedule 1 Controlled Substance" to "protect" us from using it recreationally (the cultural taboo against ecstasy) and (unfortunately) also from using it medicinally (i.e., to protect Big Pharma's profits!).

As a result, over 2 million people, mostly teens and youth in their 20s, have been jailed and thereby (often) had their lives ruined for merely taking a hit on a joint! Still, today (2019), there are many laws against its use in many states—both for recreational and for medicinal purposes. So much pain and suffering could have been avoided. Multiple medicinal uses are being discovered daily in many countries. But, jails have to be filled, and Pharma's profits protected. Don't we just love government! They're so good at "protecting" us.

Hemp is another such plant—related to cannabis but commercially used without the psychoactive aspect. Our U.S. Constitution was written on hemp paper, which is superior to wood pulp paper. Hemp clothing, too— superior to cotton. Hemp, one of the world's most useful plants, was originally spun into fibers for clothing and shoes some 12,000 years ago. So, why was it made illegal? A fast-growing plant with multiple uses, it was legal in the USA until 1937 when it was found to be competing with Dupont fibers— another triumph for Big Corporate, the owners of Big Government. (Are you getting a picture?) As with many natural substances, hemp oil has cured cancer.

Our current crazy random culture leaves so many reasons for people to take drugs, alcohol, and other substances—essentially to mentally-emotionally escape the prison of our world as it is. People want to be free to fully participate in their culture, to feel safe and secure, to not have to struggle just to survive here. These are fundamental human rights. Addictions to pharma drugs and their resultant deaths, maimings, and suicides bear witness to the madness of this rampant egoity.

Many OTC (over-the-counter) pharma drugs can become habit-forming and should be restricted. Sometimes, an OTC pain-killer drug can be useful, as in a headache brot on by a pinched nerve. Drugs of all kinds weaken and can even punch "holes" in the etheric envelope—which can be challenging to repair. Drugs, then, whether pharmaceuticals or street-types are best avoided whenever possible. More importantly, cultural changes are needed to relieve the psycho-emotional pressures that lead to drug dependency and abuse.

While prescription drugs can save lives and temporarily eliminate pain when used rightly and intelligently, they have, in fact, over the past 130 years or so, been mis-prescribed, abused, and misused, and therefore have been the cause of immense human suffering and death. We saw bumper stickers extolling the virtues of "daring to keep kids off drugs," while adults themselves go about addicted to OTC, prescription, and street drugs.

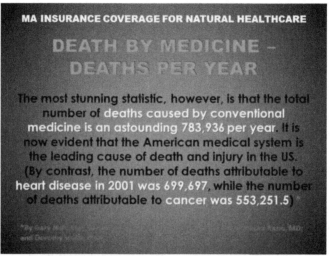

MA INSURANCE COVERAGE FOR NATURAL HEALTHCARE

DEATH BY MEDICINE –
DEATHS PER YEAR

The most stunning statistic, however, is that the total number of deaths caused by conventional medicine is an astounding 783,936 per year. It is now evident that the American medical system is the leading cause of death and injury in the US. (By contrast, the number of deaths attributable to heart disease in 2001 was 699,697, while the number of deaths attributable to cancer was 553,251.5)

Far worse is the awful practice by drug companies of advertising, lobbying, or otherwise influencing and coercing others to promote or take their products in ways that are offered as harmless but later learned to be harmful. Pharma drugs is the most lucrative and most corrupt industry in the world. It surpasses the arms industry, sex trafficking, and oil, in profits, influence, and power. The billionaire Sackler family knowingly produced the fabulously profitable and highly addictive oxycodone (Oxycontin©, by Purdue Pharma), which has destroyed so many lives.

It is important to produce drugs for certain ailments. Only a few such drugs would be truly needed in a Wisdom Culture. Not so in our crazy random culture. Nevertheless, the sheer wickedness, deceit, callousness, fraudulent science, insensitivity to human suffering and therefore patent evil of this industry move these adjectives to a whole new level of darkness. Along with some of the good it has done in saving lives, this industry has perpetrated some of the worst criminal activities in the history of the world.

The drug cartel (or "pharmafia") wants us "well"—but just well enuf to continue using their drugs…for life! These drug-pushers and poison peddlers would be the envy of any group of heroin smugglers.

Witness:

—scientifically proven (by Pharma themselves) and known-to-be-poisonous vaccinations and inoculations

—hospital errors that cause the suffering and the end of hundreds of thousands of lives yearly

—relentless advertising to mislead the public

—improperly (or negligently or not-at-all) tested drugs

—phony science research that pays for expected results (and hides negative ones)

—promotion of legislation to destroy the herb and vitamin industry

—bribery of doctors and legislators with offers of automobiles, fancy vacations, etc.

—promotion and sale of known-to-them-to-be downright dangerous medications

—outrageously high prices and profits: selling pills @ thousands of times their actual cost

—legislation to force their substances on an unwilling public

—inappropriate (conflict of interest) membership on government health and safety boards

—the creation of imaginative and false diseases in order to sell new drugs for them

—the creation of actual diseases and then frightening the public just to sell more drugs

—getting the government (via our taxes) to pay for drugs for false epidemics and pandemics

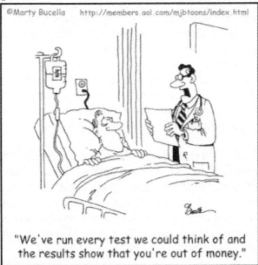

©Marty Bucella   http://members.aol.com/mjbtoons/index.html

"We've run every test we could think of and the results show that you're out of money."

The list of such sinister, insidious, vicious, and death-dealing crimes goes on and on and on. It's actually far worse than suggested here! Our recommendation: avoid these monstrous "sickness industry" companies, their purveyors, and their products. Drugs are to be used in emergencies &/or short periods only. In other words, except in emergencies, in order to be healthy, do your GLD, *The BIG 7,* and generally avoid medical doctors!

Flesh Foods

This category includes the various foods that involve killing creatures that have a separate sense of being, a separate sense of consciousness: fish, bovine cattle, pigs, deer, birds and other poultry, fish, and the like. The dead carcasses and flesh of these creatures are not necessary for human health. Granted, some people seem to do better on a diet that includes some occasional fish or chicken, or even, very rarely, red meat.

We have seen this clinically. But, these are the infrequent exceptions. They represent a very small percentage of humanity—certainly far less than is those representing what is currently eaten in terms of animal flesh. Also, these people seem not to be constitutionally like this, needing red meat. They apparently have developed certain needs as a result of disease conditions—in other words, temporary needs. This has to be determined clinically.

Huge tracts of land are denuded of trees and other natural flora and fauna to provide grassland for grazing bovine, sheep, and other so-called "farm animals" for slaughter. The worst offenders are not the small family farms that treat these creatures humanely. They're the big agricultural CAFO conglomerates that house these animals in abysmal worse-than-jail-like habitats, inject them with antibiotics and other drugs, and feed them on materials other than their natural diet. Yes, it's worse than this, and you can google it.

When we open the menu at our favorite restaurant, it never says, "Tonight's Dead Animals!" But, that's exactly what it is. True, we must kill something—including plants—in order to survive, so there's no point in being morally righteous about eating. However, we need to put this whole thing about herding, preparing, killing, and eating animals into right perspective— which means a whole hellova lot less flesh-eating than we've been doing.

Ethical arguments against eating meat include the huge negative environmental impact, the requirement for masses of grain, water and land, the harm to the poor of this world, the unnecessary suffering of the animals, and the fact that not only do we not need animal flesh to be healthy, we wind up getting sick by eating it.

Fried Foods

Super-heating foods to gain a certain quality of crispiness or other effect poses real risks to the liver, gallbladder, heart, and large arteries. Mainly, the liver and gallbladder can handle natural fats and oils well enuf.

But frying foods in any kind of oil—even coconut oil, which is the best for cooking—will cause challenges to these organs beyond their design capacity.

Fried foods leave fatty residuals sticking to the walls of arteries, increasing the difficulty in getting blood pumped thru them. This is just the short version of the problems created by the artery-clogging and heart disease-causing frying of foods. These are celebratory substances, at best. Try to keep them to special occasions only!

Genetically Modified (GM) Foods

Theoretically, it seems plausible that making certain modifications in our food might bring an increased harvest, greater resistance to predatory bugs, higher nutritive values, and better taste. All of these have turned out not to be so. Real science, ruthlessly attacked and otherwise sequestered from the public, has been done to show what such modification means to our health altogether. What remains are the possibly negative ways GMOs might affect other plants and animals that have not had such modifications. Some such results have already been seen.

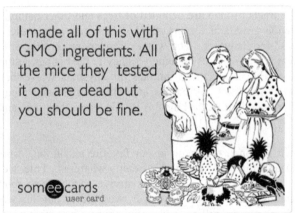

We do not know the big picture on GMO's—and yet, experiments continue, both out in the fields, where cross-pollination between GMO and non-GMO plants is occurring, and in supermarkets, where GM foods are already, for several years now, being sold to unsuspecting consumers. In view of past experiences where large companies have experimented on our health with disastrous results, we should have much reason for concern. Could GMOs in our food supply be a reason we have an ever-increasing number of people with an ever-increasing variety of diseases?

The very fact that laws have been passed protecting Bayer-Monsanto from having to label GMO foods should tell you something. If they're so damn good and "safe," why would their identity need to be hidden? The GMO lobby is extremely powerful. They have admitted a desire to control the entire world's food production. God Help us all! Fortunately, more countries are forbidding GMOs to be sold within their borders. Hopefully, this trend will grow.

Microwaved Food

In the early 1960s in Switzerland, renowned physicist Dr. Hans Hertel, working with Dr. Bernard H. Blanc of the Swiss Federal Institute of Technology and the University Institute for Biochemistry, conducted a carefully controlled scientific study of the effects of microwaved food on human subjects. Blood drawn from subjects taking the microwaved food showed that changes occurred similar to those with cancer.

Microwaved food is dangerous to health. Depending on microwave intensity and length/time of exposure, the microwaving of food effectively destroys essential nutrients at the molecular level. There is no nutritious food that has been microwaved. The microwave oven industry, of course, was more than a little upset about this discovery. Hertel and Blanc were viciously attacked, taken to court, and were threatened with harm to their families. Nice!

In separate instances during the 1980s, nurses in certain hospitals in the USA decided to take a shortcut in the heating of milk for infants—by "nuking" the milk in the microwave oven. The babies receiving the microwaved milk got sick and died. In these hi-tech, hi-stress times, where we insist on quick convenience, many restaurants comply by microwaving our food. Is this an argument against restaurants? Some, for sure.

Understand this: microwaved food looks like food, smells like food, and even tastes like food—but it isn't food! Not after being nuked. Devoid of more or less of its nutrients, it's not fit for human consumption. It shouldn't take a genius to figure out that exposing anything "live" to these microwaves will, in fact, harm it. Evidence suggests changes in the molecular structure of living things exposed to microwave energy. I don't trust it. Do you?

Refined Flour Products

During WWI, in England, the story is told of a sudden shortage of white flour to make bread. The citizenry and local institutions—including hospitals—were forced to resort to whole wheat flour. Result: hospital patients were suddenly getting well quicker.

In contemporary developing countries, there is a persistent notion that "white is better." Thus, grains are shorn of their outer hulls, then stripped of their inner and more nutrient-dense coverings, their so-called "polishings." These polishings are then fed to the pigs and other farm animals, and the resulting nutrient-poor white rice eaten by humans. Obviously, not a good idea. And, altho rice can sustain us, it isn't the best food for our consumption.

We are not advocating the use of whole wheat flour, or, for that matter, any grain. Refining grain reduces available nutrient quality. We recommend avoiding grains and grain products altogether as inferior sources of nutrients. Grains—except as grasses—have to be cooked to be rendered fit for consumption. The original bread was made by mashing sprouted grain a bit (usually wheat), soaking the pulp in pure water, and then forming it into round loaves to bake—in the sun. This would be the better way to eat grains—if taken at all.

Now, however, grains aren't prepared that way. They are stripped of most of their nutritional value in modern refining and processing. This creates real difficulties for the body, which struggles with the "non-food" results. Nutritional imbalances at the body's metabolic level occur accordingly. Cells are starved of nourishment, immunity is lowered, we are thus more vulnerable to parasites (the so-called disease organisms), and we get sick and die sooner.

A donut replaces a date or a fig on our plate, an example of using technology in a silly way, intelligence without wisdom. I've known test-measured geniuses who were quite apparently without a wit of common sense—much less wisdom. And wisdom is very different from mere intelligence or knowledge. Wisdom is the Truth of Happiness. And that is something the brain-mind cannot grasp.

Finally, re grains, Internet sources suggest that some 6% of the population in the USA have what is called "gluten intolerance," gluten being a type of protein in certain grains. It seems as tho there is an increasing number of "intolerances" appearing these days. While we can easily imagine why, it is prudent to err on the side of caution. Is it the *modern* wheat, barley, and rye *varieties* that have brot about these intolerances? Something else?

We're getting more evidence that humans are not biologically adapted to grains, that grains are not complete in vitamins and minerals, that they are irritants because they contain lectins, another type of protein that causes reactions in certain people. Then, as mentioned, there's the gluten, which is a protein even worse than lectins. Add to that, grains contain phytates, an antioxidant compound.

We're told that some 35% of the world's population is sustained on **wheat**. More than half of the world's population is said to depend on **rice** for 20% of their daily caloric intake. The USA and China are said to eat or otherwise consume more **corn** by far than all other countries. Thus, much of the world has come to depend on these and other grains as at least a part (in some cases, most) of their food supply.

So, if grains aren't all that good for you, let's say not nearly as good as the big three—fruits, veggies, and nuts / seeds—then what do we do? Do we ignore them altogether or take them minimally, like at celebratory occasions or so? Again, each of us must decide.

Diet is a very individual thing. While there are generalizations we can make—like the big three food groups—the rest is left to experimentation. Find out what works for you. But...be intelligent about it. Be honest. What causes problems and what seems to work well? Notice what happens in the moments, hours, and days that follow consumption of this or that food. Carefully notice this. How does this and that food, whatever it is, make you feel? Let this the main determinant (not this or that person's opinion) as to what you eat. You're the boss.

Refined sugar

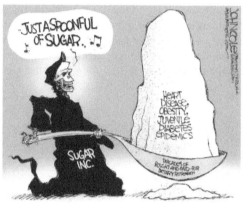

The book, ***Sugar Blues***, pretty much says it all. Refined sugar is not just "refined." It is "*super*-refined," going thru as many as 52 refining processes. By that time, it's a downrite poison! When we eat something containing refined sugar, the body tries to dilute the negative effect by causing thirst. The lack of adequate nutrition in the sugar also causes a craving for real nutrition, making us hungry, as well. So, we get fatter and sicker. In our clinical experience at Grand Medicine, refined sugar is among the very worst foods one can eat.

Refined sugar is very tasty and highly addictive. It has become ubiquitous in prepared foods. It's everywhere—canned foods, bottled foods, packaged foods of all kinds. Most Americans eat upwards of 200 lbs. of this awful substance per person per year. We consider refined sugar to be—as a "food"—the worst enemy of the heart, weakening the functional action of the heart muscle, and setting the stage for heart disease. OK, negative-reactive emotions are the main cause of heart disease. But, on the gross food level, it's cooked and refined foods. And of these, refined sugar is the very worst.

Do the research. And it can be difficult, due to laws passed centuries ago to protect the refined sugar industry. An article I trust, by Fred Rohe, is referenced below (see References). Make no mistake: the Big Sugar industry is huge and very politically powerful. Its global market is around $78 billion USD. The Pharmaceutical Industry, of course, is far bigger—near $1 trillion! Nevertheless, seeking the Net for real facts on Big Sugar can be frustrating.

When Grand Medicine first went to Brazil to teach Eyology, we were treated to something unavailable in the USA: raw sugar—as a liquid. At a roadside market, we watched as the proprietor placed a length of sugar cane into a press, which then squeezed out its liquid. It was raw, natural, and delicious. Available in the USA? Ain't gonna happen. Not as long as Big Sugar has its political clout. Not as long as so many of us have a sweet tooth for sugar.

It is not going to be easy to break away from refined sugar in all of its disguises. And it has many. But, it is just very important to greatly reduce our dependence on these highly addictive and ultimately poisonous substances. Bottom line: when buying packaged foods, read your labels. Finding anything on the *"The Many Names for Sugar"* list, we suggest you act accordingly.

Smoke

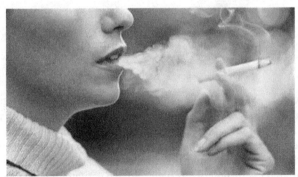

Who knows for how long human beings have been smoking, drawing smoke into their lungs for various purposes—presumably essentially to get high. It has been done for millennia for sacred purposes, then, in various indigenous cultures. Certain Native Americans are said to have been using tobacco in religious ceremonies when Europeans arrived on the scene. The rest is history, American and other companies springing up to spread this addictive substance to other parts of the world.

Insidiously, modern cigarette companies would go into developing countries, even into small towns and villages, and hand out free sample packages of these death-dealing "coffin nails." Locals would quickly become addicted, and spend much of what little they had on smoking away their health—while cigarette companies got wealthy.

Pervasive, persuasive, and shrewdly targeted advertising made smoking look like something heroes did, the young and the handsome, the beautiful and the sexy, the wealthy, and the intelligent. Foolish medical doctors accepted handsome financial rewards to smoke and advocate their favorite brands on TV. Cigarette promoters paid actors well to be seen on the big screen, smoking their way to hero status.

Smoking was portrayed to children as the behavior of truly sophisticated adults. Notice the body language: a flamboyant flick of the wrist, and a sexy tap of the finger to break off the ashes. The tobacco industry has perpetrated a heinous crime on humanity. It has already paid a price for its darkness, but that payment is still incomplete. Its crimes continue. Therefore, its most massive karma is yet to come.

**Industry funded scientists tell us GMOs
& the chemicals used on them are safe.
It's not the first time scientists have been used
to sell a business model.**

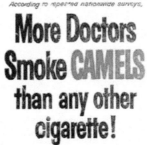
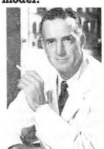

Learn more at www.robynobrien.com

The radio, TV and hi-way advertising blaring out the messages of death, the lingering smoke smell in the air, the stench of the smokers breath, the cigarette odor clinging to clothing, the smoke-destroyed air conditioning systems, the dirty ashtrays, the butts littering the ground, the burn marks on floors and countertops, the fires in beds and cigarette fire-destroyed homes and forests, the cancerous black lungs, the horrible suffering of smoke-destroyed friends and relatives. We don't see it as much nowadays, but it's still there, albeit diminished.

As children, we coffed and turned green on it, wondering how it was possible that anyone, any adult, could get any pleasure out of such a thing. But pleasure there was, from the stimulating and powerfully addicting effect of the nicotine—and the refined sugar in the paper and the other strategically-placed chemicals to enhance the whole "experience" and keep you buying this death-dealing product.

So, cigarette bashing finally happened—but not until we were overwhelmed by the awful cost in money and human suffering from allowing this insulting ugliness to become so powerful. As a society, we had to be beaten bloody before we changed, before we began to limit the progress of this monstrosity. Lawsuits were filed, legislation to force it outside certain environments, and people continue to die from it.

Yes, we need freedom of choice, but shouldn't we also be publicly informed of a wholesome, clean, and pure way of life? *The BIG 7* on national television? Who'd pay for it? Where is the profit for Big corporate? And, how does this all reflect our current attitude about life? This is about a whole culture choosing intelligent discipline and self-transcendence over gross-mindedness, bodily abuse, and self-indulgence. Is that believable?

A Listing of the LQFs
Starting with the Estimated Average Overall Worst
And Altogether most Destructive of Human Life (August 2019)

1 – Smoke (cigarettes, crack cocaine, etc.)
2 – Genetically modified foods
3 – Drugs (street, OTC, and prescription)
4 – Refined sugar products
5 – Alcoholic beverages
6 – Chemical sugar substitutes
7 – Commercial soft drinks
8 – Microwaved foods
9– Chemical pesticide-laden foods
10 – Chemicalized foods
11 – Flesh foods: red meats, fowl, fish, etc.
12 – Coffee other caffeinated beverages
13 – Cesium-irradiated foods
14 – Refined flour products
15 – Fried / super-heated fats & oils
16 – Dairy products

Having already mentioned cannabis, there is still crack cocaine and who knows what else is now being smoked. Our recommendation is to avoid any but medically prescribed cannabis. If you're going to do it, do it legally. Otherwise, remember that even marijuana will leave resin residuals in the lower respiratory tract. On that basis alone, it's better avoided—unless strictly needed for medical purposes.

Solid Foods Temptation
While on our GLD, it's generally a good practice to avoid eating more than perhaps one or two bites of any kind of solid food—especially solid foods that are not wholesome. Your resistance to the pleasure of eating solid foods will grow over time while on your GLD. You will feel stronger and

more capable of ignoring the tempting smells of a roast, a Gag-in-the-Bag hamburger, a fancy pastry, and other "fine" foods. Eventually, your restraint will grow with your lessons. Your resolve to be clean, strong, healthy, slim, and balanced, will keep you going.

Avoid people who tease you about your diet. It used to be best to not tell anyone about fasting. One used to have to say, "*Doctor's orders*." Lately, things have changed. Now, special diets are more popular, even green smoothies. When people see your meals are all liquid, tell them about the GLD. If they ask further, tell them more—including about *GLDLifestyle* membership. The more, the merrier! Let's do our part to heal the world!

Meanwhile, if you know yourself, if you know you'll be tempted by a place where a big, sumptuous meal being prepared, it's best to avoid the area, the event, the situation. Avoid placing yourself in "harm's way." Given the opportunity to go out and eat, it's best to demur, explaining that you have important work to finish. Failing in this, avoid ordering solids, choosing a bowl of veggy soup, herb tea, tomato juice or orange juice instead. (Note: food establishments by law must "pasteurize" raw liquids before selling them to the public, so unless you can be assured that it has indeed not been tampered with, forget "raw" juice.)

Avoid eating (drinking) to the point of feeling stuffed. If you've made too much of a drink, cover it and place it in the frig or otherwise where you can get to it later. If it's a volatile liquid and you've waited too long for it to maintain enuf of its nutritional value, thro it out. Learn to drink when hungry, not "when it's time." Your body will tell you when it is hungry. You don't have to watch the clock. When you feel full, stop—no matter how much or how little is left.

Toward a Clean, Green, Wholesome Environment
Don't stop with avoiding chemicals in foods. Notice how they've crept into so many other areas of our lives. Take cleaning products: we can clean almost anything in the house with white vinegar, baking soda, borax, and lemon juice. See www.NextWorldTV.com for how to clean house with these non-toxic and inexpensive products. Laundry magnets (http://mls.waterliberty.com/promo/?hop=adgu1 / 1-888-318-9445) allow us to avoid laundry soap altogether.

With vinegar and water, including for washing floors, your hands will remain soft. You won't be concerned about the chemicals that are always seen in commercial cleaning products. And you'll be amazed how effective vinegar and baking soda can be.

13—The BIG 7

A Lifestyle Reality Check

There are lifestyle factors that can seriously jeopardize your chances of success on your GLD—and perhaps even ruin your project of weight loss, health improvement, and (more importantly) harmony, balance and equanimity toward real Spiritual practice. At Grand Medicine, we spent our early clinic years working out the factors that contribute to, and take away from, well balanced health. We've narrowed these factors down to "*The BIG 7*".

Practiced rightly, these *BIG 7* qualities, or disciplined practices, can result in a state of health that is basically free from disease. On the gross level, they may be the closest we can come to leading a healthy and happy life. They are a means of making our daily activities sacred by adapting and engaging them with profound discipline and consciousness in loving remembrance of—and as our gift to—The Beloved Divine.

Let's Look into the Future—YOURS

Look at the many ways we influence each other in life. First, since everything is connected (in fact, nothing is truly "separate" anywhere in all the universes), then everything we do has ramifications, connections, ripple effects, to everything and everyone. Everything we do influences everything and everyone else. What we eat (diet) and how we live (lifestyle), of course, influences "our" health. BUT, they also affect the life and health of others!

Consider our children: these sweet little creatures have no way of rightly interpreting what adults do. Still, they look up to us to see and understand what a human being is supposed to look like and be. They want to know how an adult person eats, and otherwise what a grown man or woman does in life. If we're grumpy and moody, growling and fighting with other adults (our spouse?) like silly adolescents, they naturally think that's right to do. If we're sick, they assume it's OK to be sick. If we smoke and drink, they presume that's the way they should act.

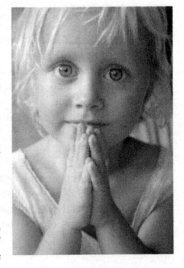

So, what kind of model <u>are</u> we, anyway? What message are we sending them? What kind of an example of a human being are we demonstrating for them? What legacy do we offer our children—and those around us? This is what shapes the future—ours and everyone else's!

Truly, the very best instruction for raising children we've ever read here at Grand Medicine is the book, *The First Three Stages of Life*. Altho specifically denominational, its basic message is universally applicable. This is true wisdom in the guidance of both children <u>and</u> adults. Everything needed is there.

The Importance of Balance in the Practice of *The BIG 7*

<u>Balance in life</u> has been touted by so many great and extraordinary people that we needn't point any further to its importance here. And yet, with food we have this tendency to "go-with-the-flow," like most people, go all-raw, like the health nut, go somewhere in-between, or exercise a little discipline here and there, sporadically. Additionally, our culture suggests to us that if a *little* of a something is good, then it's likely that a *lot* of it is better.

That's the belief of the health nut, for sure: a lot of this and none of that; exaggeration and extremes. The other side of all that is more like what most people do, except that there is virtually no discipline—or a little attempt at such, perhaps—but when the tendencies to indulge come in, the discipline goes out the window.

Take exercise: if a little exercise is good, maybe a lot is better, rite? This philosophy had baby boomers doing hi-impact aerobics during the 1960s and 70s. We wound up with improved cardiovascular systems and ruined hip, knee, and ankle joints! Whereas, moderate exercise is right—altho different—at any age.

And regarding diet, certain health nuts thot that if 70%-80% alkaline is good, maybe 100% alkaline is better. Wrong! The internal acid ash from metabolizing nuts and seeds, and possibly from the occasional celebratory cooked food, brings this balance—again, not as a strategy but as a conscious practice of intelligent eating and living.

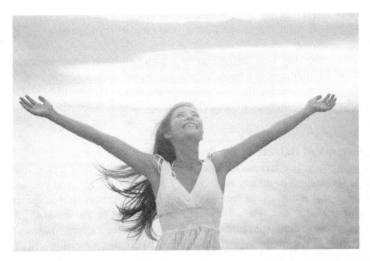

BALANCE! How to achieve it? Don't try. Just do *The BIG 7* as a regular routine, a daily program. As well as you can. You'll gain balance <u>as a result</u> of it, without making balance your goal. And when you're finally feeling clear and balanced and relatively fit, have some turkey on Thanksgiving with the rest of the folks, if you like—IF it's felt to be appropriate. Let them see that you're "one of them," a regular member of the clan—while they're wondering how you stay so young-looking and fit. It's because you don't eat the junk they eat on any regular basis.

You get moderate exercise, eat a hi-raw diet, and do the rest of *The BIG 7* as your program of health, meaning most of the time. You have a program—where you can bring discipline. They don't. Not some silly program of extreme exercise, a "don't-dare-ever-touch-that" extreme diet, or an "eat-whatever-the-hell-you-please" diet to reward yourself after some punishing exercise routine or diet avoidance regimen. *The BIG 7* is balanced and produces balance.

THE BIG 7

1—pure diet: hi-raw or all-raw natural "organic" fruits, veggies, nuts and seeds daily

2—adequate rest: early bedtime of 10 PM or so, with pure, restful sleep + daily breaks

3—right exercise: age and health condition-appropriate, rapid-movement and hatha yoga

4—natural hygiene: keeping the body clean and balanced with natural cleansing products

5—right occupation: engaging in productive, life-positive, and Earth-sensitive activities

6—life-positive environments (including people!): clean, wholesome, elegant and graceful

7—Spiritual cultivation: study and practice of the Divine Reality per to your heart-feeling

We do *The BIG 7* to create a firm foundation of balanced health so that energy and attention are free to give to God, The Divine Person, or That Which Is Great in life. Failing in this, energy and attention tend to go to "problems" in the world—that develop as disease in the body-mind. The gross physical body is a *food* body. Always take a diet of at least 80% raw fresh, natural unsprayed non-radiated in-season fruits and vegetables, nuts and seeds, <u>daily</u>—and increase that percentage upward from there.

Get to bed <u>early</u>. Get <u>regular</u> exercise appropriate to your health situation. Keep the body and your environs <u>organized, clean, and neat</u>. Do <u>life-positive work</u> <u>or activities</u> that you enjoy. Be around only positive, happy people. *Above all*, study the Teachings of the Great Spiritual Masters daily and cultivate love of God with all your heart.

Doing *The BIG 7* is so important that we finally reached the point in our clinical practice where we would tell our patients, "<u>First, do *The BIG 7* for 30 days—then we'll talk</u>." We sent people home with diet diaries after their initial intake exam (health questionnaire), asking that they return a month later and show us they could discipline themselves with these practices before we'd talk with them further about their various problems.

We weren't trying to push people away or avoiding taking them (or their problems) seriously. We knew with a certainty that (1) **if** they came back they were serious about getting well, and (2) **when** they did these basic practices for a while, the practices themselves would eliminate most of their problems. It worked! With about 70% of patients. The power of *The BIG 7*.

How Long Does It Take?

When people took *The BIG 7* seriously and put them into practice, their diseases (in about 78% of cases) would be gone within 30 days—all ages, all disease conditions, at all stages, on average. That's power! The other 23% of cases, in order to have their health issues resolved, needed to be either:

(1) dealt with immediately by specific remedial treatments <u>plus</u> <u>case-designed use of *The BIG 7*</u>

(2) given hydrotherapy, Earthing, colonics, herbs, vitamins, etc., while maximally engaging *The BIG 7*, or

(3) otherwise <u>be on *The BIG 7* longer</u> than the initial 30 days

Of course, this smaller percentage of patients also included those who for one reason or another wouldn't or couldn't follow the protocol, those who dropped off the radar (they didn't return and/or we couldn't find them), and also those who needed medical intervention.

On our old GranMed website (<u>www.grandmedicine.com</u>), we showed various protocols against a variety of disease circumstances, listing *The BIG 7* first. This way, we suggested that anyone accessing the health information for ways of dealing with health problems should—to whatever extent possible—*first* practice *The BIG 7* <u>before</u> getting into any therapeutic practices. Thus, *The BIG 7* are basic-to-good-health practices we take seriously in order to be healthy. The degree to which we take them seriously and practice them is the degree to which we will be healthy.

> **The "food-principle" is the fundamental basis for all physical healing.**
>
> Adi Da Samraj

Yes, *the gross physical body is a food body*, so diet is essential—such that (quoting Adi Da) "*...the first treatment* for **any** disorder of the gross physical body *is and rightly should be a FOOD treatment*." But there are other levels of our being that need to be considered: the subtle, which includes the emotional/etheric and the various levels of the mental/psychic; and then the causal (see the book, <u>*Conductivity Healing*</u>). All of these are taken into account when we do *The BIG 7*. Let's consider *The BIG 7*, one at a time.

PURE DIET

Pure diet means taking fresh raw ripe in-season and preferably locally-grown natural unsprayed non-GMO fruits, veggies, nuts, and seeds. Certain individuals may need some cooked foods, and perhaps even in some cases raw butter, raw plain yogurt, and kefir.

Some people even seem to need a little fish or fowl or even red meat a few times weekly temporarily toward accomplishing an improved health condition. And for most of them, this is during the transition to mostly-raw or all-raw living vegetarian food—but only a very few people (perhaps only 1% or so of the world population). The necessarily temporary need for the intake of killed food, or animal food, is rare. In our decades of clinical experience, there have never been what we considered strictly long-term needs for killed foods.

Most of us, by far, can get along very nicely on pure vegetarian foods. We've already discussed some of the many life-bringing factors of raw diet. The dietary experiment, with right guidance, can be done by everyone toward learning what is best for the body each of us has been Given. Perhaps the most important general rule about diet to remember was given by Adi Da (paraphrasing, pp22-23, *Green Gorilla*):

"The gross body is, very simply, the food-body. The gross body itself depends on and is made of food. The quality and quantity of food largely...determines the state and desire and action of the physical body and the sense-mind. If food taking is intelligently minimized, and if the food selected is both pure and purifying, then the physical body...passes through a spontaneous natural cycle...of first purification, then rebalancing, and finally rejuvenation. Therefore, if food-taking is controlled, the body-mind-complex itself...becomes...controllable."

Committing Suicide with Food

Seriously, it is a silent, deadly process. We rarely ever notice it. In our current culture, it happens three times daily during the course of our entire lives. Little by little, moment by moment, the cells of our bodies are being poisoned by the exogenous (outside source) or endogenous (inside-the-body source) chemicals of the cooked and processed foods we are eating, including by chemical processes brought on by reactions of our various body systems (endogenous) to these processed foods.

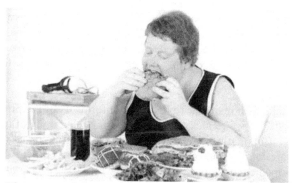

The peasant laborers in poorer countries bring home produce from the fields, eat some of it raw, and cook the rest. They cannot afford the flesh and fancy processed foods of wealthier people. Hence, they live longer! A major study done in China over several years proved this. The peasants in the Chinese countryside who couldn't afford more than a small piece of meat once per month were far healthier than their richer cousins in the city who ate dog, rat, and shark fin soup. In the USA, we have the supermarket, a "super way"

to destroy our health, with row upon row of degenerated food: death in a package!

Most of us have no sense of what we are doing to our bodily health by eating this tasty junk the way we typically do. Most of our Grand Medicine patients believed their diet was better than average. Even if it was, it was corrupt. My wealthy alcoholic friend used to say, "*Well, you have to die of something!*" Yes, but what a dark view of life! (Better to die serving God thru lovingly serving others—while intelligently practicing right life!)

He, of course, in making this statement, wished to justify his self-indulgence, his lack of discipline in the face of the stresses and frustration he suffered. And, do you have to throw away your God-Given Gift of life this way—with both hands—drinking daily, no exercise discipline, mind focused in the gross physical, and eating whatever you please, whatever tastes good? Just because you have the wherewithal to do so? Because you can?

In the wealthier Western countries, and increasingly in the East, we eat our way to death, killing the body with food. Consider the disease process this way: First, the chemicalized "food" we eat eventually leaves residual accumulated toxics and toxins in the body's areas of inherited or genetic tendency to weakness. This toxic environment destroys or inhibits the functions of cells in those and other body tissues, further weakening them. This attracts evolving parasites.

As the junk diet continues, there may be a simple "cold," with dead cells and waste products building to the point of at first acute and then chronic inflammation. Drugs are brot in to deal with symptoms. The drugs themselves cause other symptoms, and so more drugs are applied. Soon, organs and whole limbs are removed. This is the typical disease process—suicide by food, assisted by pharma drugs. It's not *intentional* suicide, of course, but it is nonetheless effective as such: digging our graves with our knives, forks, and spoons!

Who tells us how to eat right? Who informs us of the propriety of raw natural foods? If we're lucky enuf to be born into a family of intelligent raw eaters, OK. But, that's rare, and can wind up backfiring on us socially if all our friends are eating silly diets (sounds like time to get new friends!) And don't count on medical doctors encouraging raw diet. They have likely been trained in the same dietary practices as the rest of society at large: whatever tastes good, whatever is advertised as sexy or bringing us supreme satisfaction, or what's on the "food pyramid."

Worse, as we've said, drug companies—which direct the course of modern medicine—have no interest in our being well from raw diet. Good health from raw foods does not sell drugs. That's why doctors tell us we can eat whatever we want, even after having an organ (like a gallbladder, e.g.) removed! They don't see any logic in taking pure raw liquids to recuperate. Recently, however, this attitude among medical doctors seems to be turning around.

The common church won't likely direct us toward dietary purity, either—even tho the Christian bible says, right in Genesis: "*I give you the fruits of the fields and of the trees, and for you these shall be for meat.*" Television and the media? They're busy making money on ads for junk foods—and the drugs you need to take to deal with the symptoms from eating the junk!

Senators and Congressmen? They're in a board meeting with junk food industry lobbyists. The President? He's in the hospital getting an operation. So, where do we learn diet wisdom today? Wherever we happen to find it. It's on the Net from an increasing number of ordinary people, as well as open-minded health professionals, who have stumbled across the many wonders of right (raw) eating and life-positive lifestyle.

Diet While Traveling
Taking a vacation to Las Vegas? New York? Crap food is hawked in every casino, at every corner, in every line. How about Iceland? Nice! They're increasingly into natural foods. Natural produce at restaurants and buffets? In most countries, forget it! Yes, if you go a little out of your way, you can usually find a real (unheated, unprocessed) smoothie, some fresh juice, a Natural Food store, a fruit stand, or other pure food source. But not always. In some countries, it's just not there. In others, that's all they can afford! You may need to take some food you can trust along with you.

If you travel *within* the Country, you can eat whatever you bring, one place to the next. If you travel *outside* the Country, you may well have to throw out whatever fresh produce you brot along at the arrival terminal: no foreign seed-bearing plants allowed into the Country! You can bring all the crap food you like—chips, jerky, booze—but nothing healthy!

You can't bring anything that can grow and proliferate, nothing that contains the life force, the living energy of the sun. Interesting. Some of this is understandable, as with foreign weed forms that can take over local flora. But in most cases, it's not. This has to change. We, the people, need diet purity—wherever we go. One way or another.

Regarding your GLD while traveling, it is possible to bring along your juicer and blender in your luggage—at least your blender, to make the all-important green smoothies. This way, you can enjoy the local produce in whatever country you visit. Not a bad idea, unless you have to travel very lite. Otherwise, with your GLD, it can be necessary to take some solid food meals.

The GLD principle of being able to switch from liquids to solids and back will serve you in these cases.

Whenever possible, take your liquids along, making sure they are pure. Those on **Level 1** must avoid solid foods as much as possible. Taking your juicer and blender—and enema bottle—is mandatory on **Level 1**. A necessity. Those on **Level 2** and **Level 3** might wish to take along snacks like dried fruit and nuts, and also bottled pure water—which, if flying, you will have to buy after passing thru security check-in. Please read *Green Gorilla*.

ADEQUATE REST

Experiments done at various universities and other institutions have shown that "early" bedtime (especially the hours between 10 PM and 12 midnight) is—in general—important to our health. It's not merely rest we're talking about here, but real, genuine deep sleep. Great personalities of the past, such as Hippocrates, Lincoln, and Ben Franklin, extolled the virtues of early bedtime: "*Early to bed, early to rise, makes a man healthy, wealthy, and wise.*" Put into a humorous negative phrase, we might say, "*Late to bed, late to rise, speeds a man to his early demise.*"

Of course, these are over-simplifications, because several factors can influence this "early bedtime" idea quite significantly. But, in general, they make sense in terms of gross bodily health in most circumstances. The two hours before midnight (10 PM-12 AM) seem to have the sleep power of any four hours after midnight—all other things being equal. This equation seems to involve (1) the fact that we humans are not nocturnal, and (2) our bodily rhythms are significantly influenced by the pull of our moon and the planets in our sun system.

That said, in our current-time rush to get everything done, we seem to ignore such a simple health-builder as adequate sleep and rest. Getting sufficient rest and true sleep regenerates our "batteries," powerfully and primarily strengthening the immune system, the body's primary defense system. What's better than 10 PM? 9 PM!

We note that while the "average human adult" needs about 8 hours of sleep per night to feel somewhat healthy, diet is a big factor in the number of hours required to feel adequately rested. Raw diet, e.g., allows the body to work far better generally and get by on less sleep. Body systems are much more efficient than with varying percentages of cooked foods. Therefore, less food is needed. However, when we add the quality and efficiency factors of raw liquids, we up the ante: even less sleep is needed.

There's an expression Given by Avatar Adi Da: "*Eat less, sleep less, and meditate more.*" Of course, He's referring to increasing one's true

Spiritual practice. We can, therefore, benefit from Adi Da's Admonition by moving into pure raw liquids:

Average Sleep Needs of Adult Humans as Modified by Diet (in hours)
• Varied Diets = 8
• Vegetarian Diets = 7.5
• Pure All-Raw Diets = 7
• Pure Raw Liquids (GLD) = 6.5

True enuf, some people seem to need only 4 or 5 hours of deep sleep per nite to feel fine. Some can't seem to feel good without 10 hours of restful sleep. Of course, the sick need more sleep than the relatively healthy. Infants, babies, and children need more sleep to help their growth cycle. Older adults seem to need less sleep than average. Again, keep in mind that many other factors involve when, where, and how much sleep you'll need at any given time in your adult life to satisfy your body's need to maintain good balanced health.

Stress

Speaking of rest, what about relief from stress? We're told that since the beginning of the current Civilization, we technically have more time than ever for rest. This is not so. In fact, we feel like we're worked to death. Work, work, work! That's all we seem to have time for. It seems endless. If someone complains they don't have enuf time, give them more to do. Just the thot of more work to do could help them become more efficient!

But, where does the stress really come in? While it certainly is true that we need a major change in our civilization that will allow us not to work so hard to manage the basic needs of life, stress is also about how we view ourselves in the scheme of things in the Universe. The ego, the feeling of separateness, is really at the root of all this stress. Understanding the ego and doing anti-egoic activities like selflessly serving others as our gift to God, meditating on the Divine, doing daily Spiritual study—these work against stress.

Our immediate ancestors had far more difficult lives, in the gross material sense, than we Westerners do now. They had to do hard manual labor in the fields and factories. Physically, we have things easy, by comparison, with so many machines to do our work for us. OK, then, but what about the stress? There is a positive aspect to stress—like the "use it or lose it" warning regarding exercise for the cardiovascular and musculoskeletal systems. But, what about the negative aspect?

Everything we love in this realm dies. We can't get away from that fact. That's what makes this Earth realm like a hell. And if it weren't for the Spiritual Masters, Who Provide us with a Way to transcend this place, it indeed would be a hell—because there would be no way out! Essentially, as embodied beings, we can't get away from stress entirely. It's built into life in this psychophysical realm. But, by discipline and intelligent living (The BIG 7), we can minimize stress and be calm, balanced, and happy.

Stress, Problems, and Our Provable Destiny

Avatar Adi Da has defined stress as, "*The inherent discomfort of object dependency.*" Of course, there are many things—people, material items, my precious DVD collection, etc.—that we "depend on". That dependency, real or imagined, brings both comfort and discomfort. The discomfort comes in when we experience loss of those items, those objects. But, then, this is exactly what the ego does: objectifies everything.

In fact, tho, the only "thing" we are truly and Absolutely dependent on is the Divine Reality, the Eternal Person of Love. Submitted to It, turned to It, we begin to relax. The whole body-mind relaxes. The more we turn to It, grant our attention to It, the more relaxed, calm, and peaceful we are. Because the Divine IS Peace.

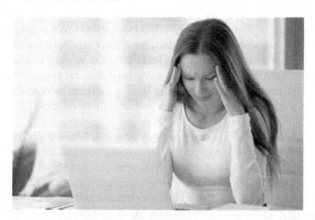

Attention is destiny! We create our destiny by the direction of our attention. Thot (the brain-mind, which is *subtle*) precedes action (body, the physical or *gross*). Traditionally, a Great Law of the Universe is: *We ARE what we give our attention to*. In other words, we become what we meditate on. Whatever we spend significant time thinking about tends to create our destiny. We tend to take on the qualities of what we grant most of our attention to. We tend to bring those thots to life. Here's how it works:

- *Activity:* Your whole life is focused on your spouse, your love (typical for women), so that you become "heavily invested" in him; he dies, gets old, sick and gnarly, or he finds some young sexpot, and he's out of there, gone, history.
- *Result:* you crash and burn.
- *Activity:* You heap attention on your child, but without directing her morally and responsibly; she becomes a drug addict.
- *Result:* you drive yourself nutty trying to deal with her craziness.
- *Activity:* Your life focus is your work/job/career (typical for men), to the exclusion of most other things in life.
- *Result:* up and down: when work is good, you're fine, but when it sucks, you're in deep do-do. If you lose your job, you could even go off the deep end!
- *Activity:* Put vast amounts of energy and attention into your place in the social hierarchy. But, there's always someone ahead of you or snipping at your heels, ready to replace you.
- *Result:* big-time stress based on fear of losing face or social significance!
- *Activity:* You're a farmer or a bank clerk or in some service job where you feel trapped.
- *Result:* you ARE trapped—by your own mind, your attitude. You are not grateful for what you already have.
- *Activity:* You learn to eat all raw foods but become obsessed with bodily purity, renewable resources, and saving the planet. Or, you're sick and determined that the only way you're going to be happy is if you get well.
- *Result:* Unhappiness! You're always struggling against the forces of negligence, wastefulness, insensitivity to life, sickness. You're always *pursuing* happiness and never simply *enjoying* it; you're never *practicing* it.
- *Activity:* You've got a great career, work that you like. But, there are your goals. A bigger home to live in, more money, a different location, a child, better sex. *"I know I can get them. They're coming. It's just that rite now they're a little out of reach."*
- *Result:* that feeling of anxiety, of non-fulfillment.
- *Activity:* You've always only wanted just to get married, have children and a nice home—which you achieve. And yet, something's still "missing."
- *Result:* It's not what you thot. The kids are hard to manage, your body starts to self-destruct, your husband runs off with a big-titty bitch, and his lawyer is better than yours so you lose the house. You want a man to be a father to your children, but now you no longer trust men—and, at age 40, you're desperately looking around for a new career to cover your expenses. Ouch!

So, the question becomes: do we want this kind of destiny? The fact is: unless we're fortunate to be raised in a Wisdom Culture (which has yet to be created), life is never what we think it is. We tend to think it's for self-fulfillment, but it ain't. It never turns out the way we imagine it should for us. No one wins this game. ***There are no winners.*** None!

Look at actors and public figures: off the screen and out of the public's eye, they're suffering their asses off with all manner of fears and anxieties, desperate for a few days of precious anonymity, and they have lung cancer from having nervously smoked themselves to the point of death. No matter how many millions they have, they're still not happy. Not really. We (you and I) could die this way, being this kind of person, always problematic, always feeling under the gun, under stress. What's the alternative?

So, when will we be happy? When we win a hundred million in the lottery? Don't count on it. Let's say we <u>did</u> win the lottery. Then, here come all the friends and family we never knew we had, all of them with their hands stretched out to us—and, of course, the IRS will want their (huge!) share, too. Now we have a whole <u>other</u> set of problems! The point: If you don't <u>practice</u> happiness, how will you ever know how to enjoy it? None of us wants always to be "a problem," broadcasting "problem consciousness" in every direction. And the alternative is…(wait for it)…

- ***Activity:*** You're in jail, or in a bombed-out hovel with no sense of where your next meal is coming from, or you're just living in middle-class heaven, a moderately upscale housing development. Wherever, <u>but, regardless, your attention is always on the Divine</u>; you have real faith, which is trust in the universe, the Divine Reality, the Great Consciousness, the Person of Love, Who is the Very Context of all life and all being, everywhere.
- ***Result***: you're calm, peaceful, and heart-happy—no matter what the hell happens. There's an old Hindu expression: "*Those who truly love God **have no problems!***" Another aphorism says, "*Fortune favors the unconcerned!*"

Mickey Mouse and Donald Duck

Donald's kids are out playing in the yard. One of them bats a ball thru the naybor's window. Crash! The naybor comes running out and angrily yelling: "*Hey! Who did that?*" Donald hears the commotion and comes out to check on things. "*Quack, quack, quack!*" It's a big problem. He ***reacts***. He egoically and emotionally contracts in the midst of what he perceives as a difficulty, a problem. To Donald, it's a problem he's stuck having to deal with.

Mickey's kids are playing in <u>their</u> yard with some friends. They bat a ball thru the naybor's window. Crash! The angry naybor comes out hollering. Mickey hears the disturbance and ventures out to see what the matter is. "*Oh, dear! How should we creatively deal with this situation?*" He ***responds***. He is "response-able," able to respond—and <u>willing</u> to respond.

Whereas, Donald reacted, drew back, withdrew from relationship, Mickey remained in place, *in* relationship with the event—and with *life itself.* Big difference. Very different life results.

Meditation

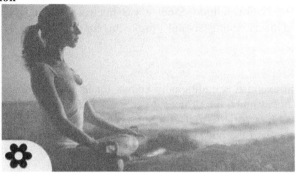

What one single activity involves the least amount of stress? Meditation (see Appendix F)! Meditation on what—or Whom? Meditating on a candle will help calm the mind. But, it won't bring you closer to Spirit or bring any higher Realization. Candles, altho they bring light, they are not, in and of themselves, "Enlightened! Remember the Law: "***You Are What You Give Your Attention To***" (or meditate on)! We take on the qualities of whatever we think about consistently.

Meditating on even a foto or drawing or other artistic representation of a great saint or sage (Jesus, Krishna, Gautama the Buddha, Adi Da Samraj) will draw us into Realization of Them, or Their Great Realization. Steadily granting the four principal faculties to Them, we will gradually take on Their Qualities. The four principal faculties are (1) **mind** (attention), **body** (sitting attentively), **breath** (the etheric), and **emotion** (feeling).

When these are all attentive to the Divine Reality (in the Bodily Form of the Spiritual Master), thus communing with the Great One, you're "There.", beyond egoity, "Home." When these are all attentive to the Divine Reality (in the Bodily Form of the Spiritual Master), thus communing with the Great One, you're "There," beyond egoity, "Home."

In the book, *The First Three Stages of Life*, Adi Da makes the following comment on stress: "*Stress in daily life tends to stimulate the automaticity of the 'fight-or-flight' reaction, the technical term for what I call the 'stress reaction'. Under stress, you want to become aggressive and angry. You also want to fall back and flee and disappear. The conflict between these two motives creates stress, a 'problem' of opposing motives in the living personality.*"

Simply giving our free feeling attention to the Beloved of the Heart moves us away from our typically stressful concerns, worries, troubles, and anxieties. Try it! Notice how we cannot be sorrowful, cannot be fearful, and cannot be angry when doing this "Siddha" (Power) meditation. Better yet, thru meditation on Them (or your chosen Spiritual Master), we gradually begin to take on Their Qualities! Strange, yes, but true—and most wonderful. You can—and most certainly should—prove this for yourself.

RIGHT EXERCISE

Right exercise is traditionally known for its health-giving benefits. Granted, it's not as much fun as sleep, or eating, or sex, but it's essential as a significant health factor. "Use it or lose it" refers to the cardiovascular and structural systems of the body—the heart, large blood vessels, and muscles, and bones. They have to move around, and not just from the bed to the couch to the computer to the refrigerator and back!

Where we used to have to move the body strenuously—and thereby got our exercise, modern conveniences have left us in a position where we must *choose* to do RM (rapid movement) / CV (cardio-vascular) exercise—or not. Choosing not to, we suffer diseases of many kinds. This is not idealistic thinking. I don't like exercise any more than many people—maybe most. But it likes me! It shows in the way this body feels every day. And that's why I do it.

The body has to move in order for the veins (venous system) to move blood adequately back to the heart and lungs for recirculation and re-oxygenation. And adequate exercise keeps other organs and bodily systems in shape and functioning well. How much exercise to do depends on several factors, like one's age and general physical condition, ambulatory capacity, immune strength, environments, and so on. The best book we've ever read on the subject of exercise is ***Conscious Exercise and the Transcendental Sun***, by Da Free John (Adi Da Samraj).

Rapid Movement, Moderate Movement, and Slow Movement Exercise

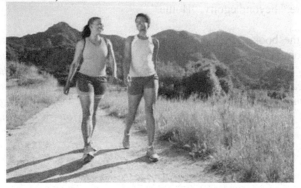

Rapid movement exercise includes most gym workouts, stair-step machines, swimming, cross-country skiing, running, jogging (not recommended, due to its stress on the spine and internal organs), and Power Walking. There are, of course, many others, with and without machines. Most adults are well to do about 20-30 minutes of Power Walking daily, or its equivalent. Most people do either more (which can be damaging) or less (possibly equally unhealthy).

Excessive exercise hyper-acidifies the body, introducing uric acids in the breakdown of bodily tissues and aging one prematurely. Lack of adequate physical exercise weakens the structural system and prevents appropriate heart and vascular activity. A brief but intense program of calisthenics—about 5-10 minutes, such as that described in the book, *Conscious Exercise and the Transcendental Sun*—can be all that is necessary for the average adult.

Here is a list of those daily calisthenics exercises:

- Windmill @ 15 each side
- Waist bends @ 10
- Jumping Jacks @ 20-25
- Walking in Place @ 20-25
- Knee Bends @ 20-25
- Running in Place @ 200-300 steps
- Deep Breathing @ 25-30 cycles
- Stomach Roll @ 12-15 rounds
- Leg Lifts @ 10-25x each leg
- Sit-Ups @ 7
- Push-Ups @ 15-20
- Relax pose

Intermediate movement exercise includes Tai Chi. This is excellent for the body in many ways, helping to keep the structural system and internal organs in balance while focusing mental and emotional energies—especially when done as real Spiritual practice. All exercise is best be done as our gift to the Divine Reality—as Spiritual practice. This brings exercise into consciousness, even moment-to-moment, and not engaging it any longer as just some merely physical activity. This sanctifies it, making it into a sacred event. (We can do this with everything!)

Hatha Yoga

The *two most important health practices* that we can do to make and keep us healthy are (1) pure diet, and (2) Hatha Yoga. Hatha Yoga is a form of **slow**-movement exercise. Rightly done, it is more than just exercise, but a genuinely religious ("re-lig" = rejoining with God) practice. However, even the simple gross physical aspect of it is quite healthful. Yoga is best done in the early evening before dinner, when the body is more relaxed and flexible. The asanas (postures) are gone into slowly and gently, never stretching too far.

These postures somehow gently massage the internal organs. The old expression, *"We're only as young as our glands,"* is a reference to the endocrine gland system. There are 20 asanas (below) we recommend as recommended by Avatar Adi Da, as described and illustrated in the book, ***Conscious Exercise And The Transcendental Sun***.

There are many local Hatha Yoga teachers currently available, both local "live" and online. A good Hatha Yoga health program should be kept simple and take only about 15-20 minutes to perform. There is no real pressing need to stretch them out into hour-long programs—unless you're just learning them for the first time. This sequence is available as a video link thru membership in **GLDLifestyle** at www.gldiet.co. While there are many asanas possible, these perhaps more important asanas include the following, done in this order:

Windmill
Tree
Neck Pull
Neck Stretch
Head Roll
Cobra
Bow
Locust
Head-to-Knee Pose
Plow
Shoulder Stand
Bridge
Fish
Forward Bending Pose
Spinal Twist
Peacock
Wheel
Headstand
Lion
Dead Pose

As we age, these yoga postures become even more important. The highly alkaline hi-raw or all-raw veggie diet does its part to keep us youthful and flexible, and our nightly hatha yoga routine does the same. Done over time, you get quite used to it, so that eventually you realize you wouldn't be without it. When or if friends and family find you doing your yoga asanas, they'll be impressed. Take the opportunity and suggest they join you!

NATURAL HYGIENE

Keeping our body and environments clean has been a significant factor in increasing our lifespan. For most of our history as humans, we bathed only very occasionally. For most of us, this has changed only in the last century or so. Our practice of bathing twice yearly "whether we needed it or not" (!) has given way to bathing pretty much daily. Modern plumbing and sewage treatment have helped this process substantially. Just the act of keeping clean and well-groomed keeps various organisms at bay that would otherwise participate in the disease process.

Pharmaceutical companies would like us to think that their products are responsible for the world's increasing longevity and the decrease in certain diseases. Altho this is so only to a relatively minor degree (e.g., via the strategic use of antibiotics), the truth of the matter is that most of our longevity in this regard can be attributed simply to *improved hygiene*, like daily bathing with plain pure soap, and to the advent of *better plumbing*.

Besides this, of course, are the obvious social benefits of personal cleansing. The "nose-gay" bunch of flowers in medieval times was used to help divert our attention from the unfriendly "aroma" attending our loved one! This is not to mention their breath! Of course, we want to use natural hygiene products, avoiding all types of chemicalized ones. Ordinary soap can be used, e.g., as an excellent toothpaste.

Dry Brush Massage

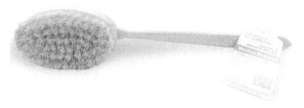

The vegetable agave plant fiber *dry brush massage* ("skin brush") often used before showering to loosen dead skin and stimulate the micro-lymphatics underlying the skin. It aids the body's natural cleansing and detox process, exercises and supports the lymphatic system, gently exfoliates and deep cleans the skin, reduces the appearance of cellulite, and thus generally promotes bodily purification. We use it as soon as we roll out of bed.

You do NOT get this brush wet. Ever! The handle is for your back. You pull off the handle after brushing your back, then use the head of the brush (the brush itself) to go over the rest of the body. The brush, used daily, will last about one year before needing replacement. We've known professional athletes who would never start their day without skin brushing. <u>We</u> wouldn't!

When the diet is relatively pure, the body takes on a different smell. It's "aroma" reflects what is taken into it. Notice the horrible odor attending the breath of cigarette smokers. Those with advanced cancer and other similarly developed degenerative diseases can have an awful stench emanating from the body. As raw and otherwise pure vegetal produce enters the body in increasingly higher percentages, and toxics and toxins leave, the body gradually takes on an increasingly light and clean aroma.

Great saints have been known to smell like flowers naturally—and that's without deodorants or antiperspirants. And, why would one wish to stop natural perspiration, anyway—unless their body "musk" was so offensive? Avoid such chemical products. Rubbing a slice of lime or lemon under the arms is just as effective and far healthier. This, then, is how to remedy any underarm "problem."

The frequency of bathing, or how often one should bathe, may be a function of (1) the degree of the body's current capacity to eliminate toxins, (2) the temperature of the body's environment, (3) body size, and (4) the body's relative activity. Large, healthy, young, and very active bodies moving around in hot weather need to bathe more often than do small, older people who eat a hi-raw or all raw diet and spend most of their time sitting in air-conditioned rooms or in cooler weather. Meanwhile, be conscious of how others respond to your personal "aromas" of breath and body, and how your own musk seems to you.

Big Pharma Medicine likes to take credit for reducing infectious diseases in the early 20th Century thru vaccination. Not so. In fact, most infectious diseases were eliminated by simple hygiene and improved plumbing—by the increasing use of soap and water for personal cleansing, including in hospitals. This simple practice is just as relevant today as it was a century and more ago. Perhaps more so—especially because of the superbugs created by antibiotic abuse.

Anal / Vaginal Hygiene

A modern essential of hygiene is the use of the bidet. Bidet models that employ a heated toilet seat, heated water, and air, are important for anal hygiene and the environment for several reasons:

- The comfort of a warm seat on cold mornings
- No need for toilet tissue (or deforestation to make it)
- The hygienic warm or hot water washing of the vagina and anus
- The hygienic drying of one's bottom

The whole process of such bidet use is hygienic, clean, comfortable, and sanitary, allowing the elimination of bodily wastes to thus be that much more of an altogether pleasurable experience. An example is the Toto© Washlet B200. Once you've enjoyed such a device, you'll never want to be without it.

The bidet (pronounced "bee-day") is undoubtedly among the more civilized health practices we modern humans have discovered (hit "bidet" on Google, or try www.totousa.com). USA Americans are just starting to get used to this clever device that have long been available in Europe and Japan. Anal washing is far healthier and more sanitary than is wiping with tissue paper. And, it's more comforting when both the toilet seat and the water that cleanses the anus and vagina are warm!

Warmer water (which many new bidet devices control) can also stimulate bowel movements (BMs), a distinctly helpful process against constipation. Once tried, there's no going back to the old method of tissue wiping. Rightly used, the bidet allows toilet tissue to be replaced by a soft hemp cloth for drying—or even by the bidet's own steam of warm air, depending on the bidet model you choose. Bidet—the only way to "go!"

Sunlight Therapy

Sunlight got a bad rap in the last part of the 20th Century. This was the result of misunderstanding perpetrated by drug and chemical companies involving excessive sun exposure resulting in skin cancer. Yes, excessive sun exposure can cause skin cancer. But, how much exposure and when? Conveniently for Big Pharma and Big Chemical, this was never mentioned on TV.

The sun has healing properties beyond what modern science has yet discovered—and we're talking far more than the very important Vitamin D3. There are many natural health benefits to moderate and intelligent sun exposure. Meanwhile, we need to avoid the so-called "SPF factor" sunscreens, which are loaded with junk chemicals which penetrate the skin and therefore and thereby interfere with many endocrine and metabolic functions within the body.

Notice how intelligent field and garden workers cover their bodies, head, and neck, with hats, lightweight long sleeves and long trousers, against sunburn. Smart! But, they are out there for hours in the sun. They need that protection. The rest of us can enjoy the many benefits of direct sun exposure IF and WHEN we do it intelligently.

Living 10 miles from the beach in Southern California, I greatly enjoy an occasional trip to the coast, where I can walk in the sand and sea. I'll spend 40 minutes walking thru the surf in a bathing suit or shorts and T-shirt, any time of the year, maybe taking a dip—depending on the weather. Very healthy breathing in the negative ions in the ocean air (positive for the health), enjoying the saltwater and sand on the feet and legs, and the scent of the sea.

Best is to get your sun exposure to both the front and back of the body for a total of 15-30 minutes daily when the sun is lower in the sky, before 10 AM, and after 4 PM in most parts of the world. This could take a while to get used to, and for some, it will be only occasional, but it is quite effective. As noted, sunlite does more than fix Vitamin D in the body. It provides forms of natural energy not yet measurable by modern technology. Among the better natural skin protectors: pure unrefined coconut oil & African shea butter. Don't use chemical crap on your skin!

Tooth Care

Among the more irritating health problems we modern humans suffer are dental caries. With chlorinated / fluorinated water, primitive dentistry, chemicalized foods, and refined sugars and carbohydrates enjoying record sales, our teeth take a big hit. Brushing the teeth *and flossing* after meals have become essential.

The best dentifrice we've found by far is Dr. Bronner's Liquid Soap© (www.drbronner.com; see Appendix B) diluted @ 7:1 with water. Place this mix into a small capped bottle in the bathroom where you commonly brush your teeth. Simply dip your brush in, re-cap the bottle, and brush.

Alternatively, rub your wetted toothbrush on a plain, regular unscented bar of ordinary soap. Dr. Bronner's© liquid soap is preferable because of its use of pure, natural oils and—when diluted as suggested—it's even more effective and very low cost.

You will quickly get used to the "taste" of the Dr. Bronner's and water mix—but, of course, don't swallow it. (It won't poison you like the fluoride toothpastes will, because it's just "soap.") Toothpastes—even the so-called "organic" ones—often use glycerin and other sweeteners as flavorings, which stick to the teeth, making re-enameling difficult, and encouraging unfriendly bacteria and fungi in the mouth. Avoid these!

Flossing the teeth takes on a whole new potency when you add a little 100% Tea Tree Oil or Young Living© Thieves Oil to the floss: simply pull out a 12-16" length of floss, wrapping each end around the last digit of each index finger but leaving about an inch or so of floss in the middle, between your fingers. Dip this part into the chosen oil. Floss your teeth with this part, using one dip into the oil for the upper teeth and one for the lower teeth. This procedure greatly enhances the floss's ability to help your teeth by killing many different types of harmful bacteria and fungi.

An ancient and excellent practice for strong teeth is called "*oil pulling*." It consists of placing about two tablespoons of pure natural cold-processed or expeller-pressed virgin coconut oil into your mouth, keeping it there, and occasionally swishing it around for about 20 minutes, then spitting it out. You don't swallow it during this 20-minute pulling process.

Of course, this process does much more than strengthen and otherwise encourage good strong teeth. Some of the oil will penetrate the mucous membranes of the mouth and do some very nice things for other systems of your body. Coconut, moreover, is one of the true SuperFoods (see Appendix C). This is just another of the many ways coconut will help your health.

Flossing has always been important in teeth cleaning. The ancients used tree twigs with edges to remove food pieces stuck between teeth. Wherever you eat your meals—at home, in the office, at restaurants—you want to carry a pocket / purse-size flosser. The best one we've found is the G.U.M. Professional Clean Flosser. At 3" long and 1" wide at the floss head, given the number of times we are exposed to food daily, I wouldn't be without it.

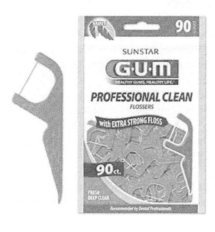

These are so handy and important to keep lodged food particles from your teeth—which particles attract the bad guys that ruin teeth and gums. Keep them in a small plastic bag in pocket or purse. Use them right at the table, then, if you like, and then either toss them out or you can rinse them in the bathroom or kitchen sink for re-use at your next meal. Very economical when you consider how they can help save your teeth and keep you out of the dentist's office.

Another excellent product to help thoroly clean the teeth is the WaterPik©, an electric-powered device that shoots a strong, fine stream of water between the teeth along the gum line. We recommend blending a piece of fresh garlic into warm water going into the *WaterPik©* and/or adding three drops of Tea Tree Oil or Thieves© Oil. Therefore, at this point in the evolution of dental hygiene technology—and given the current circumstance of food and diet—we recommend the following procedures for maximum tooth care:

1 – *Swish* around in your mouth 2 Tbsp. of pure coconut oil for 20 minutes each morning (do not swallow)
2 – *Eat* a high-raw or all-raw vegetarian diet, rightly using (or avoiding) the LQFs—especially refined sugar products
3 – *Floss* the teeth, then *rinse* with water right after meals, using the G.U.M. (pocket / purse size) Prof Clean Flosser
4 – *Brush* after each meal during the day with Dr. Bronner's© per instructions *or at least rinse the mouth with water*
5 – *Floss* after brushing (before retiring), having dipped the *floss* that contacts your teeth into Thieves© Oil
6 – *WaterPik©* last-rinse your teeth using the formula (above) to precisely eliminate food particles as described
7 – *Rinse* the mouth thoroly after each instance of food intake

Fluoride, used in toothpastes and drinking water, is a known and highly toxic poison that should be avoided whenever possible—including bathing in it. Some decades ago, when commercial fertilizer companies in Florida were penalized for dumping this toxic waste into rivers and onto vacant lots, some shrewd company man got the idea that he could foist this poison off on the people by selling it to municipal water companies. Thus, what was otherwise a big loss turned into a massive profit for the fertilizer industry—and became the doubly great expense of both health and money to us all. No escaping it, this is a modern tragedy.

Commercial mouthwashes have also had a negative effect on teeth. One of the author's alcoholic high school teachers used to drink Listerine© directly from the bottle! A more recent citrus-flavored version of this product contains ethanol, which is used as a fuel for automobiles. Most other such commercial mouthwashes are little better. Comfrey tea is an excellent mouthwash, as is chewing a small sprig of parsley. Or make an excellent mouthwash by mixing 20 drops of Tea Tree Oil into a pint of water. Just a Tbsp. of this mix will disinfect your mouth after brushing at nite. (Don't swallow.) It doesn't taste good but it really does the job!

Dentistry, as a science and a practice, needs advancement! For one thing, we need a non-chemical, non-alcohol mouthwash that quickly cleanses all materials left on, around, and between teeth, leaving the mouth fresh and clean. For another, we need dentists who understand and avoid all use of metals and other materials hostile to the human body—especially the very dangerous mercury amalgams and fluoride! We need dentists who teach the patient right use of diet and lifestyle to prevent caries, gum disease, and the various other problems associated with the teeth—e.g., to encourage good health.

Healthy teeth are strong and clean and even, reflecting good health in the body. Healthy gums are pink in color and do not bleed when the teeth are brushed. Try to brush after every meal, and floss, too—but at least rinse with water after each intake of food. Note that even certain pure liquids—especially citrus juices—tend to erode the teeth if left in the mouth without rinsing with water. Please heed this!

Brush and floss at least at nite before bed. The bacteria that cause tooth decay can be managed better by a strong body. The GLD can provide this kind of support. Pure diet, proper oral cleaning habits, Vitamin C, Vitamin D, sunlite on the skin, exercise, right use of the LQFs—these are great tooth aides.

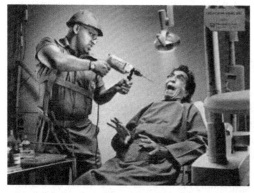

Your author has had various encounters with dentists over the years. For example, we had to have the poisonous mercury amalgams removed from a few teeth. We had a root canal (never do this!). In more recent years, the better dentists made a few good recommendations to us, including rinsing with water after each intake of food, rinsing after taking juices, carrying a toothbrush and floss on outings and for travel, and using the WaterPik.

Unfortunately, most dentists still toe the official ADA line, recommending "ordinary" (poisonous) fluoride toothpaste and mercury-filled dental amalgams. This science is still in a primitive state!

We see so many people in their 50's and 60s having teeth removed or otherwise suffering all manner of internal problems and apparently unrelated diseases just because of bad tooth care habits. And, of course, because of refined sugar intake, such sugar being the worst so-called "food" one can eat!

Neglecting these disciplines, leaving food on the teeth for hours on end (which so many of us do—or have done), plaque builds up—little-by-little, insidiously—then decay sets in, erodes gums, and settles in the jaw as infection—suggesting to dentists root canals, other surgery, or extraction. We've known friends, relatives, and patients who have been rushed to the hospital and died from infections in the jaw after tooth extractions.

Note also that the teeth are each associated with a certain organ or tissue within the body. These charts are available on the Net. Problems with teeth mean problems with the certain organ which that tooth relates to. Heed these warnings and do the disciplines of healthy teeth. It all starts with and depends on the foundation of the hi-raw or all-raw veggie diet. Believe it: it is worth the time spent—and enjoy good strong teeth accordingly.

One last item regards the **re-growing** of teeth. Soon, special stem cells will be implanted thru the gums where teeth have been removed in order to re-grow the missing teeth. Who knows when this technique—which has been known for decades now—will be allowed into the public domain? Meanwhile, we can do our life-positive oral health practices. An old Ayurvedic recipe suggests intake of ground eggshell to help promote such re-growth. Does it work? Maybe, via half a tsp. of finely ground eggshell in a smoothie once or twice weekly.

Skin Care

The skin (or integument) is nominally the largest organ of the body—an organ of protection and respiration. It absorbs and thrives on nutrients from sun and air. Substances in contact with the skin, if kept there (in some cases, even very briefly), can and will be absorbed. Clothing in contact with the skin should therefore be of pure natural materials—cotton, silk, wool, linen, ramie, jute, flax, hemp, natural rayon (pure woven cellulose/regular viscose rayon), and natural leather—in order to protect health.

Avoid any regular or (especially) prolonged skin contact by human-made clothing materials: acetate, latex, plastic, polyester, spandex, vinyl, nylon (polyamide), acrylic, Naugahyde / faux leather, olefin, etc. At least prefer natural material <u>undergarments</u> (garments contacting skin) when human-made outerwear is otherwise useful, such as against weather extremes. The same goes for shoes: only natural materials in contact with the skin.

Thousands of chemicalized lotions and compounds have been manufactured to keep the skin moist, supple, and youthful-looking. Avoid all use of poisonous human-made skincare products, including the junk-filled so-called sun protector creams and gels with their silly "SPF" factors. The best skin moisturizers include those with perfectly and exclusively natural substances. These include pure cold-pressed or expeller-pressed virgin coconut oil and African shea butter (www.naturessheabutter.com). Coconut oil and African shea butter are the best "sunscreens."

Moreover, the skin likes to be massaged by natural skin-to-skin touch. Touch is the primary sense in most life forms—including for us humans, and one's skin is the first medium of touch. The primacy of touch is essentially why we delight in being massaged, hugged, and kissed.

RIGHT OCCUPATION

Our "occupation" is our use of time, what we do with the time of our lives—whether for pay or not. A man's occupation, his job, his career, <u>his work</u>, is usually primary in his life—whereas for a woman, it's her family, her man (or woman), <u>her love</u>. But, for both, occupation is important in health. We must feel right about our work, what we do with our time, whether in the home or out.

If we don't feel good about it, our bodily health will be negatively affected. If all the while we're driving to work we're visualizing our hands around the boss's neck (!), how will this help our health? Of course, it's best if we don't have to go a far distance in getting to work—which (the travel) is itself hard on us and the environment.

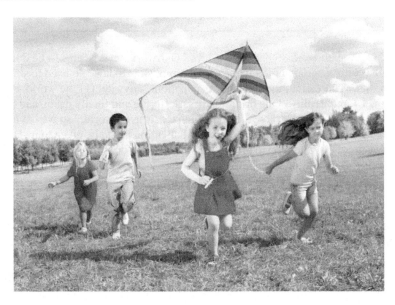

But just the work itself should be basically enjoyable and life-positive so we can feel good about ourselves and about what we are contributing to our culture and to humankind in general. Hating our job or anything else brings negative energy to the body (and thus poor health) and to everyone everywhere. Negative energy literally stores in organs, causing disease. We're talking negative etheric-emotional, mental, and even psychic energies.

Since, in these times, so many in this world have no work at all, no means of supporting themselves or their families, it's wise to offer our work to God in thanksgiving for the gift of right occupation. Work that is life-positive and that we genuinely enjoy is health-bringing—as long as we engage it in a balanced way, not overdoing it. If you do not have positive, creative work that you feel good about, pray for it, using the Devotional Prayer of Changes (See Appendix E).

Whenever you feel trapped, either by your work, a relationship, the culture you find yourself in, society in general, your community, the mind, bodily life, or whatever, do this little exercise:

> **Have you ever tried to feel to Infinity?** What would that be like? Let's try it!
>
> First, just feel to the borders of the room, then to the edges of the state, the country, the planet,
>
> out past Pluto, then to the edges of the galaxy, then…out to as far as ever there was or can be!

We all work so hard these days. Our work never seems to be done. There is only a certain amount one can accomplish in a day. No need to stress over that. There are only two basic occupations, anyway: (1) the world, and (2) the Divine Reality. One brings endless suffering and finally death, and the other Eternal Life. We have a body, which exists in a "world," so we have to work to support it. So, a certain amount of attention has to be given to it. But, can we grant that attention to the Divine Person while doing our worldly work? Absolutely! Attention is destiny!

Egoity or Unity, bondage or Freedom, conditional bewilderment or Divine-Communion. Yes, there is a way to do both; you can act in the world while granting feeling attention to the Great One. **All acts can be consciously done for the Beloved of the heart as Divine Communion.** This brings one's occupation into Alignment with Reality, transcending all bondage and unhappiness. ***Bottom line***: the right and appropriate occupation for any living being is Divine Communion—no matter what "else" you may be involved in.

LIFE-POSITIVE ENVIRONMENTS

Keeping our work and living environments neat and orderly helps keep our minds the same—and therefore affects our health. A sloppy, unkempt environment is noticed by everyone—even our self, the perpetrator. Is it a breeding ground for bugs and germs? Maybe we know where everything is, but the chaos and disorganization reflect our mind. Will people looking at our room or work area ask, *"Hey, was anyone hurt in this wreck?"*

Los Angeles is one of the great cities of the world, with some 19 million people (2019). But it was never rightly planned from the beginning. It does not exist on a human scale (see Appendix G). Even with its beauties, its positives, it is random chaos. Ever notice how stressful it is to drive thru such a large city—like Los Angeles (and I don't mean just the traffic)? On the other hand, notice how you feel when driving thru the countryside, out on the open highway, viewing forests, mountains, and deserts. It's calming—and therefore healthy.

It is possible to design a city that does not feel chaotic. But, when the design motives are money and power, monetary gain and egoic control based on gross materialism, the result is going to be something less than fully human. It isn't taking the holism of humanity and the natural environment into account.

Beings thrive in natural environments: seashores, mountains, deserts, flowers, with plants of all kinds. Private homes, commercial buildings, and whole cities can be made this way, as proven by design professor Ian McHarg (*Design With Nature*) and the great architect Frank Lloyd Wright. Habitat can be designed to flow with Nature, seeming to grow out of the landscape— like trees, e.g. They can be beautiful. It is healthy to live and work in such lovely, quiet, peaceful, and happy environments (see Appendix G). Let's get together and create them!

Sunlite

Life-positive environments include those that provide natural sunlite. Getting out in the sunlite does more than help fix Vitamin D in the skin. It can even nourish the body to the point that you don't need to eat at all! In recent years in the USA, much has been made of the "dangers" of sunlite, of skin exposure to ultra-violet rays, and of skin cancer. So-called SPF creams and lotions (already mentioned) have been offered to help against sunburn.

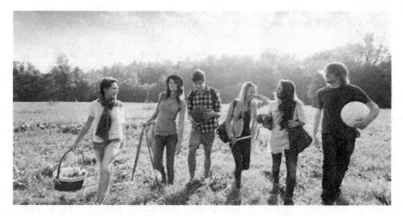

These chemical-filled creams and lotions do far more harm than good. One is better off using the original protector, pure coconut oil. Prefer extra virgin expeller-pressed or cold-pressed organic raw unprocessed coconut oil (see Appendix C). Moderate exposure to the sun is generally very healthy—15 minutes or so on each side of the body before 10 AM and after 4 PM in most Earth locations. Longer is OK for a covered body, but try to get some sun exposure on some body part daily or otherwise whenever possible.

When the sun is between 1° and 10° off the horizon, we can look directly at it without harm. Start with just a few seconds and, if you like, gradually, add a few seconds per day, building up to long minutes. This process brings the various energies of the sun into the body for increased health overall. It also lessens the need for gross food!

The sun is a primary form of gross and etheric energies, like the Earth's oxygen envelope, but prior to Earth-grown foods. Otherwise, when the sun is anywhere in the sky, glance at it briefly each day, just for a second, to allow its energies to penetrate the body thru the eyes. This stimulates higher endocrine functions—at the level of the pineal gland—toward longer life and better health.

Breathing

One of the observations made by native Hawaiians when first visited by Captain Cook and his "howlies" (white men) was that "they don't breathe!" Their breathing was shallow and uneven, reflecting their mental makeup, their concerns and worries, their fears and anxieties—basically, their egoity, their sense of separation from The Divine Consciousness. Whereas the native Hawaiians were, in some sense, far more relaxed and settled in themselves.

Breath is "spirit." As such, it can be used as a vehicle to move and manipulate prana, or etheric energy, in and thru the body to enhance health. Deep, relaxed breathing is basic to good health. As suggested, our breathing reflects what is in our minds. Attention on the Beloved Divine brings a calm, serene mind. A calm mind allows for this deep, slow, relaxed breathing.

Breath is also intimately connected to emotions, to feeling. Our breathing reflects what we feel at any given moment. Attention to the Divine Person, the Person of Love, allows for deep relaxed breathing. The body needs to take in oxygen thru the lungs to the blood and thence to the rest of the tissues. Long, slow, rhythmic and deep breaths relax body, emotions, and mind.

The in-breath and the out-breath symbolize nourishment and the very flow of life. We take in food, and we eliminate waste. We receive positive energy and release the negative: assimilation and elimination. Avatar Adi Da calls it "Reception and Release." This is a basic principle of life. Notice how the breathing becomes interrupted, uneven, shallow, and with sudden big loud gasps when we are emotionally upset. We even approach new tasks thus.

Notice also how the breathing slows way down and becomes inaudible and even—and can even become suspended—when we sit in meditation on the Spiritual Master. What does this say? There's nothing more important, balancing and settling on which to place one's attention.

Now, notice the air quality in your environments—inside and outside. People have died from smog in certain cities, and from poor air quality in their own homes lacking adequate ventilation. Buildings in which we live and work need circulating clean air. In interior environments (home, work), living plants can provide health-giving oxygen, an etheric connection with another living being, and a gentle unmoving friendship.

Sound
Plants are also sensitive to our moods and to sound. By actual scientific measurement, we have learned that they don't like "heavy metal" or "acid rock" music, preferring classical and sacred music instead. Apparently, our bodies also enjoy classical music. Studies show our IQ increasing in a classical music environment. Calm and quiet surroundings are conducive to improved concentration and general good health.

Imagine serene and uncluttered home and work environments where soft music is playing in the background, flowers growing, lovely plants are tastefully placed, with harmonious décor colors. Art is stylishly displayed, a sense of understated elegance pervades the space, and an air of peace and tranquility abides. Notice how only the finer restaurants have classical music playing in the background—because it's considered "fine art." But it's also more conducive to good digestion!

SPIRITUAL CULTIVATION

It is said that the Divine Blessing and Grace are always falling from Heaven upon us, upon the world. However, the only way the Divine Reality can "get to and into" both "us" and the world is via our attention on It (the Great One) by humans and other beings—as many beings as possible—the more the better. If we only think of God, The Divine, occasionally, the Blessing will be minimal. If we held up a thimble, a thimbleful is all we'd get!

The non-humans (so-called "wild animals") already spend most of their time with their attention on the Divine. Just watch them—the wild ones out in Nature—and you'll see. They look around to see if there are any predators. If they're already eaten, and sexed, they look for a quiet spot and…meditate, contemplating the Divine!

In these "Dark Times," we humans are distracted by the various aspects of the psychophysical domain, the world, in strictly gross-level terms. Our attention is virtually exclusively on the gross physical plane. In our egoity, we're like the "monkey with its hand in the candy jar," unwilling to let go of the candy—and therefore trapped. Hence the world's current dilemma. Avatar Adi Da says, *"...in this gross ego-culture now...humanity has disconnected itself from the field of energy in which the cosmos exists and which it (in fact) is."*

He goes on, *"Matter is energy. To make a global culture of people who are only thinking and perceiving in terms of sheer physicality is to have established a gross culture that is going to destroy itself. To understand and correct this is critical. It is critical for the sensitivity to be restored, the balance restored, the responsibility restored by humankind as a whole— because its gross-mindedness is the basis for self-destruction."*

As egos, with attention on ourselves as separate entities (as tho all we are is a "separate-from-everything-and-everyone" gross physical body), we always tend to do four things:

(1) **objectify** everything
(2) **surround** whatever or whoever it is
(3) attempt to **control** it or them
(4) wind up **destroy**ing it (or them)

This is what we've been doing to the world. You can see it in the activities of government and Big Corporate—even in our movies. As egos, this is what we tend to do with everything. Attention on the Divine Reality, on the other hand, is counter-egoic. It is our very freedom, bringing compassion, harmony, and love to every thing and every one.

172

Genuine Spiritual practice, cultivating the relationship with the Very Divine, is the most important activity in life. Nothing takes away our stress like feeling to the Beloved of the heart. This is why the Great Spiritual Masters (Rama, Krishna, Mohammad, Jesus, and the most recent God-Man, Avatar Adi Da Samraj) have turned about to Teach us—mainly to teach us out of our egoity, our "sin," our sense of separateness.

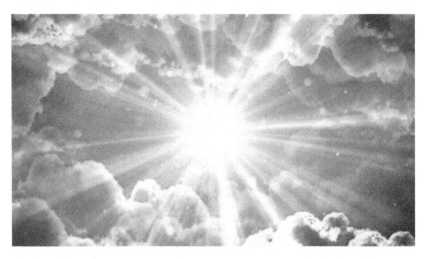

The Wonderful Unity that These Great Ones Teach is Music and Real Food to our hearts. It is our Perfect Nourishment, and therefore our best Healing Balm. Beginning our day with prayer, meditation, and Spiritual study of divine scriptures sets the tone for our day and encourages the Divine Reality to be the core of our lives.

In these "Dark Times," where egoic self-interest comes first, and the focus is material life, we feel the stress of egoity more than ever. The world is currently mad with it—with egoity. Turning to the Divine Person relieves us of this awful burden—at least to some degree. One cannot be fearful, sorrowful, or angry when meditating on the body of the Spiritual Master. Continuing such cultivation, with and by Divine Grace, we move into the higher stages of life toward true Divine Enlightenment. We enjoy the very purpose of our embodiment: Blissfulness, Freedom, and Happiness.

Avatar Adi Da Samraj calls God "*The Transcendental Consciousness and Radiant Life that Pervades the body, the mind, and the world.*" Many great books encourage attention to God. Besides the Christian **bible**, the Muslim **Quran**, and the Hebrew **Torah**, there are many Great ancient scriptures, such as the *Lankavatara Sutra*, the *Platform Sutra* of Hui Neng, and the *Diamond Sutra*. More recently, in our modern idiom, we have *The Knee of Listening*, **The Dawn Horse Testament**, *The Pneumaton*, *The Gnosticon*, and *The Aletheon*.

173

Summarizing *The BIG 7*

Therefore, while on your GLD, be encouraged to not only take pure food but also to get to bed early as often as possible. We get better results with exercise appropriate to your specific health circumstance. Improve more rapidly by right grooming and bathing, engaging in right occupation, and keeping environments clean and neat—and this includes keeping good company: avoiding negative, quarrelsome and otherwise problematic people, and spending our time in the company of positive, intelligent people who insist on continuing to grow as human beings.

And finally, and most importantly, managing the mental-emotional factor (considered by many as over 70% of the cause of disease) by cultivating your relationship with Real God, not the "god" the human mind dreams up, but the Great Consciousness, the Matrix, Reality, or Context within Which everything appears, the Very Beloved intuited by every heart. Do your prayer, meditation, and Spiritual study daily, *making and keeping the sacred as (rightly) the core of your life*.

Service

Service is *right use of the body*. In the Words of Adi Da, the bodily human form is an opportunity. In utero, the fetus trusts its environment, its parent. Born into the world, we begin to feel frightened, vulnerable, separated from our source of nourishment and safety, identifying with the body as a separate entity. The body-mind becomes "me," "I," separate from all "others." We must learn to rightly connect with the world *in relationship*, to surrender, trust, and love. This is the Law of Divine Life. It's also the Law of basic human life.

Love is surrender into God, sacrifice, feeling-radiance. Faith is trust in the Universe, in the inherent Unity of All. Ecstasy requires this trust, acceptance of everything, even death. Fear is lack of trust, lack of faith. We must have compassion for all of existence, not just loving cooperation, the blessing and help, locally, for other human beings with whom we are close, but for all beings. They are all struggling to survive within the Divine Radiance.

The cosmic reality is all about **sacrifice** (Love, surrender, submission), so there must be a fundamental acceptance of death and suffering as part of the cycle of bodily life. We can, therefore, intentionally use our lives as a sacrifice, as Spiritual practice, minimizing suffering, bringing love, trust, and faith to all. Use yourself up in service. We have to die of something. Rather than of some disease from self-indulgence, it might as well be service to God as Spiritual practice, in love, in positive participation in Reality.

174

Finally, we can think of life without Spiritual practice as the typical approach of Pharma medicine to disease: treatment of symptoms—whereas, life with and as true Spiritual practice is like Radical Healing: it's about going to the root of the "problem," the disease of egoity. It's about understanding it and transcending it altogether in Real Happiness.

Wandering the Realms of Possibility

There are only two general directions we can go with attention, only one of which we can do in any moment: the conditional realm or the *Un*conditional realm, the profane or the sacred. The conditional realm is about shift, flux, constant change, paradox, repetition, wandering the realms of possibility. The Unconditional realm, or the Divine Domain, with attention on the God-Man, the Spiritual Master, is about Eternal Freedom, Perfect Peace, and Absolute Happiness. Since we are what we give our attention to, it's then easy to choose between these two exclusively. The choice becomes simple—and obvious.

In the current world culture, the young look for adventure, excitement, searching the realms of possibility. At some point, in some lifetime, usually in older age, we realize the futility of all experience. It all just leads to more experience, an endless cycle. Life is difficult here in this yellow-red realm under the best of circumstances. But, even when things seem to "work out," they don't! There is no final satisfaction here. This is a place of suffering.

Still, you can be happy here. Even "Divine Awakening" Happy. The wise tell us the heart can be truly and finally satisfied—even all thru life. They say it's very difficult and takes profound dedication. They say the best thing one can do with one's life is to turn most fully and profoundly to the Eternal Consciousness within Which we all appear and disappear, our true Source of health and Happiness.

A Suggested "Solid Foods" Healthy Daily Routine
(incorporating The BIG 7)

5-6:00AM – arise, meditation / prayer / **Spiritual study**

6:35 AM – **exercise**

7:05 AM – herb tea, study work-related / pleasurable / informative reading material; **dry brush massage, shower**

7:30 AM – **breakfast**: keep meals small; chew all food thoroughly; pray, invoking Divine Blessing on your food

8:30 AM – start work, doing **work** you enjoy and feel entirely right about, that your efforts serve humanity and the Divine

10:00 AM – Green smoothie, RMVJ or other fresh-squeezed liquid fruit or veggy juice

1:00 PM – **lunch**: a big mixed salad; try to make your diet mostly raw or even all raw, natural, ripe, in-season, and locally-grown

4:00 PM – maybe a lite snack of chopped fresh fruit, nutmilk, chopped dates and nuts, perhaps dried fruit

5:30 PM – Arrive home, change clothes; tend to your **environments**, keeping them orderly

5:45 PM – stretches or (preferably) **yoga** helps the body stay youthful, supple and flexible

6:00 PM – check the Net to stay current with world and local events

7:00 PM – **dinner**: bowl of raw granola fruit, berries, with rich nutmilk, sprinkled with shredded coconut and raw sunflower seeds

8:00 PM – evening entertainment: **interact with moral, intelligent and responsible friends** and family

9:30 PM – prepare for bed; **meditation, prayer**, thank The Great One for the Gift of life, the opportunity to Realize the Divine

10:00-11:00 PM – latest **bedtime**; after prayer and meditation, your head hits the pillow for sleep

Justifying *The BIG 7*: Hedging your Bets

Those who carefully observe their life will see the importance of at least most of ***The BIG 7***. Those with no real connection to life as sacred activity won't be involved in #7, but will at least be able to help their life by doing the first 6—with the understanding that if the body isn't well, this puts a damper on our enjoyment of almost anything.

Even the sick can love—and turn to The Great One. With good health, we can enjoy both the world of possibilities (the profane) and the Divine (the sacred). And if the Divine is Real—and the Matrix within Which all of this life and world appears—then a little daily Spiritual study won't hurt. So, hedge your bets and get into the daily **BIG 7** practice for the fundamental practicality of it. This is just basically intelligent.

Transcending Failure

Occasionally failing to do this or that part of our **Big 7** is common. Life is not about perfection. It's about the gesture. It's about purification. Now, at least we have a program! Even a program to fall off of, if need be. Most people don't even have that. Miss something today, and you just start again tomorrow. No biggie. You'll get better at it as you go along. No one is perfect at doing **The BIG 7**. Not always.

Something always comes up to prevent us from doing it perfectly every single day. A persistent gesture to The Beloved is shown in this image (shown at right). It is the gesture of mutual giving, the Sacrament of Universal Sacrifice (Grand Medicine's company logo). It represents our gesture of surrender and self-sacrifice, of offering ourselves to the Divine.

So, no concern about "failure." We're all in the same boat together, helping each other, cooperating with each other, serving each other, and encouraging each other in love. Sincerely making this feeling gesture of surrender and submission to The Divine, we are already transcending failure and everything else.

THE IMMUNITY-HEALTH CONNECTION
Love and Emotions

Have you ever been in love? It's some kind of magic! It's like you're walking on air. Everyone and everything looks just fine to you, even beautiful. You want to kiss everyone—or at least hug them or shake their hand. You're happy all the time. Everything seems to sparkle with light. You feel a kind of numbness or invulnerability all over the body. Your appetite is diminished: "Who needs food when I feel like this?!"

OK, we're talking about romantic love—not Real Love (sacrifice, surrender), which is a whole other subject—and even better, even happier. But the point is that being in love is a definite immune booster. Consider other emotions. Every positive emotion—kindness, gratitude, happiness, thankfulness, etc.—all of these boost immunity. <u>Negative</u> emotions—hate, anger, jealousy, fear, sorrow, etc.—reduce and lower immunity.

At some real level, immunity is health. A strong immune system protects the body from almost anything harmful. Besides emotions, **gross food**, of course, also powerfully affects immune protection—and therefore, health. When the body tissues get what they need in terms of nutrients (from raw, living foods), the immune system is strongly benefited.

Mind

Then there is the **mind** connection. Consider the two parts of mind—*conceptual* and *perceptual*—which constantly come into play in the moments of waking life. <u>*Perceptual*</u> mind is the part that "touches" things—e.g., as we walk along the street seeing whatever is there to see. In this sense, seeing is touching. Perceptual mind does not think nor does it judge—it simply notices—patterns, colors, textures, shapes, etc. Perceptual mind is holistic, then, non-linear.

<u>*Conceptual*</u> mind, however, is what takes over when, as we're walking, e.g., we visualize ourselves at the office hearing the boss's voice telling us we're late on that report. There's the trouble, then. The conceptual mind is like "a fat, adolescent idiot" (Adi Da's description). Conceptual mind is ego-mind—which can be useful when rightly guided by attention.

The conceptual mind seems always to be focused on some "problem" or other. Conceptual mind tends to see life this way—linear, in a "problem-solution" fashion. The average human adult thinks some 82,000 thots daily, and most of these thoughts, by far, are negative! This is the <u>conceptual</u> mind, the part of mind that gets us into all the trouble. So, how to deal with the conceptual mind?

Managing the conceptual mind has been the subject of philosophy and religion for millennia. You can <u>distract</u> that part of mind in various ways with something extremely *physical*, like skiing, bungee jumping, or dangling yourself over a cliff by a rope! How about a *mental* distraction, like meditating on a candle, doing a crossword puzzle, or watching an *emotionally* engrossing movie?

Or, you can engage the conceptual mind in a positive way, like working out a dress-making plan, or visualizing the details of a fix-it project, planning a wedding, or considering a surprise gift for someone. That's better, more creative! Or, besides doing these positive mental activities, you can <u>transcend</u> the mind altogether in Divine Communion by meditating on the Spiritual Master. This activity can finally bring the mind under control.

The trouble with the first two practices (distraction and engagement) is that "the problem" is still there when you're done. Conceptual mind remains to do its worst. And it doesn't care how dark the subject matter it may torture you with! With Divine Communion, or meditation on the Spiritual Master, mind is immediately (and even progressively) moved beyond, transcended, and otherwise brightened and made wise—precisely because of (and by) What (or That Which) it is meditating on. Grace!

We become what we meditate on (or otherwise give significant attention to)! So, what (or "What") is the subject matter? It will be either "problems" (real or imagined by conceptual mind) or Happiness, difficulty or Perfection, stress or Peace. One lowers immunity, while the other raises it. Now, mark this carefully: it is a choice we can make in every moment of life. However, attention is a mighty force. Grace is necessary to overcome it— which is why Real Spiritual practice (transcending mind) is so difficult.

Immunity and *The BIG 7*

Of course, other gross level life choices enter into the immunity picture. These include the rest of *The BIG 7*: exercise, rest, the company and environments we keep, our work, and how we spend our time, and our hygiene. The same with attitude/mind/emotions (as Spirituality) and diet. So, it always comes down to these practices. When done as God-Communion, as our gift to The Divine, they become happy play.

Humorously repeating a media advertising phrase, Adi Da once said of our use of these disciplines, "*You can pay me now, or you can pay me later!*" —From a Talk called, *The Location of Happiness*, Given at the Mountain of Attention Sanctuary on 28 November 1981, available as a DVD of the same title from The Dawn Horse Press.

14—The Disease Process

Its Causes and its Source

Avatar Adi Da says, humorously, *"Disease is a crime punishable by death!"* Disease (dis-ease, ill-at-ease) occurs as a result of egoity, the sense we have of being separate, our separateness, separation from everything and everyone. Egoity is the source of all disease. Of course, the ego is a lie, entirely false, but also an activity we wrongly engage in—in every moment! In fact, however, we are living in a Perfect Unity—all the time!

There isn't one speck of separation anywhere—only apparently. We are breathing the same air Jesus breathed 2000-odd years ago! Everything is intimately connected to everything "else." It's all one "Thing." How and why? In our egoity, which implies inherent unhappiness, we attempt to become happy. But (and here's the problem), the attempt to become happy is the confession of **un**happiness! The activities of the ego are therefore the *cause* unhappiness and disease.

Happiness (living in the Body of The Divine) is our Native Condition. But, we don't notice this because we are not connecting with The Divine—moment-to-moment. Most of the time, not at all! Unhappiness **is** disease, the dis-ease of egoity. That makes egoity, and all its attempts to become happy, the *source* and the *cause* of disease. Source is prior to cause. Ego is our sense of identification with the body. But in Truth, the body is just a temporary mechanism—that will die—while "we" (as Consciousness) continue on.

With food (as egos), we're sure we can eat our way to happiness. There's gonna be some great meal, some super sandwich, that'll finally do it for us. We're certain that once we get the right partner, we can perhaps sex our way to happiness—better sex than we've ever had. Or, as is so often the case these days, we tend to think we can earn our way to happiness thru getting more money and material things: we can buy happiness. Or, we may think we can do it thru social status. Many of us actually believe this—for real! But, it just isn't going to happen!

We may disagree with these ideas philosophically, but they are nonetheless true in fact for most human beings in these Dark Times: we try even desperately to become happy via money, food, sex, and social life. The frustration we feel in all of this struggling to become happy is actually our state of dis-ease. It certainly contributes to physical disease, disease in the body. This is traditional knowledge and ancient wisdom.

Therefore, the *cause* of our disease is our attempts to become happy. The *source* of our disease is our egoity, our activity of separation. Again, source is prior to cause. Consider this: everything you can "become," you can *and will* lose. Death makes its claim on us in these material terms. In fact, in gross physical life, the only thing we can count on is death.

This being so, what is the "cure?" How can we cure this pervasive disease of egoity? Everyone is in the "cure" business. Everything is sold as a "cure" to unhappiness—food, land, marriage, sex, social position, power. What is the cure for the loveless heart? What is the cure for egoity? If the highest Law of the universe is, *"We are (or become) what we give our attention to,"* then obviously we should give our attention to That Which is Great!

Granting attention to (or meditating on) stocks and bonds, in and of themselves, we take on their quality, our mind and emotions going up and going down with market ebb and flow—like the changing weather. Then, what <u>doesn't</u> change? Change is the nature of the conditional realms (including Earth). The Change*less* is the Spiritual Divine: Perfect Happiness, Absolute Freedom, and Eternal Peace. Doesn't it make sense to take on these qualities rather than those that constantly change? This brings with it a level of wellness beyond the merely physical.

Some healers think that preventing disease is simply about eating all raw food. Others believe that certain organisms (germs, parasites, etc.) cause disease, so health would therefore be a matter of killing the germs with drugs or herbs—or otherwise avoiding contagion. There are variations on these two themes, and there are other ideas as to how disease occurs, how to treat it, and how to prevent it. However, there are many causes of disease—if only because there are many planes of existence.

This means that disease can come from simple genetic inherited tendencies that quickly become expressed as disease. Or, one's "disorder" can express at the physical level as a result of a profound emotional event from long ago, or of a mental attitude, feelings of long-held hate, or of a psychic occurrence long since passed. Any of these and many more such possibilities and events can manifest as disease at the gross physical level.

The true healer approaches the patient's situation with this understanding, and does not try to cure or heal the so-called disorder. He or she understands that the natural condition of the body is Radiance, and that it is always appropriate to place the body into a position to enjoy that condition—which requires responsibility on the part of both the healer and the healee. Each has responsibilities relative to the body-mind and its health.

It is inappropriate for a patient to expect the healer to work some magic with an herb, pill, tablet, drug, potion, process, or procedure of some kind or other that will relieve their suffering. It is equally inappropriate for the healer to struggle to find some remedy, magical or ordinary, that will bring such relief. Both of these attitudes assume and represent the "problem" approach, the Donald Duck approach to health and disease. The body is not a problem to be dealt with. The ego is the problem.

The <u>Source</u> of all disease – *Egoity*

The <u>Cause</u> of all disease – *The egoic struggle to <u>become</u> happy.* In our egoity, we attempt to become happy via money, food, sex, and social life—and every other means. Therefore, since we are always trying to <u>become</u> happy, happiness is always out of our reach. Our <u>search</u> for happiness is thus our <u>confession</u> of <u>unhappiness</u>.

The <u>Cure</u> of all disease – Happiness, love, surrender to The Divine, the Beloved of the heart, via Spiritual study, chanting the Divine Names, constant worship of Real God, prayer to The Great One, meditation on the Spiritual Master—and engaging all the disciplines (*The BIG 7*) that support our attention on, and otherwise worship of, the Divine Reality.

Owning Disease

At Grand Medicine, we've heard patients refer to the disease process they suffered as, "My cancer," or "My diabetes," in some sense "owning" the disease. This as opposed to "the cancer," "the arthritis," or "the disease process in this body." It's almost as if they don't want to give it up, like it's their possession, and "you can't have it; it's mine!" In some cases, it's very much like that, people even getting a hit off of the disease, getting special attention from others while suffering the disease.

There is no intelligence in identifying with bodily disease any more than there is in identifying with the body itself—a temporary vehicle Given to our care while we grow in Real understanding and love of God. That's precisely what the body is—and an opportunity to awaken in intelligence and understanding for Real human growth.

Additionally, we've heard patients say they were "in excellent health—except for my malignant tumor." What?! How can you be in excellent health while suffering from a chronic degenerative disease? You cannot. Health is relative, and no one is in perfect health. The body always has some genetic tendency to weakness or a disorder or dysfunction of some kind.

The body is always going thru various changes, and there's always something "wrong" with it, some at least small irritation or imperfection. There's no sense in making these into a "problem" —just something to be responsible for—namely, *The BIG 7*, or right care of the body. Given the right care, the body does its own thing, which is self-organizing, self-correcting, and self-rightening. If you're always messing with it, how can you expect it to do this?

Bottom line: you can't perfect what is inherently imperfect (the physical body), but you <u>can</u> allow the body the opportunity to rightly manage itself (which it will), and you can ***transcend*** the imperfections of the body and everything else by turning to the Perfect (the Very Divine Reality).

Disease as Opportunity

Within Adidam—the Way Taught by Adi Da—is a guild of healers and healing that is guided by the Divine Wisdom of the Avatar relative to this area of life. It is called *Adidam Radical Healing,* as described in the book, <u>*Conductivity Healing*</u>. In Adidam Radical Healing, disease is not a negative or problematic condition. It can be seen as the result of egoity, our activity of separating ourselves from the All-Pervading Life Force.

Disease can thus be seen as an opportunity to inspect our lives, and happily relinquish the ego-driven life-negative habits that cause disease, that cause bodily systems to dysfunction and fail. We can take on more life-positive habits (***The BIG 7***). This makes a substantial part of the process of healing <u>our</u> responsibility, beyond that of the doctor, healer, or other external authority. Thus, we must learn these habits, these bodily responsibilities, so we can work with the body and the healer to bring the body back to some semblance of purification, balance, and well-being.

True healing requires a change of action—mental, emotional, and physical. The individual's participation is necessary in this process. The four principle faculties of body, emotion, mind, and breath are interdependent. A disturbance or frustration in one will tend to manifest as symptoms in the others—unless habits are consciously made, and thus the disease process transcended and released. Therefore, with the help of the true healer (rightly a teacher), we must inspect all of our psychophysical activities and discover the roots of the symptoms.

Food as Poison

As noted, the gross physical body is a <u>food</u> body. Most of the health problems we suffer at the gross physical level are due to the way we eat, the amount and quality of the food we choose to consume. In these current times, so much of it is tainted with chemicals and otherwise abused by heating and other degenerative processes. Except for the emotional, mental, and psychic (see below), this is where most physical disease comes from. What we eat!

It is estimated that, on average, approximately 73% of overall human disease is mental-emotional based; 17% is diet-involved; 10% involves other factors. "We are what we eat," the expression goes. It's true at some real level, and we feel guilty about what we eat and even the way we eat—because we know in our heart that the body is designed to eat pure raw natural and untainted food. The guilt is part of this mental-emotional disease factor.

Consider this: there are ways of eating and living that are life-positive and ways that are life-negative, each way with its own speed. How can you progress by taking one step forward and two steps backward? Smoke and drink, flesh (killed) food, sugar and other refined, processed and chemicalized foods, are life-negative. Cooked food is essentially life-negative—in the sense that it's not our natural diet or what otherwise brings natural life-energy to the body-mind.

If raw vegetal food is essentially our natural diet, how can we expect to know what the body is supposed to look like, feel like, and be healthy unless we eat that food? We've got to at least try this and see how it works for us. Do it for a few months and find out for yourself. If cooked and processed food has such a negative effect on our health, we must do the experiment with raw food—at least to learn the truth about this raw diet "theory."

The Bank of Disease
One darkly humorous way we can think of this disease-developing process is to picture a big bank where we people are making deposits. Every time we eat junk, we deposit at the Bank of Disease. It's quite a large bank— weirdly opulent, gigantic, and bizarrely impressive in its sheer size, but basically gross and truly ugly—inside and out. It's just that we don't want to see it as ugly—even tho we know it actually is ugly.

We want to think the big Bank of Disease is really OK, because…it's so much fun to go there. We've learned to enjoy hamburgers and French fries. We take our money for our burger and fries to the disease bank to "make a deposit." It's not even a Holiday, but we're eating turkey, chocolates, ice cream, and all manner of teased-up, chemicalized, and processed foods. More deposits in the Big Bank of Disease.

Little by little, unnoticed as it happens, our dark account at the big Bank of Disease builds up. Before long, maybe by our 30s, our huge "account" is showing the signs: Disease! Our doctor (teller) gives us our first diagnosis—but not to worry," he's got some drugs (bank fees) for us. We're finally starting to "cash in" on our deposits.

And, oh!, the tellers at the bank (the medical doctors) are delighted for us. We're paying their wages. We're paying for their son's education with our surgeries, and for their daughter's new Mercedes. Why shouldn't they be happy with us? And—whoa—the owners of the bank (the drug companies) are just gonna love us! All the drugs we're consuming and being injected with. We're sick, sick, sick, and they're rubbing their hands in glee!

You can take this analogy a lot further by adding lifestyle factors. We smoke a cigarette, and they shout, "Hoo-ray!" We stay up late drinking, and they jump up in the air, "Yahoo!" We develop cancer, and they have a major celebration! They hear, "ka-ching!" The pharmafia doesn't want to cure cancer. Cancer, to them, is not a disease. It's a business. Why would a good capitalist company want to end a multi-billion-dollar-a-year business?

Make no mistake about it: these folks are in the *disease* business, the *sickness* business, not the *health* business. They've been trained in disease and the treatment of symptoms. They tout health and their so-called "health maintenance organizations" (HMOs), but those are just places where they poison you with drugs, burn you with radiation, and cut you with surgical scalpels. Yes, there are times when one actually needs these treatments, but those times **should be rare**—far less often than they've ever been happening since Rockefeller "bought" medicine.

The disease business is a big and terrible business, with all its awful suffering. And it's all unnecessary. It's a bank. It's a money and power game, essentially. They are not there to make you healthy. The Medical Industrial Complex exists to treat your disease with their abusive, intrusive, back-door approaches. Get this straight. Be very clear about this. Yes, there are lots of sincere doctors, and especially nurses, who truly want you to be well. But the cards are stacked against anything like wellness. The whole system is rotten to the core.

If you want to be healthy, learn from those who are already healthy—those who actually practice The BIG 7. Stay away from the Bank of Disease. Avoid these people as much as you possibly can. If you need their tests, go and get the tests, and then get out of there. They are not going to teach you *The BIG 7.* They have no financial stake in teaching you genuine well-being, health self-responsibility. Eat pure foods and do the rest of *The BIG 7.* Learn this life-positive way and *do it*—at least for the sake of being free of disease...if not for God's sake!

The Role of Drugs in the Disease Process

Pharmaceutical drugs have a function in certain disease processes. They can be useful in situations of hi sudden and chronic pain, accidents, and injuries. They can help stabilize certain other circumstances, including (temporarily) chronic diseases, until balance can be restored via pure raw food and other natural methods. But, can you imagine a medical doctor telling you this?

Without combined natural therapies and patient cooperation, participation, and instruction in the health and disease process, drugs are at best mere temporary, palliative. They're OK for acute care, for temporary (palliative) relief of symptoms—and for little else. Other than accident and injury, for those who simply refuse to accept the discipline of adult life, there are drugs.

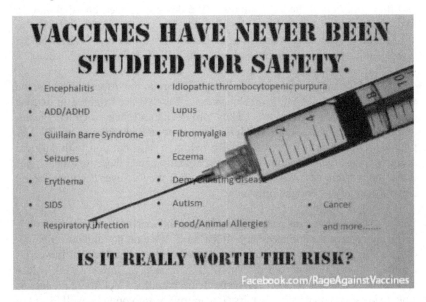

VACCINES HAVE NEVER BEEN STUDIED FOR SAFETY.

- Encephalitis
- ADD/ADHD
- Guillain Barre Syndrome
- Seizures
- Erythema
- SIDS
- Respiratory Infection

- Idiopathic thrombocytopenic purpura
- Lupus
- Fibromyalgia
- Eczema
- Demyelinating disease
- Autism
- Food/Animal Allergies

- Cancer
- and more......

IS IT REALLY WORTH THE RISK?

Facebook.com/RageAgainstVaccines

Terrible abuses have been heaped on the unsuspecting public the world over by unscrupulous pharmaceutical companies for over a hundred years (see the book, *The Hundred-Year LIE*; www.hundredyearlie.com; also the book, *Medical Armageddon*). To learn even a small part of this story leads any sane person to understand that Big Pharma's behavior is (or should be considered) nothing short of criminal. Vaccination is but one example.

Of course, we in the USA are supposed to have various protections against drug and medical abuses, against harmful substances, procedures, and prescriptions. The Food and Drug Administration (FDA), for example. The history of that institution is one of increasing scandals, of collusion with drug company interests, of being bot and sold by the pharmafia. Big Pharma lobbyists have instigated legislation protecting themselves from the harm their vaccines continually cause to innocent infants, children, and adults. This is patently evil.

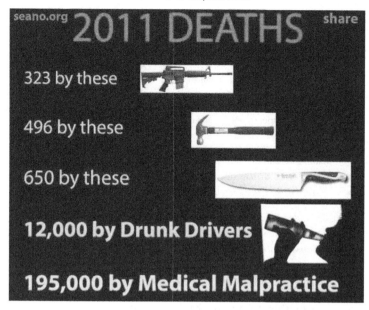

During the latter half of the 20th Century, with citizens dying of lung cancer, a movement finally developed against the abuses of tobacco companies, their TV and other public advertising, and smoking in public places. Tobacco, cannabis, peyote, and other such substances, were used in sacred ceremonies by Native Americans. Obviously, it's stupid to use these substances otherwise. The sins of the tobacco companies have been documented elsewhere. But, drug company policies and activities have been far worse.

Whole populations have been poisoned by legally required and government-sanctioned mass vaccination—paid for by our tax dollars. Heretofore unknown diseases have developed by these modern "miracle drugs." There will come a time when this whole misuse of medicine, this domination by drug-controlled allopathic, will be looked upon as a monstrously immoral chapter in human history.

At some future time, traditional and otherwise natural therapies will be combined with intelligent use of technology—including certain drug-type medicines—so that Hippocrates' original medical admonition to "first, do no harm," will once again be the watchword of all healers.

The Leading Health Risk Factors Globally

- *Negative-reactive emotions (the NREs)* (stress from fear, sorrow, anger, sadness, depression, unhappiness—i.e., **egoity**)
- *Dietary insult / nutritional deficiencies* (underweight, starvation, iron / other anemias, and various other disorders and diseases related to inadequate supply of nutrients; obesity and other diseases and disorders related to abuse of diet)
- *Poor hygiene* (poor sanitation, polluted water, unsafe sex, inadequate bathing / cleansing / food prep)
- *Substance abuse* (tobacco, alcohol, drugs—OTC, street, prescription—etc.)
- *Environmental factors* (indoor smoke from solid fuels and poor ventilation; other toxic physical environs; ugly human-made or otherwise depressing & debilitating mental, emotional and physical environments)
- *Doctor-caused* (iatrogenic) and/or *hospital-caused* (nosocomial) *disease & death* (kill hundreds of thousands yearly)

Together, these account for more than 97% of all deaths worldwide.

The Mental-Emotional Component

Psychologists tell us that *negative-reactive emotions underlie some 73% of all disease*. Of course, accidental injury, war casualties (mostly of innocents), or chance irradiation are not emotion-caused. But, our attitudes and reactions to the various events of life are the biggest factors in our disease. We at Grand Medicine have certainly seen this proven clinically. Many others have, too.

After careful study of the subject, J. I. Rodale, the progenitor of Rodale publications, wrote a series of articles entitled, "*Happy People Don't Get Cancer*." So, happiness is a real factor in health. And <u>lack of happiness</u> is a factor in *disease*—the biggest factor. Disease is the result of diet abuse and the other lifestyle factors of wrong use of rest, exercise, environments, hygiene, occupation, and the Divine—<u>combined with</u> negative-reactive emotions. *Disease is the wrong practice of life.*

BTW, we are always being led to believe that we, as individuals, are the cause of all our "problems," and therefore the only way out is for us, as individuals, to get it together and find our own private solutions. WRONG! While we all must be individually responsible for our lives, there are cultural, political and economic reasons for our problems. We eat junk food because it is cheaper than pure organic food and gives us a little bit of enjoyment in the midst of our depressing and frustrating struggle to survive—while our rich corporate "owners" rob us of our freedoms.

It all begins with this feeling of separation, the activity of the ego. Attempting to eliminate this feeling and get back to the sense of One-ness, of basic native happiness, we get into all kinds of difficulty. <u>Seeking</u> happiness is not <u>practicing</u> happiness. We are always "going to find happiness"…someday. We don't have it now, and we know it, and that's "the problem." Not only can we *practice* Happiness individually, but we can gather in small groups, work together, share our resources, and do much more than merely survive (see Appendix G).

The TWO FRONTS of our Problems

(1) **egoity**, which is the *source* of all our problems, real or imagined

(2) **sociocultural**, as main *cause*: living in a "crazy random" culture within a declining civilization

> In a Wisdom Culture—which we now desperately need—egoity would be identified and understood by everyone, worldwide, in the midst of Sacred practices as our foundation of life.

As with sex, food is a handy way to stimulate temporary small-"h" happiness in the midst of our frustrations. We tend to eat these teased-up, unwholesome, sugary, salty, cooked, chemicalized, processed, degenerated food because…

(1) we see it on TV; others all around us eat this way

(2) it's cheaper, less expensive than organic natural food

(3) our jaded taste buds say it's tastier than the purer, more wholesome foods

(4) it tends to be easier to prepare, quicker, more convenient—often with no prep time at all

(5) we are taught, trained, propagandized by our crazy random culture, to eat this way from birth

(6) of feelings of hopelessness, despair, and frustration under corporate and government tyranny

So, when we first try to eat more of the wholesome raw natural food, we don't like it. We don't want it—because it doesn't taste as good as the crap. We need to spend some time getting used to what is truly good for us—and what always has been our real food. We need to "phase in," to get into it a little at a time—but for real.

How, then, do we handle the emotional part of us? Mentally, we can easily agree on the importance of staying positive about life. But, emotional issues can subvert our best mental intentions. The emotional is deeper than the conceptual mind. For one, at least some **mental-emotional support** of like-minded or otherwise sympathetic others is critical. Talk with others, do the Devotional Prayer of Changes (see Appendix G), and otherwise reach out and find these people. You don't have to take this all on yourself. We need each other.

For another, by consistently granting as much of our attention as we can to What is Higher in life, the emotional and everything else is transcended. Our Grace-receiving "cup" is widened, enlarged. And then, to whatever degree possible, there is maintaining positive emotions such as gratitude, joy, compassion, and love. This way, the immune system is greatly boosted against disease, and the emotional body altogether is strengthened.

There is much in this Earth realm life to disillusion us—the death and suffering of loved ones, the frustration of our plans, and the wars, starvation, lack of cooperation among governments, corruption, and so on. There is strife within the human family, even tho we're clearly all one family, one race—the Human Race. But, the Divine is here.

We have a lot to be grateful for—even tho our governments only rubber-stamp the continuous wars we all suffer (and finance and pay for with the lives of our young men and women) for the benefit of the Surveillance-Military-Industrial Complex that calls their tune. There are so many people around the world who can't afford a power blender or juicer, who have no access to much in the way of solid food—much less pure raw liquids.

The Divine, plus working together and cooperating with each other (see the book, _Not-Two Is Peace_), is our "way out" of this suffering. Adi Da suggests that we can be *"positively disillusioned"* with the crazy part of the world, being positive in worldly life while tolerating our petty differences, cooperating, and relying on and having faith in the Beloved Divine. This turns everything into loving, intelligent, compassionate, and most positive living. We can do this.

Eight Principle Health Influences

Consider how these eight items impact the health of the body-mind, or bodily being. The mental and emotional aspects are subsumed within items #2, 5 & 6. We estimate that, in the average person, they each significantly influence human health to the following degrees:

- *Diet* = 37%
- *Spiritual Practice* = 18%
- *Rest* = 18%
- *Exercise* = 9%
- *Occupation* = 8%
- *Environments* = 4%
- *Hygiene* = 3%
- *Psychic / Karmic / Cosmic* = 3%

Our Dance of Death Ritual

We learn to stay up late at night playing cards, watching TV (it's such junk, now, that it's hard to imagine people still watch it), working on various projects of business or entertainment, trying desperately to be fulfilled, trying to stimulate fulfillment, happiness. We see others smoke, and we want to look good and be accepted into the "in" crowd, so we smoke. We see our parents drinking alcohol, so we drink. We try different drugs, noticing that at some level, they take us out of our minds and into some pleasurably stimulating place—hopefully even permanently.

But after years of smoke and drink, late hours, and diet insult, the body starts to show symptoms. We go to the doctor, who gives us drugs against the symptoms. We feel better. We go on with our abusive lifestyle until more and worse symptoms appear. This cycle persists over time, with more drugs that themselves cause symptoms—for which still more drugs are given. The symptoms worsen until the doctor informs us we have a chronic degenerative disease, organs need to be removed, and other organs are malfunctioning.

Then, sometime after the pain has been "managed" by drugs, we learn that we have cancer and are given a death sentence: 6 months to live. The doctor wants to irradiate us and give us more drugs—"chemotherapy," the "cure that kills"—after the surgery. So, it's the usual drug, burn and cut. Let's say we don't like this prognosis, so we seek out the services of a Natural Health practitioner.

We must understand that it took a while to get ourselves into this mess, so it's going to take a while to get out of it. It's not magic. Unless it's already too late, our only real shot is (essentially) Natural Health therapies. In most instances, the GLD can play a major role in recovery—IF recovery is to occur.

Some very revealing studies on DNA were done at *Heart Math Institute* by quantum biologist Dr. Vladimir Poponin, and reported by Gregg Braden, Ph.D. These studies have shown that when we practice feeling such positive emotions as joy, love, gratitude, and compassion, our immune system gets a gigantic boost—by a factor of up to 300,000! This is immune protection at a whole other level. It can prevent all manner of infectious processes, and propel us beyond whatever negative disorder is preventing the immune from getting the upper hand.

A famous example of the power of mind and emotions over bodily illness is the story of the former editor of *The Saturday Review*, Norman Cousins. As recounted in the *New England Journal of Medicine*, and in his subsequent book, *Anatomy of an Illness*, Cousins apparently healed himself of medically diagnosed ankylosing spondylitis in 1964 by reading humorous books and watching comedy movies. Cousins concluded that 95% of diseases can be eliminated by mind energy. He apparently laffed his way to health, beating the disease and bewildering his doctors! Check out the documentary, *Doctored*.

The Disease Personality

There appear to be certain personality traits and otherwise personal characteristics present in people who are (1) susceptible to and who consequently develop chronic degenerative diseases, and (2) those who also have developed diseases but are willing to make changes and take responsibility for their disease—and therefore are more likely to get well.

You have the "Disease Personality" if you...

- Worry for others
- Are people pleasers
- Tend to suffer in silence
- Tend to carry the burdens of others
- Have an extreme need for approval
- Have difficulty expressing emotions
- Are reluctant to accept help from others
- Are opinionated; have an inflexible attitude
- Lack of closeness with one or both parents
- Derive their worth from being a caretaker
- Harbor long-suppressed negative emotions
- React negatively to stress / traumatic events
- Feel great loneliness and deprived of affection
- Tend to internalize problems, care, & conflicts
- Need professional help to make major changes
- Find it very difficult to make diet/lifestyle changes

You are Ready to be Healthy to the degree that you demonstrate the following...

- Have a positive attitude
- Are accepting of Divine Help
- Want to be health unexploitable
- Are willing to take charge of your health
- Have confidence & faith in your course of action
- Learn to say No! to others laying burdens on you
- Actually make the needed diet and lifestyle changes
- Accept responsibility for how your disease developed
- Are willing to work to reverse a self-destructive lifestyle
- Are willing to be accountable to a trusted health professional
- Understand that mind & emotions powerfully affect immunity
- Are willing to participate in your general and specific wellness
- Are grateful to have a plan of pure diet and life-positive lifestyle
- Reject that conventional medicine is your only hope for survival
- Accept radiant health as your birthright & are willing to work for it
- Are skeptical of conventional medical approaches to disease treatment
- Reject the prevailing concept that death from your disease is inevitable
- Are interested in Spiritual growth & developing your relationship with God
- Learn as much as possible about all your treatment options and your disease
- Choose a healthy course and apply it with dedication, discipline & common sense

---

Much of disease is emotional and held deep beneath the surface. Counseling is almost always needed to reach these emotional depths—and this should be done along with the GLD and other therapies, whether conventional or alternative or both. This is part of the real nature of healing, which is both scientific and artful. Compassion and love are part of the practice of the true healer, who looks at the healee as a whole person. These qualities are beyond the scope of common scientific studies, and also why the current system of medicine is in such need of repair.

One excellent reference on emotional and Oedipal healing (early life relationships with parents) is Richard Silk. We met Richard many years ago in Northern California and were impressed with his work right from the start. His fees are reasonable, and he can work with you at a distance. His comlinks: richardsilk@newfamilynetwork.com; h/w707-928-6932; c707-227-4903.

Allergies

If you wonder about allergy, about what foods you may be allergic to, you may wish to test by checking your pulse after drinking the juice, smoothie, or nut or seed liquid. If your pulse races, it's likely you are allergic to the food item or to a specific food within a mix. Keep testing, learn what it is, and temporarily eliminate this item as soon as you find it. Eventually, on your GLD, your small intestine—which is the food allergy center of your body—will be cleaned out, and the allergies will diminish and may even disappear entirely.

Levels of Understanding Disease

There is *treatment* (palliative, therapy, or remedy) and then there is *cure*, or resolution. There is addressing *symptoms* (which is essentially what is done in Allopathic medicine), and there is addressing *cause* (basically the approach of Naturopathic medicine). Deeper than symptoms is <u>cause</u>. Deeper than cause is <u>source</u>. Symptoms arise from cause, and cause arises from source. Disease is the wrong practice of life.

In ignorance, symptoms arise from life-negative habits. Life-negative habits (including diet insult) are the <u>cause</u> of disease. Egoity is the <u>source</u> of disease. Ignorance is cured by knowledge, and knowledge is cured by wisdom (which is Love—the Truth of Happiness). Allopathic is about the treatment of *symptoms*. Naturopathic is about the treatment of *cause* and bringing a cure. Adidam Radical Healing is about health beyond cure (Wisdom).

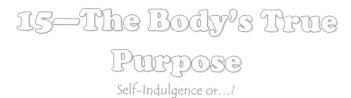

15—The Body's True Purpose

Self-Indulgence or...?

The gross physical body is a Gift to us from the Divine, and, as such, an opportunity to grow in Real Understanding, in Real human terms. It is not an excuse for self-fulfillment nor a means of pleasurizing ourselves into oblivion. Of course, it's fine to have fun, but with consciousness, not stupidly. The body is an opportunity to Awaken to the Great Happiness of the Heart, the Permanent capital "H" Happiness of the Sacred One. This Awakening is Accomplished thru hard (albeit happy) work, disciplining the body-mind, and by Divine Grace.

What we do with the body is truly our choice. For the most part, in these so-called "Dark Times" predicted by all the Great religions, where egoic self-interest dominates virtually every culture on Earth, and where the Divine, is on a "back burner" (if considered important at all), we tend to abuse the body variously. We tend to use it for self-pleasuring, for even absolute self-fulfillment (as if that were actually possible)—even to the point of death.

We can do something else, something different, something better and more intelligent. We can show our respect for the body. We can show our thanks to The Beloved Transcendental Reality for the bodily Gift, for this opportunity to transcend our "selves" (the body-mind). We can do this by learning about the care of the body, now that we know its primary function. We can notice how, as egos, we tend to abuse money, food, sex, and all kinds of life activities in a vain attempt to *become* happy—instead of simply being Happy, practicing Happiness.

Face it, any happiness that we can gain we will necessarily lose, at least when the body dies—whereas, the True Happiness that every heart desires is the Eternal, Which we intuit at the heart. The body can be a vehicle for Awakening to this Happiness. It's mainly a matter of caring for it properly and using our Divine Resort.

Notice how the body feels when it's young and healthy. Young, we tend to think we will live forever as the body. The great English poet, Wordsworth, wrote, *"A simple child, that lightly draws its breath, and feels its life in every limb, what should it know of death?"*

Infants and children are "life signs" in the sense that they have this attitude or sense of Eternity. Their energies are clean, flower-like. The vital force or etheric energy propels them into life. They have little sense of death.

They don't worry because those mental functions haven't developed in them yet. However, they can get sick—mainly, depending on how we treat them, what we *feed* them, and how well we love them and bring them intimacy.

When a little older, we start to feel the stresses of life. We notice the frustration inherent in being alive in a body. There is culture, civilization, business, livelihood, career, relationships, goals, and the institutions of marriage and family. We learn about death. Eventually, we notice how the world isn't designed to please us or satisfy our every whim. This is frustrating. We aren't getting happy. We struggle to remedy this. More frustration.

Three times a day, we try to eat our way to happiness, but that isn't working, either. No matter how good the meal, how jaded our tastes, or how capable we are of getting whatever kind of food we want, food still never makes us finally Happy. This includes the "health nut," who thinks he is superior to others by eating all raw food. He thinks a sandwich will enlighten him! But, that just ain't gonna happen.

Notice how, after a great and delicious meal of fine rich food, you at first just feel full, gratified by the delectable tastes. Then, there are the hours and days that follow, the irritation, pain, and suffering from overeating, from indulgence in food that serves not the health of the body but the taste of the tongue. So, food isn't going to do it for us. There is merely a right way to eat, and that has to be learned.

Sex is the same. It can be good, even excellent, but no matter how good or how many times we do it, it never really gets us to that final capital "H" Happiness. And, mind you, it's only the capital "H" Happiness that will finally satisfy our heart. Therefore, there's just a right way to use the body. The childish approach is to do whatever you *can*. The adolescent approach is to do whatever you *want*. But the adult approach is to do what you *need* to do to bring real balance and equanimity to the body-mind.

SUMMARIZING: Why Are We Here?

In a brilliant Talk called, "*Submission To The Self*" (available at www.Adidam.org), Avatar Adi Da Samraj Describes in exquisite detail the age-old reason why human embodiment is traditionally so highly valued: **purification!** The body provides us the perfect vehicle to move beyond the two karmic structures (brain-mind and deeper or higher mind) to enable us— via the Grace of (and in the relationship with) the Spiritual Master—to transcend everything in Divine Enlightenment or Awakening.

In general, here are the crucial qualities in this sequence of events:

- Human birth
- Finding and making the connection with the Spiritual Master

- Recognizing that this Earth-realm is currently (has been and continues to be) dominated by the activities of the brain-mind—and, as such, life in this realm is essentially painful, suffering
- Recognizing that the main function of the brain-mind is to block the activities of higher-mind, the deeper personality, commonly and culturally referred to as the sub-conscious mind
- Altho a large part of the brain-mind (which involve higher-mind functions) is not being used, that part is all about mechanical functions, psychism, mysticism, and is not about Divine Awakening
- Recognizing that altho higher-mind and its activities are the goal of some esoteric religions, it is only more karma, just as with the brain-mind—and, as such, it only represents more to be transcended; it is therefore better bypassed in and via the relationship with the Spiritual Master
- Since both body and mind are to be transcended, our best activity is the focus of attention on the Spiritual Master (the incarnated Divine Person of Love) as The Awakener

We can see, then, that our true purpose of life, of being born into this Earth realm, is Divine Enlightenment, God-Realization. The ego, while it would like to think so, cannot accomplish this Awakening. It can only happen by the Grace of, and in the Relationship with, the Spiritual Master—the most profound relationship in life.

It is in this greatest of all relationships that our purpose in life occurs. The devotee (or disciple) turns to Him and He does the rest. It is all about purification. Life represented by higher mind is only a distraction. And at the level of the body and brain mind, it is also about purification.

This is where the GLD comes in. In some sense, it is relatively homely by comparison with Real Spiritual practice, yes, but it is necessary **purification**, nevertheless. This **purification** prepares the functions and energies of the body-mind for Real Spiritual practice. Without such **purification**, the body-mind vehicle cannot receive the Grace needed for our true purpose: Divine Awakening.

16—The Food Sheath

The Body's Right First Treatment involves Disease States

In His book, **_Santosha Adidam_**, Adi Da describes the gross physical body as a "food body":

> "*The quality and quantity of food taken in largely or very basically determines the state and desire and action of the physical body and the sense-mind. If food-taking is intelligently minimized, and if the food selected is both pure and purifying, then the physical body and even the entire emotional dimension of the being, and the total mind, passes through a spontaneous natural cycle that shows progressive signs of purification, rebalancing, and rejuvenation. Therefore, if food-taking is controlled, the physical body itself (including its desires and activities) becomes rather easily or simply controllable.*"

That's a pretty big statement. And mind: you're not gonna hear this thru the MSM (no commercial potential)! The statement is easy to prove. Eat six candy bars for breakfast and notice how you feel! Also notice how such a meal influences your mind. The cells of the body are genetically programmed to receive only pure raw ripe untreated fruits, veggies, nuts, and seeds as food.

Yes, we can eat some cooked foods and animal products and still remain essentially healthy. But our diet should rightly be at least mostly raw but preferably all raw <u>produce</u>—in other words, basically vegetarian as found directly in Nature.

Healers take note: Since the gross physical body is essentially a food body, the <u>first treatment</u> for *any* disease of the gross physical body is and rightly should be a <u>food</u> treatment! (Imagine this principle being taught in medical schools and practiced by the physicians of the world! Hospital visits, deaths, and injuries from medical mistakes, and overall costs of diseases, disorders, and so-called "health care" would plunge dramatically!)

The Battle of the Diets

There are so many diets out there to choose among, some still going, some gone. Why should we do the GLD over any of the others? There's Jenny Craig©, Weight Watchers©, Paleo Diet©, Keto Diet©, Mediterranean Diet©, the Zone Diet©, and so on and on. They seem to work for some, but not others. And of those they "work" for, how many stay with it indefinitely—much less are healthy while on it? Look at the kinds of food some of them recommend, foods with their long list of chemicals or processed foods. How can one be healthy on that junk?

Yes, you can lose weight by counting calories, but does calorie restriction alone bring health? Can you lose weight and be healthy at the same time? Not by their methods, you can't. It's not that they have bad intentions. They're just playing to the crowd: most people want to continue to eat whatever they like best, what they're most familiar with, most enjoy, and that bring them the most pleasure: the popular processed, chemicalized junk.

Food is so important to us because (1) it's necessary to health, (2) most of us are obsessed with it, and (3) it is an immediate source of pleasure, of gratification. We'll try any number of diets in order to look good, feel good, be healthy, lose weight, gain longevity, and so on—especially those that promise to allow us to enjoy our favorite dishes and continue to indulge our food passions, habits, and tendencies.

The food industry is the largest in the world—bigger than drugs, bigger than oil, bigger than anything else. Because people have to eat. The industry plays to this—knowing we'll buy what sounds best to us, the most fun to eat, the most convenient, the least expensive, the most delicious, the sexiest!

But, knowing that diet has to do with health, and that what we like is not necessarily good for us, we're complicated and problematic about food. We're not completely satisfied with what we eat or the way we eat, so we resort to "dieting"—meaning food restriction. And, the bad word, the "D" word: discipline!

Some people find their way to vegetarianism. This is intelligent for many reasons. It takes enormous amounts of land to feed cattle to make steaks and hamburgers. Whole forests need to be cut down to create pastureland for cattle—whereas, if that land were put into food directly for human consumption, far more people would be fed.

And then, there's the killing of the animals. Nice! These are sentient, sensitive creatures who want to live, have families, and enjoy life—just like us. Plants have a different consciousness. Not that plants want to die; they just don't feel the sense of separate consciousness that the so-called higher animals do. In any case, something has to be sacrificed for us to eat. Plants or animals of some kind. We kill many microscopic creatures in the very acts of breathing and bathing. Sacrifice is the basic law of life. Sacrifice is…love!

So, we have to kill something at the gross physical in order to eat and survive. Something has to die for us humans to live. It's just a matter of us being intelligent and humane in how we go about this killing, this harvesting of life. If you take the time to investigate how these non-humans—the pigs, chickens, and cattle—are kept penned up (often in despicably small enclosures), drugged, then inhumanely slaughtered, you'd become a vegan on the spot!—i.e., if you have any humanity left, any moral sensitivity left, after living in this current ego-mad culture. Therefore, for an infinite number of reasons, it's better to harvest plants than animals!

Vegans and the GLD

Some of us become even more refined with our diets, avoiding not only flesh but dairy—the products of animals. We become "vegans"—even all-raw vegans (raw food only). This is good for essential physical health. One big difference between raw dieting and the GLD is the fact it takes a lot of energy to chew all that raw food when eaten whole. It can be hard on the teeth—especially compared to the GLD. Now, how to get around that?

The GLD involves all raw or mostly raw foods, but liquefied. So, one can be a vegan and use the GLD selectively. The liquefying of these raw foods makes a very big difference in health. *Less energy* is expended in taking liquids—in chewing, digesting, absorbing and assimilating them, and even in eliminating their waste products. This means far *more energy* freed up for purification—which means getting healthier faster.

The Health Nut—Being Silly with Food

We've all met them. They're usually thin, even skinny. You know, the ones with the orange skin from drinking a gallon of carrot juice daily. They think they're healthy, but they're really not. Maybe a little healthier than the average. They are like the 75-year-old same-teeth-I-had-when-I-was-15 idiot! They may even have freed themselves from most illness—physical illness. They still have a problem: themselves! It's their attitude. They have this attitude of being superior to the rest of us because they eat "superior food" (all raw).

What the health nut doesn't understand is that food will never make us Happy. Physically healthy, perhaps, but never finally heart-deep capital "H" Happy. That's not the purpose of food, so food shouldn't be burdened with that responsibility. *A sandwich will never Enlighten us!* (—Adi Da Samraj) There is simply a right way to eat: consciously and intelligently, not requiring food to do more than provide basic psychophysical health.

Our best understanding suggests that the correct percentages of raw food in each category should be approximately:

—45% raw greens, especially including green leafy veggies
—35% raw ripe fruits
—20% raw nuts and seeds

Dietary Factors Influencing Health

In modern times, several qualities or factors influence health thru diet at the gross physical level. Among these are the following, including the estimated percentage of the average overall influence or difference each item makes on health:

- *Praying over food* vs. forgetting the Divine at meals – 100%; prayer positively affects <u>all levels</u> of being
- *Raw* vs. cooked – 93% difference in significant nutrient presence and availability
- *Natural* vs. non-natural / GMO – 86% difference involving relative help or damage to bodily systems
- *Soil quality* – 78% difference in nutrient presence and bioavailability
- *Pure unadulterated* vs. food processing chemicals added – 71% difference on average
- *Radiation exposure* (incl. microwave) – 67% average damage differential
- *Pleasant environment* vs. hostile, noisome, ugly, etc. – 66% difference in effective processing by the body
- *Vine/tree-ripened* vs. picked early – 59% nutrient availability difference
- *Equanimity while eating* vs. eating under emotional stress – 53% difference in effective food processing
- *Local grown* vs. shipped in from afar – 36% difference; many factors are involved in location/transfer
- *Blended with cold or room temp water* vs. with hot water – 7% loss of nutrients with hot water
- *Eaten whole* vs. blended – 6% loss of nutrients on average from the blending process itself
- *Drunk After Juicing/Blending vs. Refrigerated* – % nutrient loss if refrigerated = average 20% per day

<u>Therefore</u>, based on the above, *the best foods for optimum health are* those that are (1) prayed over, (2) raw, (3) natural / non GMO, (4) grown in pure mineral-rich composted soil, (5) unadulterated, (6) un-radiated, (7) taken in pleasant environments, (8) vine/tree-ripened, (9) eaten while content, (10) locally grown, (11) blended at room temperatures or with cold water, (12) preferably eaten whole, and (13) if blended or juiced, drunk immediately after preparation.

Nutrient Availability in Liquids

In certain health circles, it is a well-known and established fact that *nutrient availability* is greater in foods that are liquefied than in those taken whole. Of course, softer natural foods, including bananas, don't need to be liquefied to be better digested (for their nutrient availability). It's also true, of course, that cooking breaks down the cell walls of food, thus making certain nutrients more available that would not be digestible if taken in the raw state.

Potatoes and yams are an example of this. However, the cooking process also destroys many, most, or even all nutrients, depending on the type of food, the length of time cooked, and the cooking process employed. In some cases, the cooking process renders certain nutrients—like some proteins—into poisons. On this basis alone, it's prudent to make at least most of one's diet raw natural.

Calories, Registered Dietitians and Nutritionists

We at GranMed have been called to hospitals to visit relatives of patients dying of cancer. In comes the food tray—with Salisbury steak, ice cream, and Jell-O! Now, what could possibly be the rationale for serving such a meal to someone with cancer? Or to anyone else, for that matter? It surely cannot be to help them be healthier. Maybe as a gesture to the tastes and pleasures of one who is dying anyway? You don't feed this kind of food to someone in need of the highest quality of nutrition. Not if you want to help them survive in any healthful way. Not if you know anything of any importance about food.

The registered dietitian (RD) has been the darling of the medical industry. As such, many are seen haunting the halls of hospitals. RDs, in general, don't know shit about diet! Nothing of real importance. They can tell you the RDA's of vitamins, describe the FDA food pyramid, and list the exact calorie count of any food—as if any of that were important. They trump MDs when it comes to what hospital patients eat. Could it be that the drug companies thrill at these diets that serve to keep people sick—and thus keep them coming to hospitals, bringing in more profits?

Hospitals are hotbeds of germs of every nature. People get well there despite the germs and the food, more because of the loving care of the nurses. The very fact that people get well in hospitals is more a testament to the resilience of the human body than to any efforts on the part of these Big Pharma-operated sick houses. The old-fashioned nutritionists know about food. They know that raw foods heal. They know that there is a time to avoid solid foods to allow the body to heal itself. It's called "fasting," a word seldom heard in hospitals.

Registered dietitians are taught to tow the party line, kowtow to people's tastes, go along with the so-called need for animal products and grains. Taking pure foods on a hi-raw diet, most people can ignore calories completely. Those who don't, the fast metabolizers and thin-body types, need only focus on (1) eating more often, and (2) nuts and seeds—how to get these into the body in productive ways. Generally speaking, calories are not a significant marker or indicator of the healthful value of food. There are many so-called "foods" these days, substances that are passed off as foods—hi-cal and lo-nutrition, packaged, processed, GMO, etc., all recommended by dietitians.

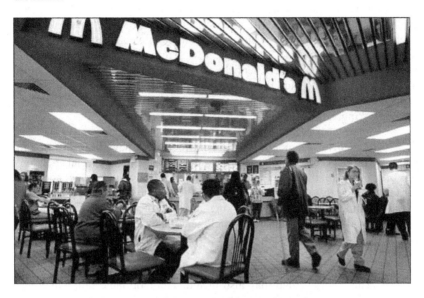

To be fair, there are some dietitians who seem to be coming around to understanding the importance of pure foods and the avoidance of junk food—including the junk food sold in hospitals. However, as of this writing (September 2019), fully 23 states are listed as having McDonald's©, Chick-fil-A©, or Wendy's© fast food service facilities in their hospitals.

Can you believe this? Note the white coats. At Mickey Dee's, it's just business as usual. Hey, wherever we can get a foot in the door—even if it's places of wellness. Hell, if they could set up a counter in churches, you bet your sweet ass they would!

Levels of Dietary Purity
Before Human History, there was only "natural" food. No such thing as "process-tainted" food existed. Yes, there was vegetal food that was unripe or spoiled, and animal food that was diseased, rotten or decayed. Taking these simple precautions of appearance and smell, we could rather easily select pure foods.

Perhaps around 140,000 years ago or so, some character kicked a potato into a fire and noticed that it tasted OK. Cooked food eventually became a staple—perhaps 70,000 years ago. The current Civilization (which began about 11,000 years ago) brought with it the influences of contamination by contact with various metals (lead, gold, silver, iron, copper, etc.) and—eventually—the chemicals of food processing. So that now we can arbitrarily distinguish various levels of dietary toxicity as well as purity.

Lowest Quality Foods

If we consider whatever is taken into the body orally as "food," we can list, at the lowest level, such items as alcoholic beverages, smoke, and street and pharma drugs. We can add the commercial cola beverages, refined food products ("Twinkies®," "Ding-Dongs®," refined sugar and refined flour products, etc.), and the other chemicalized "triumphs" of the food processing industry. We can also add the various chemicals used to preserve, add shelf life, give the desired color, alter the taste, stabilize, hold ingredients together, prevent caking, and so on.

Genetically engineered foods and foods that have been exposed to the waste products of the atomic energy industry come in for special attention. It is only by a rare stretch of the imagination (and almost utter lack of common sense and integrity) that such concepts can be conceived by the human mind to be healthful: by tricking, working against, or improving on Nature. Nature's work can be enhanced by intelligent action (as thru composting and adding ground glacial rock), and even (ultimately) transcended, but not improved by phony science.

This lowest group may also include common table salt, which has been chemicalized and heated to the point of being poisonous. Pesticide-contaminated food can also be included here. And then there are the fried foods, with their super-heated fats and oils, and the hydrogenated and partially hydrogenated fats and oils, which coat the linings of arteries and give an impossible task to the liver and gallbladder.

Leave it to the morally bankrupt psychopaths working in the Big Food industry, and the poor suffering factory workers there who are just happy to have a paying job, to give us ever new versions of non-foods designed to get us hooked and have the illusion of ecstasy with every bite. Whatever brings in more profits and titillates the shareholders. And if people get sick on their products and they get sued, well, it's just part of business operating expenses.

Increasing Levels of Quality

Next higher on our list could be ordinary bread foods, made from grains. *Grains are not needed in human nutrition*—and we're talking about the grain-based diets of Asia, Africa, and the Indian Sub-Continent. Moreover, as processed grain (flour), bread foods, including (for some) their gluten, have caused much harm to human health. They can be prepared in many tasty ways, but taken on any regular basis, they can hurt you. As starchy foods, bread foods and grains encourage pancreas metabolism dysfunction (the so-called hypoglycemia and diabetes disorders).

The caffeinated beverages, foods grown in chemical fertilizers, and even animal products that have been variously processed (meats containing sodium nitrates and nitrites, etc., and milk that has been pasteurized, "ultra-pasteurized," etc.) can all be listed here. Taking it to the next higher level, we can go to specific cooked food preparations, like soy products (many or most of which are GMO these days), which have come under fire recently as not only unneeded but also harmful for various reasons. Fermented soy is a different story.

Next up on the scale of somewhat higher quality food products are the whole-grain sprouted flourless breads, the fresh-frozen and freeze-dried food products, the natural-style snack crackers and rice cakes, certain naturally-sweetened granola bars and such, perhaps raw unsalted butter, plain yogurt, certain soured foods (natural pickles and sauerkraut without the chemical preservatives), steamed, cooked and baked veggies (potatoes, yams, squash), honey, rice syrup and other natural-style sweeteners (especially coconut sugar and date sugar), and perhaps some of the flake cereals and granolas. Various fermented foods are good, like natural sauerkraut.

Hi-Quality Foods

At the highest level, we have the fresh raw ripe locally-grown in-season unsprayed naturally fertilized natural fruits and veggies, nuts and seeds, sprouts, and grasses (wheatgrass, barley grass, and the like—and the juice of these). We can include unsulphured, unsprayed, and otherwise untainted sun-dried and home-food-drier-dried fruits and vegetables and dried vegetables, some of which may have subsequently been powdered.

Sprouted grains and seeds are here, as are pure waters. This food group is the smallest and simplest. Raw natural coconut sugar—which tastes great and is exploding in popularity—can be included, as well as Celtic and Himalaya salt. Pure food may cost more at market these days, but pay the money! Do whatever it takes to get it. Grow it, if you can. It becomes the body. You'll be healthy and wind up spending far less in the long run.

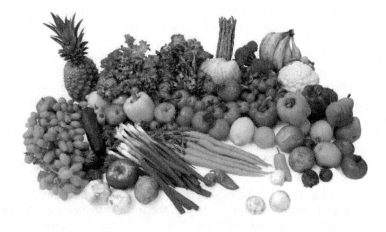

Water itself is a whole other issue: how to get genuinely pure water these days. We must resort, in most cases, to filtering it by various means. In prior times, we simply took the water from streams that bubbled over the rocks in the sunlite—the purest of all. Where is that water now? Where are those pure streams—now that we all need them? Altho a few streams on Earth may appear to be pure, we humans have, to one or another degree, polluted them all.

Back in the 1960s, we used to hear this silly argument about drinking only "room-temperature" water—as if such were available to us thru-out our history as humans. The water in Earth's streams and rivers is almost uniformly cold. So much for that argument. Meanwhile, several well-filtered waters are good, but steam-distilled and placed in the sun is best. (See Chapter 36, "Water," for further information.)

Eventually, we will get back into growing only pure foods. Many of us will be creating backyard natural gardens, like the "Victory Gardens" of WWII. We must come full-circle in this sense, getting back to purity. Yes, we're going to lose a small amount of nutrition by liquefying foods on the GLD. But the tradeoff is well worth it for the enormous number of benefits gained.

The Effect of Diet on Our Physical Appearance
Various factors affect our physical appearance in life, the way our face, skin, and body look altogether. In general, these factors include genetics and (mostly) environment. On the genetics side, we can inherit various levels of what is considered natural beauty. Toward the other end, we can also inherit debilities and tendencies that require medical and cultural help.

On the environment side, we can be fortunate to have no serious accidents, smoke exposure, extreme weather exposure, prolonged stress, poverty, or other such events that cause "negative" structural or cosmetic changes in our appearance. Then, there are the factors that are—in general, at least in Western countries—more under our control: our thots, feelings, lack of social / community support, constant frustration, and actions with food and lifestyle.

Little imagination is needed to sense the quality and amount of food all these people we see around us are eating. Their bodies are fat, exaggerated, cartoon-like. Forget imagination when we are next to them in a grocery line at a supermarket. Their baskets are filled with junk and processed foods of all kinds. We want to talk with them about this, but are hampered by the inhibitions our culture suggests to us about what constitutes polite communications with others—especially those we haven't yet met personally. We want to help them, intervene somehow. It's frustrating.

Meanwhile, what about you? Have you gained some extra fat-type weight? Has your body gotten frumpy and lumpy? Cellulite? Are there significant areas of that body that displease you, that you know very well don't have to look that way? Have you tried various diets, only to get frustrated and gone back to at least some of your favorite not-so-healthy foods? We can say for a certainty that the GLD will help you!

It takes an estimated average of 90-120 days (3-4 months) on an all raw foods GLD to learn what the body is actually supposed to look like (in its physical appearance) by nature. By doing this dietary experiment, we can see for ourselves if this is true. Of course, in this equation, we must take into account genetics and environment, what we were born with and what happened in our life 'til this diet experiment happens. Interesting? And you don't need to be on the GLD that long before seeing the positive changes— in both health and body appearance.

What are you really supposed to look like at this time in your life— as opposed to what you've created or has otherwise happened to your body thus far via diet, lifestyle, and life events? Ready for what the GLD can show you? Worth a try? Go for it! Of course, the body is also reflective of, and appears to anyone's physical view as, whatever the person entertains in thots and feelings, psycho-emotionally. Our thots and feelings help make us look this way!

Real meditation on the Divine Reality also helps our physical appearance. (Don't believe it? Then, here's another experiment you'll have to try!) Applying all three of these ideas (diet + action + emotional feeling) into one concept, taking genetics and environmental events into account, the body takes on the appearance of *what we eat (57%), do (26%), and think (17%).*

Concern for the Body

The esoteric Teachings of the ancients and (especially) the saints and sages provide a different impression of what the body is, different from what we usually or commonly think. Adi Da Samraj has Spoken of the body many times in His Adidam Teachings. Consider these Instructions of His (from two separate talks) to give us a better sense of what this body is really all about:

"The body is replication with minor modifications, constantly changing, a process of aging, a pattern. Sameness is never achieved, just constantly changing replication. It is patterns patterning on the basis of two, male and female, complexity and simplicity—always one of these undermining the other, back and forth from one to the other. Time and space are part of this patterning.

"By learning how the body works in certain circumstances one can extend its life. Concern for the body-mind is misplaced. You are not the body-mind. The body-mind is not the feeling awareness self nor the True Self (Consciousness Itself). Therefore, concern for the body-mind is of no use because the body-mind is a doomed pattern. Why be attached to it? Give it what it needs in order to be balanced and forget about it."

Based on this amazing and profound esoteric description, the GLD can be most useful simply to promote the balance the Avatar suggests!

17—The Role of the Healer

Healer / Healee Responsibilities in Health and Disease

Good News and Bad News

[Dr. Leonard reviews the patient's Intake History, then her Eyology images, and finally considers the "live" interview notes. Then, he turns to her and addresses her with the prognosis:]

Dr. Leonard: Betty, I've got good news and bad news.

Betty: Doc, can you give me the good news first?

Dr. Leonard: You can eliminate your disease completely. The GLD liquids are a major part of the process.

Betty: Great! But what's the bad news?

Dr. Leonard: You're going to die, of course, as we all must do at the gross body level. Meanwhile, tho, for this body to be symptom-free and genuinely healed, you can stay focused while those around you are eating whatever they damn well please—and getting sick as a result. Given your tendencies, this won't be easy. At this point in our consideration, you know how you got sick, and you know what to do about it. Now, it's just a matter of kicking ass and doing it. Your body is your baby. You don't allow a baby to do whatever it wants. Just require your body to do it.

Betty: That doesn't sound so hard. Do you think I can handle it?

Dr. Leonard: Others have. I have. Just keep a picture clearly in your mind of your body being healthy. See yourself happy with your liquids and **The BIG 7**. Keep saying, "*It's happening. I'm getting healthier and stronger by the day. Thank You, Lord, for Your Wonderful Wisdom and Guidance!*" The adult in you knows the importance of discipline, of turning to the Divine for Help, and it can and will take it on.

Betty: Thanks, Dr. Leonard. I'm going for it!

Ignorance and the Accidental Creation of Disease

It takes years to develop chronic degenerative diseases. We know this inside, yet we are being told that some mysterious disease organism has victimized poor innocent "us." We are led to believe that we had no role in creating this process. But in a real sense, it was us all along. Despite the awful pressures, stresses, and frustrations of living in this crazy world, and being led by our culture (and even by doctors) to believe that junk and processed foods (the LQFs) are OK to eat, we can be responsible for our life-negative diet and lifestyle regarding this disease.

Some well-meaning "experts" say that parasites are the cause of all disease. Wrong! Parasites are only along for the ride. They are the undertakers of the body, awaiting their big day when the body gets sick and dies so they can finally take over (unless we have the body cremated). That's their job. Like any other living thing, they just want a life. And if we're silly enuf to junk up the body with smoke, drink, junk foods, late hours and lack of exercise, the parasites will gladly have a family of 45 million at our expense! Before we die!

The Role of Parasites

Health is about responsibility. No "Book of Health" telling us how to live right is placed on our tummy at birth. No one comes on commercial TV to give us instructions on how to live a pure life and be healthy. No one informs us that Radiant Health is our birthright, meant to be enjoyed thru-out life. Living a relatively balanced life, the parasites are kept below "clinical levels," meaning that our body systems handle them, manage them, and keep them from destroying bodily life. Above clinical levels, there are symptoms. That's when we need professional help against the parasites. That's when the GLD is particularly useful.

What are parasites? The categories we are currently aware of include the somatids, viruses, bacteria, fungi, protozoa, and worms. Some family members of these, the commensals, are helpful in the body. Certain bowel bacteria, for example, as in yogurt, help us stay healthy. But the rest need to be managed. The Law of the body has us eating pure natural foods. Living the Law, our body has the best opportunity to get and stay balanced—lifelong.

The Healer's Responsibilities—and Ours

Enter the healer. He or she is responsible for teaching us about our disease and how to be healthy. He or she is our coach, and we are the team. We must learn from the healer how we got into the mess we're in in the first place. And not just how to get out of it. The healer instructs us on how to be responsible for our health. The healer is thus a teacher and an example, doing what he or she teachers, empowering us to be straight with our diet and lifestyle.

The true healer doesn't try to heal us. First, they rightly ask us questions that help us understand how we got sick, what we did to develop our disease *so we can be responsible for it*. They first focus on the activities we engaged that brot on disease—including the negative-reactive emotions. We consider with the healer our life-negative patterns of diet and lifestyle. Then, they interest us in *The BIG 7*, the ways of being healthy. Right practice of *The BIG 7* keeps our immune system strong, and therefore and thereby keeps parasites below clinical levels.

The healer is not responsible for our health, per se—only our health *instruction*. The healer did not make us sick. We made ourselves sick—with the help of our sick culture! The true healer requires us to change our act, to do something different, something life-positive with our diet and lifestyle—which will help us AND our culture. And this health and healing process is something we must consciously participate in—not just take an herb, pill, tablet, surgery, or whatever. Healing, therefore, is participatory. Without our participation, no real healing takes place.

The true healer brings good energy to us, loves us, and demands that we be responsible and intelligent with our actions. The true healer, then, requires us to be strait. He or she knows that the only person that can heal us is <u>ourselves</u>—thru our right relationship to the body and to the Divine Person. The true healer is an example to us of good health and balance in life—and is not him/herself dallying in gross life-negative habits. The true healer is a healing presence.

Ancient Healing
In primordial hunter-gatherer times, the young men were out searching for animals to kill and bring home for food. Meanwhile, the women, children and elders gathered whatever local vegetal edibles were available—our "insurance" food. From those earliest times emerged our first doctor, the Traditional Naturopath, the barefoot healer, most often a woman. These ancient healers collected the herbs, roots, and leaves we found useful in healing.

Thru the ages, the healer was revered. He or she may have been a shaman. In ancient China, it is said that this barefoot healer would occasionally visit each family in their area. If all were well (by his earlier instructions), he would be paid. If not, no pay! Today, the healer (doctor) wears a white coat. We are expected to trust him or her—by virtue of their office (healer, doctor) if not their education. But they are not trained in Earth Medicine.

Today, trust itself is a rare commodity. The talents and abilities of some entrepreneurs far outclass the education of some well-trained. We all know some doctor we would never refer anyone to. So, we must do our research, vet them, ask others what they experienced with this or that doctor. Especially when our health and that of our loved-ones is involved. Especially when all the healer knows is drug, cut, and burn.

All forms of medicine have their right application. There are times when surgery is definitely needed. And a drug—like with temporary acute pain. But, more often than not, this type of medicine is wrongly applied. Perhaps the best example of this wrong application is with chronic degenerative disease. This is where Earth Medicine shines. The forms of Natural Medicine need to be brought back into the mainstream.

The Highest Level of Health and Healing

Adidam Radical Healing is the highest known level of health and healing, the teachings on the subject by Adi Da. In Adidam Radical Healing, **disease is not a negative or problematic condition**. Disease is the result of egoity, our sense of separateness and separation from others—which sense takes many forms. Egoity is our actual moment-to-moment activity in which we objectify everything and everyone and thus separate ourselves from not only "others" but the All-Pervading Spiritual Life-Force. This is the source of all of our problems.

In Radical Healing, disease can be seen as **an opportunity to inspect our lives and happily relinquish life-negative habits, taking on more life-positive ones**. This makes healing <u>our</u> responsibility, not that of the doctor, healer, or other external authority. **True healing requires a change of action**—mental, emotional, and physical—and <u>only the individual can do this</u>. This principle also takes the fault away from "germs" (the ubiquitous parasites) and places the responsibility for health squarely on…us! Which, essentially, is where it belongs.

The principle human faculties of (1) body, (2) emotion, (3) mind, and (4) breath are interdependent. Any disturbance or frustration <u>in one</u> will tend to manifest as symptoms <u>in the others</u>—***unless consciously transcended and released.*** Therefore, we must inspect all of our psychophysical activity and discover the roots of the symptoms. The real healer knows how to accomplish this. He or she helps the patient with this understanding.

Two Approaches to Healing

Finally, most people approach the healer (whether medical doctor, Naturopath, Nutritionist, or other practitioner) with clinical level symptoms, meaning symptoms that are out of control or otherwise not able to be understood sufficiently for the patient to deal with them without professional help. This is common and appropriate. The healer usually considers the circumstance "objectively," applying logic and reason to the situation. This is looking at the problem "from without," doing an objective analysis—the ***analytical approach***.

A certain amount of this analysis is fine, but to depend on such exclusively is to avoid something far more fundamental and appropriate: the knowledge of the body itself—beyond testing of any kind. In Radical Healing, as Described by Avatar Adi Da, this is what we call the ***body systems approach***. You make sure the body is being given what it needs to right itself, and then leave it alone. You don't spend enormous amounts of time desperately searching for all manner of remedies. Most often, the body just needs to fast and rest from the food cycle.

We can think of the GLD as a version of this "fasting" process. This body systems approach goes directly to the cause of the problems and eliminates them outrite. This approach doesn't obviate testing, but simply deals with the pathology directly. So, testing is good and useful, but this body systems approach is primary. The problems are usually particular stoppages, blockages, congestions, imbalances, subtle inflammations, toxic deposits, and so forth, that our various tests are unable to precisely describe or show us—especially if such obstructions are on subtle levels.

So, when we give them the opportunity, the various body systems already and automatically deal with these problems directly, eliminating the underlying difficulty. This is the more basic and intelligent approach. Whether it is a fast, a juice diet, a liquid diet, or a mono whole food diet that is recommended by the healer, this is what gets the job done quickest and best. This gives the body the ability to organize, correct, and righten itself. It beats the hell out of merely treating symptoms—whether with drugs, acupuncture, herbs, vitamins, or whatever else.

Surrender

Sometimes, a disease appears whose presence is a total mystery to everyone. The patient can be doing everything "right" in terms of life-positive living practices, dietary and lifestyle-wise, and yet the disorder persists. The healer can be doing his or her role responsibly, and still, the dysfunction remains. This could go on for days, weeks, months on end. We have to be ready to accept that some disorders occur for reasons that may never be known.

So, what is our position relative to such conditions? Doing our best to serve the body is merely appropriate. Turning to the Divine Person, the Person of Love, too, is entirely appropriate. It is our submission, our surrender to the situation, to the Divine, that heals us at the heart. The body has its way, its destiny, which ends in its death, and bodily death is only a natural part of the cycle of life. Meanwhile, it is always ours to surrender to and into the Context In Which we appear and upon Which we absolutely depend.

18—The GLD vs. Fasting
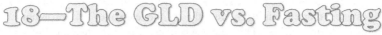

Similarities and Differences

Is the GLD the Same as a Fast?

No. But there are similarities. On your GLD, you will get hungry, especially during the first few days. Then, your body will make certain adjustments to taking all liquids. The hunger will quickly die down, and you will settle into taking less food in quantity and more in nutrient-dense quality. Altho the principle is the same, the GLD is NOT a fast. The GLD is not even a juice diet, which is all fresh juices only, taken as they come. The GLD is essentially mixed liquids, so, technically, it can embrace and include both fasting and juice dieting within it.

Fasting involves taking either thinned-down juices (thinned down with pure water, as in juice fasting), or just herb teas with a few drops of lemon and honey (water fasting). There are certain other important differences between the GLD and fasting. One can fast on thin juices or water (and perhaps herb tea) for up to 40 days or so without starvation occurring. If continued, the body will self-digest, even to the point of death. The GLD can be taken indefinitely—meaning years, decades, for life. Here is a list of more of the differences:

FASTING	*The GREAT LIQUID DIET*
Limited to 40 days or so before the body self-digests	Can be engaged indefinitely
Purification is most rapid ("faster")	Purification is slower than on a fast, but quicker than on solids
Can be done in moderate stages of health	Can be done in all stages of health, including the worst disease states
Stringent, with possibly irritating purification episodes	Easier on the body, purification events are less disturbing
Weight loss is rapid, obviating thin-body types	Weight loss is more gradual; GLD can be done by all body types
BMs stop, frequent bowel cleansing needed	BMs slow down; only occasional or no bowel cleansing needed
Only thin juices/water/tea/broth allowed	OK to use thick smoothies, undiluted juices, blended soups, etc
No banana, avocado, coconut, other nuts or seeds	These items and more are fine on the GLD
No supplements allowed while fasting	OK any and all appropriate nutritional and herb supplements on GLD
Hunger pangs are more acute during fasting	Hunger pangs, when & if there, are less irritating, more easily sated
Energy focus is internal, & heavily on purification	Energy focus is also on purification, but is more available elsewhere

The GLD and the Fasting Principle

As noted, the principle of the GLD—**purification**—is the same as in fasting. On taking a solid food meal, an average of about 25% of the body's available energies are needed to break down the food within the gastrointestinal tract. These energies come to bear first on the stomach, then on the small intestine, and finally on the large intestine, or colon, as nutrients are taken up and the waste products are processed.

The pancreas and liver also come into play, and then the spleen. Eventually, over time, while on the GLD, every system, organ, and tissue will be positively influenced thru the principle of purification brot on by the power of the raw liquids. With liquids—on your GLD as compared to taking solid meals—far less energy is needed (average 11% per meal on the GLD), freeing up all that extra energy for purification and healing.

In general, the thinner the juice or other liquid, the greater the purification. The purer and fuller of Life Force (Universal Life Energy, or etheric energy) the liquid (we're talking raw juices, smoothies, and herb teas), the greater the purification and healing. Yes, the GLD involves some thicker liquids, and perhaps even some cooked liquids (when used appropriately), as well. But the principle is generally the same, altho some think liquids pack high nutritive power. Smoothies, e.g., can include several SuperFoods (Appendix C) and be thick and quite tasty.

A main point here is that on the GLD, the purification and healing takes a little longer than on a fast—but in many disease circumstances, longer is better. There are no sudden shocks to the body—as on initiating a fast. And, again, not all bodies can sustain a fast. The GLD is gentler on the body than is fasting. And the GLD, in terms of purification, is a lot faster than any solid food diet.

Fasting vs. Pain—Two Stories

Traditional Naturopathy is our oldest form of medicine. One of its basic principles is that when sick one should rest and fast. This is ancient knowledge. Unfortunately, it has been marginalized by (and contrasts with) Big Pharma's principle of calling your doctor and getting a drug. We have gotten so far away from being healed by walking barefoot on the land.

Once, while visiting friends in Mississippi, I was playfully tossing a young boy up in the air when a vertebra in my neck was tweaked. Barely noticed at the time, as I drove toward my Florida Keys destination it became increasingly obvious—and painful. By the time I arrived, the pain was at the "exquisite" level. In other words, I couldn't think of anything else.

The next day, a Sunday, I could find neither an Acupuncturist nor a Chiropractor who's office was open. Finally, that nite, I tracked down an MD. After a brief examination, he suggested I travel to Miami the next morning for surgery! I begged for a pain killer drug to get me thru the nite until I could take the next step. By morning, my intuition silently shouted "fast".

Within 24 hours, half the pain was gone. In another 24, it was down to a quarter of what it had been. By the third day, it had completely disappeared. I took the opportunity to do my first 30-day fast. In retrospect, it was more like a combination of a juice fast and a juice diet, with herb teas, several thinned-down juices, and a number of juices taken straight.

Some years later, while in my late 50s, I was in a hurry to get to the office. Instead of walking around the building per usual, a shortcut was to leap the fence. I had done this before, but this time I felt something in my back. Later in the day, the pain came on. And it got worse. Remembering the earlier pain event, I decided to get right into a fast. This time, the pain was gone within 24 hours.

Of course, there are many factors to consider in these events as in any event of pain. Fasting will not necessarily alleviate every instance of pain. But when accompanied by proper rest, by my estimate it will eliminate or significantly alleviate some 90% of cases. Please consider this if pain is a factor on your GLD. In general, the more the pain the more likely GLD Level 1 is appropriate—until resolution.

Hunger and the GLD
You're going to get hungry on the GLD just as you get hungry on solid foods. *It's OK to be hungry!* "Lean and hungry"—hungry for life, not just for food! Always maintain your appetite for life. (As Adi Da says, "*Never eat to the point of fullness, or make love to the point of emptiness.*")

During the first few days on your GLD, you will likely experience more hunger pangs than usual. This is part of the normal adjustments the body makes with any new dietary regime—especially one that suddenly moves from solids to liquids. Just wait a few minutes, and the hunger pangs will go away. They will likely return, but then, as appropriate, just drink something. Even a small amount will eliminate the pangs.

During these first few days, especially, your stomach will grumble, and your bowel will make various noises. This, too, is normal, as your Nutritive system (stomach and bowel) makes certain adjustments to the liquids. YOUR STOMACH IS SHRINKING to adapt to this new dietary administration.

The GLD is a *delivery system*, a way of taking foods that is far more efficient than the chewing of solid foods. In this case, the juicer and blender accomplish most of the "chewing." Add to this the fact that the GLD is mostly raw or (better) even all raw, and you see why the GLD allows greater cleansing and purification than do any of the solid food diets. On the GLD, hunger pangs gradually diminish. You get used to them, when and if they do appear, and even in some sense welcome them as signs of purification and improved health. You will feel better.

19—Natural vs. Non-Natural

These Days, a Big Deal

"Natural" means different things to different people. Here, we are referring to produce that has been grown in relatively pure, healthy soils (no artificial or chemical fertilizers), not sprayed with chemical pesticides, not irradiated by anything other than the sun, and otherwise not processed or treated by or with human-made materials.

With natural farming, gardening, and horticulture, soils are nurtured by adding natural matter, such as shredded paper, dead leaves, sawdust, kitchen wastes, animal manure, worm castings, ground eggshells, earthworms, compost tea, and ground glacial rock powder. Besides this, food quality is increased by rotating crops and by planting beneficial cover crops.

In modern industrial or "conventional" farming, soils are replenished with chemicals and synthetic additives. This degrades soils and local waters. Meanwhile, natural "organic" farming works in harmony with Nature to sustain a healthy, fertile, and biologically active environment. Scientific studies show that natural produce is higher in nutrients. While natural produce typically costs more than non-natural, what price do you place on the health of your body? Are you willing to pay more for the health of your body? Buy and grow natural.

How the GLD will save you money and make you healthier:

(1) yes, you'll be paying a bit more <u>for produce</u> (unless you grow it yourself!)

(2) you'll be eating more—or mostly or even all—<u>produce</u>—living foods

(3) you'll be eating less packaged and processed food in bottles, cans, and boxes

(4) packages cost money to manufacture, whereas living produce comes in its own no-cost package

(5) chemicals (preservatives, coloring agents, surfactants, etc.) cost money to manufacture

(6) You won't be spending that money—or very little of it—on your GLD

(7) Bottom line: you'll save money on your GLD—and, you'll be getting healthier in the process!

Natural Junk Foods

Let's differentiate between natural produce and naturally prepared food. True, many foods are labeled "natural" that are also packaged foods. There is "naturally grown" rice, for example, and "natural" flour, "natural" fig bars, "natural" soy products (most soy products in the USA are now GMO), "natural" veggy burgers, "natural" potato chips, "natural" vegetable chips, and so on and on.

We currently have a whole pantheon of "natural" processed foods—even "natural" junk foods. How do these "natural" foods enter into the picture of our use of the GLD and the new way of life (**GLDLifestyle**) that the GLD represents altogether?

This question is answered by deciding where we are currently with our diet and our state of health. In disease processes, all foods less in quality than pure living natural produce need to be minimized, eliminated altogether, or at least temporarily stopped, accordingly. While on our GLD, the more severe the disease condition, the more strictly we avoid anything that is not living natural produce (See Chapter 7, "GLD *Level 1*").

During our GLD, if there are no significant symptoms, we have room to use some natural snacks. These can range from a few veggy chips with hummus dip (on the lower end of quality) to natural figs, a little sauerkraut, a few untreated banana chips, and a tablespoon of raw almond butter (on the higher end). We don't have to use snacks. It's a judgment call on the part of our health professional if we have symptoms, and on our part, if we do not.

As noted, it has been scientifically proven that natural foods contain higher amounts of nutrients than those found in non-natural produce. Fruits tend to emphasize vitamins. Vegetables tend to emphasize chlorophyll. Nuts tend to emphasize fats and oils. Seeds tend to emphasize minerals. All fresh produce—raw, ripe fruits, veggies, nuts, and seeds—contain food enzymes, arguably the most important of all nutrients at the gross physical level. Natural produce has higher available amounts of all of these nutrients than non-natural produce.

The Costs of Eating Poorly and Eating Well

This is just a very brief sketch, an overview of a major problem in the Western way of eating. We tend to think that because those natural foods "cost more" than the non-natural, why should we bother shopping for them? After all, we're trying to save money, right? But, what are the actual expenses to us all of natural produce vs. processed foods? Eating more raw foods is actually far less expensive, and cuts way down on many other costs, especially if we choose natural. We and the planet are going to be healthier and with less waste to eliminate.

Consider all the actual steps in food processing vs. whole food prep. Google it! You won't believe the difference. But that's just the beginning. How about packaging? We're always bringing home all those packages that need to be thrown away. Eating poorly involves purchasing food in plastic, paper, and metal foil packages, food that has been corrupted to varying degrees by baking, cooking, chemicalizing, and other types of processing. This is an enormous expense to industry, the producers of the food, the consumer, and the environment.

How much of our landfills involve food packaging? How many trees have to be cut down? How many hamburger and fries wrappers do we see along our streets? (Alternatively, how long does it take an apple core to decompose?) Compare these expenses with those of pure raw foods grown at local farms and (best) in our own garden, and you start to get the picture. We've just been talking about produce. Add the cost of killed and processed animals, and you go off the "eating poorly" scale!

20—Fresh vs. Frozen

The Difference Might Surprise You

This brings up the question of freezing foods to be used later in making liquids. Freezing destroys, on average, 25% of the nutrients of foods! Depending on the method of freezing—which includes freezer temperature, packaging of the food to be frozen, freezing method, and the state of the food being frozen—the food will lose at least some of its original vitality.

Think about it: what would happen to your "meat" if you were suddenly flash-frozen! Not a lovely thot, right? So, in general, it's best to *avoid using frozen food whenever possible*.

In most circumstances, by far, we choose fresh over frozen. However, notwithstanding, some foods, like blueberries, live in climates that require them to survive the natural outdoor freezing process, become frozen, then thawed out, then frozen again, and still continue to grow and ripen. Blueberries, therefore, can handle freezing without appreciable loss of nutrients. While there are a few other edible foods that can do that, it's best to avoid frozen foods.

If you live in a location where fresh produce is hard to come by, you are left with little choice but to use frozen foods—at least to some degree. If you are facing tossing out (wasting) otherwise wholesome bananas, e.g., better to peel them and quickly place them into a sturdy well-sealed air-free container and then into a very cold deep-freezer.

When taken out and blended into a smoothie, bananas can taste fine and bring the chill to your drink. When run thru certain juicers, you get an ice cream-like effect. Large batches of vegetable soup can be frozen for use much later, but, again, try to avoid this: they won't taste quite as good nor be as nourishing as fresh-made.

Finally, we are not yet in an age when Real CoOpCom (Cooperative Community—see Appendix G) is sufficiently valued to create it en masse—worldwide. But, we CAN start creating Espheria Units one-at-a-time! In an Espheria Unit, the GardenDome provides some 95% of your community's food needs in its three climate-controlled divisions. Espheria Units can be constructed almost anywhere in the world, in virtually any climate—wherever water is available. The design is there. We only await the interest and financial energy.

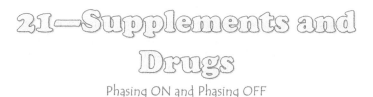

21—Supplements and Drugs

Phasing ON and Phasing OFF

Can nutritional and herb supplements be taken on the GLD?

Yes, you may continue to take your nutritional (vitamin, mineral, enzyme, herb, etc.) supplements on your GLD. Because of the high intake of nutrient-dense foods on the rightly done GLD, you will need, under most circumstances, fewer and fewer of these as you go along. In other words, the amounts of the various required supplements will necessarily change as the body undergoes positive changes and gets healthier.

Your body will continue to purify on the GLD, and so nutritional supplements will likely need to be reduced in number and amount as this purifying metabolic process progresses. Therefore, ask your Natural Health practitioner to check your supplement needs frequently—usually monthly: your dosage will—again, under most circumstances—need to be reduced— and often rather rapidly!

What about prescription medications? Is it safe to continue them?

Your need for pharmaceutical medications, both prescription and OTC (over-the-counter) drugs, very often diminishes on the GLD, depending on the specific drug and how long it has been taken—usually to the point of not needing them at all. Again, this is due to increasing health and the diminishing of disease processes.

Therefore, periodically check with your prescribing physician as your health improves, symptoms diminish, and you feel the need to lower your prescription(s). In most cases, meds will all be eventually eliminated on the GLD. This is desirable, since most drugs have adverse effects (so-called "side effects") on body tissues, at least becoming embedded and otherwise causing lowered function, loss of function, destroyed tissue, and even malignancy.

It is inappropriate for practitioners other than the prescribing physician to direct the course of a patient's drugs, especially medications that can cause negative health effects in the body if withdrawn suddenly or otherwise inappropriately. However, patients have, by themselves, successfully phased off their medications by (e.g.) carefully shaving tablets down by hand over a sufficient period of time. This is best done, of course, with the blessing of the prescribing physician.

Moreover, when the doctor sees clear evidence that the patient is getting well, he or she will have little choice but to follow this obvious course of action. If the symptoms are sufficiently diminished or eliminated, but the doctor refuses to acknowledge the improvement and needed change of prescription, he or she may need to be fired and/or replaced by one who is more open-minded, has sufficient understanding of natural health practices, and is more sensitive to the realities of diet and health.

At GranMed, we have encountered doctors who refuse to believe their patient no longer needs their prescribed medications—even when the patient has no symptoms and feels fine. These are often those who have been sufficiently brainwashed by, otherwise convinced of, the standard Big Pharma philosophy that drugs are the only viable option in most disease processes.

Cancer alternative advocate Ty Bollinger recently quoted the World Health Organization (WHO) as estimating that 80% of the world's population relies primarily on traditional medicine. Of these people, 2 billion depend on medicinal plants as their primary treatment option. *"Plant-based natural medicines are often just as effective—and sometimes more so—than the toxic drugs that Big Pharma manufacture. Plus, they are far more affordable and less prone to negative effects than pills produced by the pharmaceutical industry.*

"So, why don't we hear more about natural medicines and remedies in our part of the world? Good question. The answer lies with the **trillion-dollar-a-year** *Big Pharma industry (yes, that's "trillion" with a "T"!) This global pharmaceutical juggernaut spends billions of dollars each year advertising their products.*

Of course, they'd rather you don't veer from drugs to more natural solutions—it would eat into their profits."

A General Nutritional Supplement Protocol for Those on the GLD

The following supplements and lifestyle habits can be useful for most people engaging the GLD. Please note that the supplements are necessarily rather general. People can have very different health conditions, one person to the next. Altho the list below will fit most adults on the GLD, it is necessarily a broad-spectrum outline only, designed for the average person taking the GLD. Your qualified Natural Health professional will guide you toward supplements that may be appropriate and specific to your case.

Note that you may pull apart capsules and pour their contents into the blender with smoothie ingredients. Tablets may also be blended into smoothies.

—Amino acid caps @ 2/day

—Vitamin A Mycelized @ 4 drops daily

—Vitamin B Complex tabs @ 1/day

—Vitamin C crystals (ascorbic acid or L-ascorbate or sodium ascorbate) @ 4gm/day, separate doses (2x2gm)

—Vitamin E Mycelized @ 6 drops daily

—Vitamin Q (CoQ$_{10}$) caps @ 2/day

—Digestive Enzymes caps @ 1/meal

—Astragalus liquid @ 2 droppersful daily

—Milk Thistle Liquid @ 2 droppersful daily

—Dry Brush Massage @ daily before shower

—Rapid Movement Exercise as appropriate to your specific case

—Extra Virgin Expeller-pressed Coconut Oil @ 1 Tbsp. orally in liquids, plus ample amounts rubbed into the skin and hair daily after shower or at other times of the day

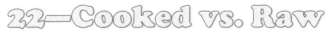

22—Cooked vs. Raw
The Difference is Instinctive

Hippocrates said it: *"Let your food be your medicine and your medicine be your food."* Jesus of Nazareth is said to have Recommended raw food (notes translated from the Dead Sea Scrolls suggest an understanding apparently tot to Jesus by the Essenes). The Christian bible says (in Genesis 1:28), *"And look! I have given you the seed-bearing plants throughout the earth, and all the fruit trees for your food."*

Avatar Adi Da has Said, *"Diet is about participating in Divine Activity. Taking gross food is rightly a sacred practice. The gross physical body is a food body. Make your diet maximally raw, even all raw. Food is medicine."* So, we at Grand Medicine say, taking these expressions of these Great Ones into account, and from our long clinical (since 1972) and personal experience, eat food the way it comes in Nature and be healthy.

Raw food dieting is a challenge in these junk food times. It is a confrontation with the ego. It confronts our memories, tastes, and preferences for all the foods we have learned to like—unless we were fortunate to have been eating raw foods from childhood (which these days is exceedingly rare). We are fearful of losing the ability to reach for all those nice tasty food items we've gotten used to over the years—and are, perhaps, still being introduced to.

We don't know yet (until we make the change) that our tastes will change while taking raw foods. Our palates will accept the new flavors, textures, and aromas of raw living foods. We'll feel better, and our health will improve. Soon, on a hi-raw or all-raw diet, we notice that our body no longer feels well whenever taking cooked and otherwise degenerated foods. We absolutely MUST learn these things via personal experiment.

The Formula for Good Health is Simple
The formula is *simple*, but not *easy*: eat raw foods and be healthy. What's the difference between **simple** and **easy**? Taking raw foods, while everyone around you—even your own family, and even your spouse—is destroying their health and insulting the God-Given Gift of the body via lesser-quality food—that's not easy, it's hard.

Mainly, it's hard to watch when you know the difference: that what we eat, the way we eat, how the food is working in the body (being digested and assimilated, and the waste products eliminated) makes such a profound difference in our health. It's hard to watch others, and it's hard—especially at first—to do the raw practice ourselves. But, it's necessary—and the result, the payoff, is big: good health.

Appropriate Percentages of Raw and Cooked Liquids

Appropriate percentages will vary with the health circumstance of the individual. Your Natural Health Practitioner will make suggestions in your case as to what percentage raw you should start with. On solids, it should never be less than 55%. In general, always *keep the raw liquids above 90% of your GLD daily*, and increasingly higher, depending on the severity of your case and/or how quickly purification, rebalancing, and healing are needed.

The cooked percentage may be as little as 5%—or (better) none at all! In most cases, a cooked meal (blended soup, e.g.) is more for psychological nurturing value than for gross physical nourishment. Those who actually need a cooked solid foods diet of 20% or more are those with very special medical circumstances, disease conditions that, e.g., involve certain exceedingly rare bowel conditions. Only specialized medical professionals practiced in these natural health principles can properly assess such cases.

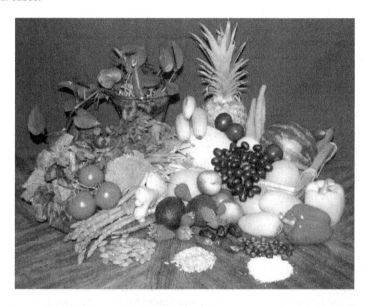

The consideration of fresh raw vs. cooked also applies to the whole question of bottled juices vs. fresh-made, and raw vs. cooked sauces and soups. Of course, it is best to prepare your own fresh juices and soups, simply because they are more wholesome and do not need to be pasteurized to be legally sold to the public.

The basic rule is: Never take more soups, broths, and other cooked or prepared items (including bottled juices—which have been "cooked" via pasteurization) than fresh raw juices on any given day. The raw juices accomplish most of the weight loss, tissue nourishment, and purification.

Always emphasize them over all other liquids—unless you need to maintain or even gain weight.

Make your own fresh raw juices whenever possible—and drink them the same day as made. ***The more severe or serious the health condition, the higher the percentage of immediately taken raw that is needed***. The 100% raw GLD is appropriate in most cases by far—especially in cases of chronic degenerative disease. Herb teas and hot cacao (cocoa), which use boiling water, are fine at any time on the GLD.

The Cooking of Food Destroys Important Nutrients

The cooking or "firing" of food destroys certain nutrients in food to the point of rendering some of them as actual mild (slow) poisons. This especially includes certain proteins. ***The cells of the human body were genetically programmed to receive food in its natural raw state—and essentially in no other way***.

Consider the quoted passage from the book of Genesis: "*I give you the fruits of the fields and of the trees, and for you, these shall be for meat.*" One interpretation could be an admonition for us to be vegetarian. Most of us, by far, can easily handle vegetarianism. Only a very few people seem to need a little animal dairy or some small amounts of flesh foods now and then (red meat, fowl, or sea flesh—fish) in order to be healthy.

On cooking food, the very first nutrient to be destroyed (by the cooking process) is food enzymes. There are three kinds of enzymes involved in the processes of being healthy: (1) *food* **enzymes**—found in raw foods only, (2) *digestive* **enzymes**, located in the mouth and stomach, and (3) *metabolic* **enzymes**, found thru-out the body. When <u>food</u> enzymes are missing (via cooking), the <u>digestive</u> enzymes must over-produce to make up the deficit.

<u>Metabolic</u> enzymes also suffer from excessive amounts of cooked foods by not being able to speed enuf essential nutrients to their cellular destinations. Besides this, we all have our own separate enzyme *quotient*, which is used up much quicker when we eat cooked and processed foods. When this quotient is at an end, we die! Taking raw foods enhances the enzyme quotient and extends it to its maximum length—thus lengthening our lives.

Avatar Adi Da puts it this way: "*The reason that the cooking or firing of food is generally not optimal is that heat destroys the enzymes, heat-sensitive vitamins, and other heat-sensitive nutrients naturally present in raw foods, and it also changes the chemical structure of proteins and sugars in raw foods such that these proteins and sugars become less usable by or even harmful to the body.*" —Adi Da, in <u>*Green Gorilla*</u>

The GLD vs. an All-Raw (solid foods) Diet

If whole raw foods are so great, why do the GLD? When patient Ina described her condition and asked for our help, we knew whole raw foods would be too slow to deal with her tumor. And fasting wouldn't allow her the high volume of hi-quality nutrients her body needed to deal with the situation. But, other factors enter into the picture when we consider whole vs. liquefied.

Make no mistake: whole raw natural in-season locally grown in quality soil foods are excellent and vitally important to health. When it comes to solid food diets, they're the very best. You simply purchase (or grow it yourself or get it from your nayborhood) natural unsprayed fresh raw produce, take it home, wash it and eat it. So, why compare? Read on.

The GLD involves the strategic use of technology for improved health: the juicer and (especially) the blender. *Pure liquids made from whole raw natural produce are easier on the food processing organs and structures of the body than is the same produce eaten whole.* There is less chewing, so the teeth are spared all that grinding. How much grinding? Check out the recipes at the end of this book and see! And liquefying foods saves time. Yes, there is the possibility of blending *cooked* foods, like soups. These are used strategically only.

Here's the test: how long would it take you to eat the produce in a typical Green Smoothie? We're talking a big handful or two of greens, e.g., which is typical for a green smoothie—the standard daily drink on your GLD. OK, now add the other ingredients—the whole fruits (and possibly nuts, seeds &/or oils, if they're added). For that matter, how long does it usually take to prepare a tasty gourmet cooked meal? Including at a restaurant?! And then, add the cost, restaurant or not. Now, you begin to see how efficient, effective, and inexpensive the GLD really is!

When making up your Green Smoothie, get some variation into the mix by occasionally including a leaf of kale, maybe a few beet leaves, sometimes a few little broccoli trees, even a little cauliflower. **It's the greens** that you especially want to vary now and then. But always include the greens! They're the most essential ingredient—especially because of their chlorophyll.

The Green Smoothie, the key and most important liquid in the GLD

- A BIG handful of mixed greens (e.g., kale, beet greens, celery, chard, baby spinach or mixed greens)
- 1 cored apple (or pear or peach)
- 1 peeled orange
- Possibly add 1 peeled banana (if more sweetener is needed)
- 1-2 cups pure water (prefer steam-distilled & left in the sun 3 hours)—or nut-seed milk (see Appendix A)
  Blend on medium speed and serve

Most of us aren't going to eat the amount of food in this recipe raw and whole—but we mite, if it were liquefied and tasted good when mixed together. And that's another factor—the taste. Who is going to take a bite of raw broccoli and then a bite of apple to make the broccoli taste better? The point:

(1) Not only will you be taking in the amount of greens equivalent to six salads (wow!), but also...
(2) Liquids in combination can taste better than many single solid foods (raw broccoli, raw cauliflower, e.g.)

Then, there's the nutrition factor: the GLD liquids contain higher concentrations of nutrients, in part because the vegetable fiber is removed (in juicing) and reduced in size and yet still effective (by blending). Such change conserves precious body food-processing energy for purification, harmonization, and rejuvenation—instead of having to use that energy for processing all that whole food bulk and ruffage.

The age and longevity factor tops the list of superlatives for the GLD: as we get older, we become more vulnerable to disease organisms, stress, genetic weakness tendencies, weather changes, and frustration. The GLD clearly reduces these stresses by providing easeful processing of highest quality nutrients with minimum energy expenditure by the body.

Full vs. Satisfied

What is the difference between "full" and "satisfied" as regards eating? When full, you don't want to move the body. You just want to sit there in a big soft, comfortable and relaxing lounge chair and "veg out." This happens when eating *cooked* food, but never with *raw* food. One can always move the body easily after a raw food meal, and the feeling is one of satisfaction, satiety, but not stuffed-fullness.

An excellent example is the Green Smoothie as a meal. Notice how long the body feels satisfied and not hungry after taking your drink 16-20 ounces of a Green Smoothie. It is usually something like 4 hours or so, often more. Compare this with a meal of pizza, and you get the picture.

And notice this: how many bananas do you think you can eat before they don't taste good anymore? And yet, you NEVER lose your appetite for pizza! Pizza *always* tastes good—even when you're stuffed with it! Why? Because the human body has an innate instinct for living foods (the bananas)—but not for cooked foods!

Eating to the point of fullness shortens life. In ancient Rome, senators and others, indulging themselves at the baths and at feasts in orgiastic eating and sexing, would gorge themselves and then purposely vomit up the meal so they could continue the pleasures of gustatory indulgence. This, of course, is quite stressful on the body.

While fasting is a rest from the eating cycle, liquid dieting provides such a rest that can—unlike fasting—continue indefinitely. Both of these practices extend life, as recent research has clearly shown. This wisdom regarding amount of food taken at meals has been known since ancient times: hence the Hindu expression, *"At mealtimes, one's stomach should be half full of food, one quarter full of water, and one quarter full of Love of God!"*

23—Packaged vs. Live
Toward a Longer Shelf Life

Is it OK to drink bottled juices on the GLD?

Bottled juices may be taken on your GLD—IF they are all you can find available, BUT…they should be avoided if at all possible. They are not preferred over fresh raw self-prepared juices. By current law in some countries, bottled and otherwise packaged juices must be pasteurized. Therefore and thereby, they have lost a significant amount of nutrients, especially food enzymes, which are much more important than vitamins or minerals. Especially avoid bottled and canned juices that contain chemical preservatives and additives.

To be sold legally in the USA, liquids must be heated to varying temperatures for varying amounts of time. E.g., 145°F for 30 minutes or 162°F for 16 seconds, etc., the higher the temperature, the shorter the time for Pasteurization (HHST = higher heat shorter time). So-called "ultra-pasteurization" requires the liquid (usually cow's milk) to be heated to 280°F for two minutes. How much real nutrition will be left? Damn little!

Worse, there are inherent dangers associated with drinking pasteurized and (especially) ultra-pasteurized liquids. It masks the use of low-quality milk, it destroys nutrients and enzymes, it causes asthma and allergies, it promotes lactose intolerance, it weakens bones (bone density), it weakens antibiotic effectiveness, it promotes IGF-1 (the cancer-involved hormone), and it takes cows out of green pastures and puts them into concrete pens.

Cow's milk is designed by Nature to make calves grow very big, very fast. It's not for humans. After being weaned from our human mothers' breast, let's (as adults) make our milk from nuts and seeds. Clinically, I spent years teaching new mothers who couldn't nurse to quickly make coconut milk to feed their infants. (And, BTW, whatever you do as a new mother, NEVER feed your infant commercial canned alternative "formulas"!)

Read your labels! It is by far best to make your own fresh raw juices (or have someone make them for you)—and drink them the same day as they are prepared, or as soon thereafter as possible. The natural surfaces and flesh of fruits and veggies have been infinitely compromised by liquefying them, so they are now quite vulnerable to nutrient loss. The longer they sit, the greater the nutrient loss.

Try to consume fresh-made juices the same day they are prepared. And when not finished drinking them, place them in the frig for longer life and nutrient maintenance. When you cut an ordinary natural apple in half, how long does it take to "brown"? Cut it into quarters or eights, it seems to brown faster. The more cuts, the greater the exposure. A few minutes after it has browned, you don't want to eat it. Blending it or juicing it exposes it infinitely—a good argument for drinking it right away!

Most packaged foods have been prepared, processed, added to, subtracted from, preserved, colored, stabilized, and otherwise variously broken down and compromised from their original natural state. The original fresh raw living food, as it comes in nature, is wholesome, full of life, and containing the sun's and Earth's energies and other natural energies and nutrients, many of such energies that have yet to be measured by current technology.

When foods are cooked, food enzymes are among the first vital nutrients to be lost. As cooking proceeds, various other nutrients, including vitamins and (finally) minerals, are drawn out of them. What is left is without the nourishing and healing power of the original fresh, raw, ripe food. Practice seeing packaged foods this way: devoid of various levels of nourishment; entertaining, but without the nourishing and healing power of raw produce. Think of them as for special celebratory and entertainment purposes only—if then.

When our diet contains higher percentages of cooked foods, the cells of the body are not being nourished, so they gradually weaken. Since the gross physical body is essentially a <u>food</u> body, and since fresh raw ripe locally grown natural produce is the best food for the gross physical body, then obviously, this is the best food for us to consume. It's not that we should necessarily never touch cooked food to our mouths. There can be times when cooked foods—including cooked liquids—can be useful and appropriate.

Excessive amounts of cooked and processed foods is among the main reasons our #1 protective system—the immune—gets weakened, setting us up for disease. There are many other systems, of course, that are negatively affected by this process of taking cooked foods. We humans are supposed to be living upwards of 200 years—according to Adi Da Samraj. This inappropriate intake of cooked and processed foods is among the reasons we don't!

Possible Appropriate Times to Use Cooked and Processed Foods (LQFs)

- Parties
- Holidays
- Birthdays
- Anniversaries
- Sacred Occasions
- Family Gatherings

Of course, it is not strictly necessary that cooked and processed foods be used on these occasions. The question of whether or not to use them at these times or at all is really up to us as individuals. Use your good judgment. We must learn to use these substances intelligently: a few times per year, if at all, and always in the company of others. Otherwise, they will bring disease and suffering. Again, the rule: *appropriate use and intelligent abstinence.*

Note that packaged foods are, in some sense, even worse than homemade cooked produce, since they have already been cooked and otherwise processed—so they'll need to be re-heated, which will cause even more loss of nutrients. If you're going to eat cooked foods, better to buy or otherwise collect whole foods from local gardens and prepare them at home. And, in liquefying foods, prefer raw—in and as increasing percentages of your daily fare.

Notice the physical appearance of people who eat significant amounts of processed foods: in a word, ugly! They are fat, or, if slim, they look sallow, sickly, aging rapidly, prematurely gray, wrinkled, paunchy, sagging before their time, tired, with fluctuating or low energy, diseased, negative, uninspired, and dark. There are, of course, other factors in people looking these ways—and we have mentioned them.

"No praise, no blame," says Adi Da. If this is what you want to do with your life, OK, so be it. This doesn't make the person evil or wicked— just needing to learn something important about diet, food, and eating. These are our brothers and sisters, friends and family, acquaintances and colleagues. They're our people, and they need our love.

Observe the hugely fat woman at the grocery counter. Now, look at what she's got in her shopping cart: commercial soft drinks, boxed cereal, white bread, hot dogs, donuts, cold cuts, chicken, a box of candy bars, canned veggies, and a gallon of ultra-pasteurized milk. She also has a couple of fat, anemic, sick-looking children tagging along behind her.

You can see the medical bills passing to the insurance companies. You can see her in the hospital, and her children suffering, as well. Oh, the children! What an example of humanity she is! She is...you...and me, our sister, our mother! Her health understanding and discipline are vanished.

24—Animal vs. Vegetal
What the Consequences Imply

Anthropologically speaking, for perhaps hundreds of thousands of years, we humans roamed the Earth in small groups. The younger men would go out hunting for any animal dumb enuf to stand around long enuf for them to club them over the head or spear them with a lance. Meanwhile, the women, children and old folks would gather the "insurance" food: fruits, nuts, berries, roots, and other vegetal foods.

When the young men came home from the hunt, more often than not, they had nothing. When they did bring a dead animal, whoever was nice to them would get some meat. So, we didn't eat much meat for the longest time—actually for most of our history as human beings—until we started keeping and herding animals, called animal husbandry. That was perhaps 14,000 years ago, not very long in terms of our evolution—which, BTW, includes pattern response to our environments.

Our dentition, the length of our bowel, the design of our stomachs— many factors suggest more of a vegetarian diet for us humans—or perhaps leaning just a bit toward omnivorous. But, definitely not carnivorous. We can eat meat, yes, but what happens when we make it a more significant part of our diet? We get diseased. Our lives are shortened. Human populations that eat meat as the largest part of their diet have among the shortest lifespans— e.g., the Eskimos, the Inuit peoples, and certain African tribes.

Dietary Percentages of Vegetal and Animal Products

As individuals, we modern humans take varying percentages of vegetal and animal products. Not that we need to, but mainly out of cultural direction and habit. Some individuals seem to get along better on a little animal product—some yogurt, a few eggs, some fish. Some people—a very few—even seem to work better with a very little or occasional red meat. At Grand Medicine, we estimate the *appropriate percentages of real dietary needs that would bring good health for human beings* (not the amounts that people actually take) as the following:

- Vegetarian – 88%
- Some soured dairy (yogurt, kefir)– 3%
- Some sea flesh – 4%
- Some fowl flesh – 4%
- Some red meat – 1%

Therefore, we feel that most of us humans, by far, should and can be eating far higher percentages of vegetal foods than we likely thot. Some of us seem to get along better on a little occasional (not regular) soured dairy, including yogurt or kefir, which bring beneficial bacteria to the bowel. *The only way you'll find out what is right for you is to do the dietary experiment.* Spend some time trying out varying percentages of animal and vegetal foods and see what happens. Remember, it's not about how the food tastes—it's about how it makes the body feel.

The Acid/Alkaline Connection

Consider body pH (acid/alkaline): most vegetal products (fruits and veggies) in the raw state are *alkaline*. Other vegetal products (nuts and seeds) are essentially *acid*. All animal products, flesh or dairy, are (on the other hand) inherently *acid*. *Our bodies thrive on about 75% alkaline and 25% acid.* Certain foods that are "*acid*" outside the body (lemons, e.g.) are *alkaline* inside the body.

The acids in animal products are far harder on the body than are the acids of nuts and seeds. The residuals left in the body when animal products break down—the purines and uric acids—are fiery and aging to the body. Therefore, for these and many other reasons, animal products should be minimized in the diet or avoided completely.

For some of us, those who are more sensitive to the suffering of living things—including the non-humans—all we need to do is investigate such phenomena as CAFOs. These are the Concentrated Animal Feeding Operations. This is a tragedy of global proportions. CAFOs are industrial animal factories where these innocent creatures are confined for weeks at a time. Do just a little investigation and it'll turn your stomach.

The adverse effects of these operations on the environment are horrendous. Huge tracts of land—including in the Amazon Rainforest area—have been and continue to be cleared to raise cattle so we can have hamburgers. The slaughter of animals just for the pleasure or tastes of humans has karmic consequences we do not like to contemplate. In fact, we are already suffering them.

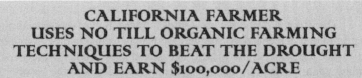

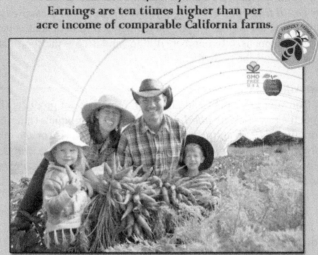

These animals, these non-humans, want to live. They have feelings. Keep one as a pet, and you'll see. Their love is very direct. Show them just a little compassion and kindness and they'll give it back many fold. They want to roam freely in pastures, not forced into pens (concentration camps) where they can barely move. I lived in the country where factory hens were kept in tiny wire cages, never enjoying the sunlight or pecking on the ground.

Again, just do some investigating. It'll break your heart—unless your heart has already turned to stone. Unless you are used to rationalizing away the suffering of billions of animals just so you can have a tasty meal you don't even need, one that acidifies your body and darkens your soul, your psyche. If we had to kill an animal to survive, that's one thing. But that ain't the case here. That is definitely not the case!

The food industry is the biggest in the world—bigger than oil, bigger, even, than drugs. Everyone has to eat. But...we have given over the production of food to huge monstrosities, big corporations governed by psychopaths—unfeeling, uncaring, unsympathetic characters lacking in empathy, unable to feel the suffering of others, humans and non-humans alike. We need to take back our food production—and keep it in the hands of normal adult humans!

One option is a design for living described near the end of this book called Espheria (Appendix G). This involves small community units that grow at least most of their own food. Getting back to small organic farms is another way to solve our current food situation. Organic gardening and farming are far more productive and economical than the big chemical-laden operations (industrial farming). This has been proven many times over.

We don't hear much about this because of the enormous power and money involved that buys advertising in the media—and thus supports and in some ways "owns" the media. But. Again, we can change this situation. There is strength in numbers. When enuf of us want to do this, it will happen.

25—Local vs. Distant

Serving the Body, the Community, and the Planet

Notice how each geographic locality has its own special qualities. Rome is heavy with art. New York has hi culture. Paris is known for its romance—and fabulous cuisine. Las Vegas…well… Each location has its special charm, even Las Vegas. The plains of central Texas are so different from the beaches of Western Australia. Settling in and living for periods of time at any of these or other Earth locations, one begins to get the full flavor of the area, what it has to offer in terms of people, food, weather, and its various energies.

We have been given to understand that herbs from China can heal virtually all ailments if provided at the rite time and in the rite potency. But there is another understanding we can have of geography and the quality of herbs—and foods. Local-grown foods and herbs have the local energies in them, and therefore properties that are most healing for beings living in the local environment. This understanding has been largely lost on modern people.

Any area of the world where plants grow contains healing substances that are most effective to the local inhabitants, the animals, and people who dwell nearby. Animals seem to know this instinctively. They do not need to travel across oceans to find the grasses or shrubs that will help them heal. Humans may have lost the instinct (if we ever had it)—or at least the knowledge—of such healing substances. But they are available to us locally, nonetheless.

The lore of local herbs, plants, and foods that heal has been passed down thru the generations in every area and culture on Earth. True, natural disasters, cultural events, certain groups, and individuals have erased such lore from time to time. Technology advances culture in specific ways. Wars have come and gone, and with their passing, certain plant wisdom has also vanished. In this sense, one of our most painful tragedies of antiquity was the burning destruction of the vast library at Alexandria, where one-of-a-kind books were lost forever.

At various times in our history—especially during the Middle Ages—adventurers, churches, and religious fanatics have set out purposely to destroy whole civilizations, burning their artifacts, books, art, paintings, and records of their cultures. This, of course, is despicable, erasing our heritage, our common human history. This is a way to control people, to move us in a philosophical direction desired by the plunderers, the "victors" (read "savages"!).

Our current technology allows for infinite numbers of literary copies to be made. Better still, helpful health knowledge and wisdom can be spread electronically worldwide instantly over the Internet. This is a significant advantage, especially when it involves genuine health wisdom. Adidam Radical Healing is an example of such Wisdom. And traditional and ancient health wisdom is also coming online and being made generally available.

Altho there may be some 200 nations currently existing in this world, many more languages than that are represented therein. The confusion that persisted thru the ages from lack of understanding each other's speech has recently been fading by the emergence of English as the tongue that finally connects us all as a human family in these crucial-to-survival times and in this critical area of life—communication.

Instant translations on the Net also help significantly. We have the opportunity to communicate our great desire for peace and freedom, for tolerance and cooperation, and for sharing the joys of life. This makes every place on Earth and every people close-by. This is so important to our sense of being a single human family. (see the book, *__Prior Unity__*).

Food-taking is among the oldest ways we humans share good energy in peace. Only relatively recently in our history have we been able to transport food over long distances. Most of our food was gathered from our local environments. We would join with family and friends to enjoy the local harvest. This cultural event continues in smaller cultural areas of the world.

In more recent times, where cultural development shows evidence of advanced technology, large markets have sprung up with foods from countries all over the world. In the process of transporting and consuming these foods, there are health and economic factors we have not fully accounted for—factors that are quite negative.

Yes, oranges from Florida are tasty and healthy. But, why are people in California eating oranges from Florida when oranges grow readily and plentifully in California? Can this involve the trucking industry, trade unions, and politics? It certainly involves enormous wastes of energy, the horrific expense in dollars, the wear and tear on human life and machines, pollution via gasoline, oil, diesel fumes, and brake dust, and people and animals killed on roadways.

Of course, people in Canada need to have fresh produce during the winter season. And what's wrong with them enjoying dates from California's Imperial Valley—or from Saudi Arabia, for that matter? Nothing, but where's the balance? Certainly it's something more intelligent and less polluting than the system we have now.

At Grand Medicine, San Marcos, California, we've been growing carob, guavas, and cherimoyas along with veggies in our backyard garden. With a rightly structured greenhouse, people from virtually any part of the world can grow their own food. Everything from apples to avocados, from coconuts to cacao (see Appendix G). Every human being should have easy access to locally-grown pesticide-free natural produce. The point is…we can!

A significant part of this high toll on our environment and on us altogether can be alleviated by resorting to local farms, and to community and private gardens, restoring flora and fauna to their original forms and locations. During WWII, we planted "victory gardens" out of necessity. There were food shortages developed from sending so much food overseas to our soldiers, so we had to plant our own food in our back yards. It worked.

Many of us find it hard to even conceive of being involved in such activity at this point in our hectic lives, even tho we want to. Others can. Creating cooperative community (CoopCom—see Appendix G) is one sure way to help solve this situation of great waste, and at the same time bring *human scale* stability, sustainability, and order, to our culture—and to our planet!

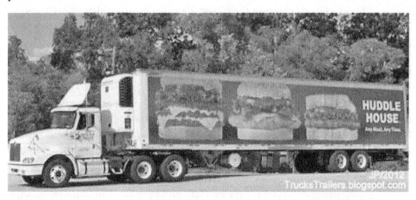

The energies of the local area where we live are shared by plants and animals, and this includes humans. We're talking all kinds of energy, including physical, vital, etheric, emotional, mental, psychic, astral, mystical, causal, and Spiritual. These energies blend in a meld of harmony that nourishes us at all levels of being. *The herbs that grow in our local environment are the best ones to heal us at the physical level*. We needn't go to China or other countries—altho herbs from these various other areas can be helpful in certain instances.

Please note, BTW, how our present world cultural model is steeped in and stuck in gross pseudo-scientific materialism, dismissing the many other levels of the human sensorium noted in the last paragraph. This effectively denies us a huge and important part of our native humanity—another human tragedy being sustained by the "powers that shouldn't be". We can and must turn this picture around (see the book, *Not-Two Is Peace*).

In past times, local healers and shamanic medicine practitioners had a repertoire of only ten local herbs for all the maladies that could attend life in their tribe. This was fairly common among such groups—and among indigenous people everywhere before the current civilization. Now, we seem to need medicines of a bewildering variety. Why? And our medical texts describe hundreds of never-before-seen disorders. Why?

Because we have built enormous complication into our lives. We have, as the Native American term puts it, Koyaanisqatsi: "life out of balance." We must find ways of simplifying our lives. Is CoopCom an answer? At least one answer? Can CoopCom pre-solve so many of our current cultural, social and economic ills? Will locally-grown natural foods and herbs be enuf to handle the many new maladies our complex and toxic culture has developed? Maybe we need to do an experiment here and find out. What do we have to lose?

Don't Just Buy Local—Buy *In-Season* Local

Increasingly, we as "consumers" are beginning to understand the enormous environmental and economic benefits of living, staying, and buying local. We're talking about food that is grown nearby. Industrial agriculture and long-distance food transportation and processing now generate up to 25% of all climate-destabilizing greenhouse gases. Massive amounts of CO^2 are produced when the average often highly-processed and wastefully-packaged store-bought food item travels 1500-2500 miles from farm or processing plant to our plates.

Meanwhile, farmer's markets across the country are reporting record attendance and sales. We do the planet and climate an enormous favor when purchasing items grown by farmers in our area, by encouraging and developing community gardens, and, of course, by growing our own food in our own back (and front!) yards. This is bringing things back to human-scale (16-25 people), a scale of life we can trust—and be and hold others accountable in!

Buying foods *in-season* can be as valuable as buying locally. A bag of tomatoes grown locally has less of an energy impact on the environment than those shipped from Peru. But tomatoes grown out of season in a heated greenhouse can have an energy impact exceeding those imported. We're not suggesting buying tomatoes from Chile in winter, but looking for foods that are grown locally in season or that were grown or otherwise prepared locally.

We can, in truth, create human-scale local environments where life can be far simpler and less expensive to ourselves and the environment than the current chaotic circumstance. True, things could get worse—far worse. But, why wait for that? We need more balanced, Nature-harmonious systems of food production that are currently available. And we have all the talent and technology available to accomplish it.

Meanwhile, until we do get together via the Internet—everybody-all-at-once—as described in the book, _Not-Two Is Peace_, and create a true Wisdom Culture, we can do so many little things individually to—as Michael Jackson sang—make the world a better place. I'm not talking idealistically. No! I'm talking very practically and realistically.

26—Liquids vs. Solids
Strategies for Regaining and Maintaining Health

Most of us, by far, while on the GLD, are not consuming many of the foods we would normally eat—likely much more on the "raw" side, right? Pizza, pastries, bread foods, animal products in general, and virtually all processed foods—these all fall away on the GLD. Some of us may be taking cooked foods like blended soups (or at least hot raw liquids) at some point or points on the GLD. These are not from cans, bottles, and boxes—in other words, they are fresh raw, and not processed foods. They are *wholesome*, made of living produce.

This higher percentage of wholesome quality food is much of what makes the difference between the GLD and other diets. The fasting principle (*liquefying* before intake) is what does the rest. The dietary *parameters* of the GLD (i.e., mostly or all raw liquids) are far clearer and easier to follow than those of most diets. These and other qualities make the GLD easier to do and otherwise superior to solid food diets.

Water is the perennial and perfect liquid for living beings on Earth. Water *quality* is another subject that always arises while on the GLD. For many, the best waters to drink are often those purchased in plastic bottles in local markets (see Chapter 36). Of course, plastic isn't the healthiest carrier for water—and we urge you to avoid it. Waters that are appropriate to drink, whether on the GLD or not, include variously filtered waters, especially including multiple filtered and (most especially) steam distilled.

Perhaps among the better filters currently available are **Mr. Water Filter®** and **Pure Water©** steam distiller units. Tap waters can be of varied quality, many containing poisonous chlorine, and others with fluoride, an even worse toxin. If tap water is your only resort, use this remedy: up to 45% of the chlorine can be dispersed by placing uncapped glass containers of the chlorinated water in the frig for 40 hours each. But, try your very best to avoid this crap! Bypass the whole mess by purchasing a **Pure Water© Mini-Classic II** steam distiller unit.

GLD Allowable Liquids

- Amazaki
- Herb teas
- Pure water
- Smoothies
- Homemade veggy broths
- Homemade blended veggy soups, cooked & (especially) raw
- Sips from natural-style pickle & sauerkraut jars (salty/sour)
- Homemade raw nut and seeds milks (see Appendix A)
- *RMVJ* (or other single or mixed raw veggy juice)
- Carob and cacao hot drinks (Appendix A)

Right Use vs. Indulgence

Eventually (usually quickly!), on your GLD, you will come face-to-face with your tendencies regarding food and how it is typically used (or otherwise <u>abused</u>) by you—no praise, no blame. You will have favorite liquids, favorite individual recipes, and favorite combinations (and favorite snacks!). You must become sensitive to and aware of this process of indulging taste desires and tendencies and how it works with the actual needs of the body—which needs to include only fresh raw <u>nuts and seeds</u>, fresh raw <u>veggies</u>, and fresh ripe raw <u>fruits</u>.

As Adi Da says, *"There is no law that says food has to taste good or to give you the illusion of ecstasy."* Food needs to be able to truly nourish the gross physical body. That's it. And, of course, raw living foods do this best—tho they may not taste as good as the great cuisines of the Chinese or the French. This is, of course, a very good point to keep in mind during your venture into the raw liquids of the GLD—and also for when you're finished with your GLD and getting into the hi-raw or all-raw *solid food* diet.

Some of us tend to like fruits more than veggies—i.e., e.g., those who have genetic tendencies to carbo metabolism dysfunctions, toward so-called hypoglycemia or diabetes. In these more extreme cases of this tendency or pattern, they may select only fruit juices for whole days at a time. Others prefer veggies juices, so these will tend to be emphasized. Still others, savoring the rich, thick smoothies with their nuts and seeds, will focus on them.

Except for the veggie preference, this is very likely mere indulgence. Notice this and immediately go back to including the three primary food groups—daily. Maintain this *three-basic-food-groups-daily* balance, and keep the percentage of raw liquids intake at or above 95%, and you'll be fine.

Of course, one or the other of these three food groups will inevitably be emphasized on any given day. However, you should always try to (1) be aware of your tendencies to be self-indulgent, and (2) be sure to get all three groups in daily. One way to do this: get your Green Smoothie (always!) maybe adding some RMVJ. Note that if and when you do your GLD as your gift to the Divine, the whole process will be easier and bring you greater self-understanding. That conscious connection with the Divine makes a huge difference!

Liquids vs. Solids

It is essential to minimize solid food intake on your GLD because of the effectiveness of pure liquids vs. solids. Liquefying foods allows for their easy passage thru the alimentary tract (stomach and bowel), which involves the events of digestion (mouth and stomach), absorption and assimilation (small intestine), and waste processing / mineral re-uptake (large bowel).

Liquids require less energy to process than do solids, first in the mouth, then in the stomach, and finally in the small and large bowel. Thus, with the juicer and blender turning the solid foods into liquids (instead of your jaws doing all that work), there is far less need to process solid wastes. This means that more bodily energy (and reserve energy) is available for purification, healing, and rejuvenation.

GLD Snacks are Not Liquids

Some of us are so fixed on food, so dependent on gross food for pleasure, so devoid of connection with The Divine Person, that we tend to think of food many times daily. We think of the frig, the pantry, the secret area next to our desk where we have our "provide stash" of our tastiest treats. So, when we learn we can have snacks on our GLD, we think, '*Yahoo!*' Each day, we get into a few chips or pretzels, a "natural-style" dip, nut butter, etc.

Checking our weight, we notice that the number and degree of our snacking equates to little or no weight loss. "*Ouch! What have I done? OK, no snacks for me today.*" Many of the snacks allowed on your GLD (nut butters, guacamole, chips, pretzels, crackers—see the list in Chapter 7) are solid foods. The rest are sauces, gels, and thick, rich nut or seed butters. These require a lot more digestion than the liquids. That energy could go to purification.

The suggestion here is to consider your actual need for snacks—e.g., if you're a thin-body type, a fast metabolizer, and needing to gain weight. In that case, snacks can be beneficial. If you are obese, are a very slow metabolizer, or have cancer or some other (or combination of) chronic degenerative diseases, you want to be on GLD *Level 1*—meaning no snacks. For the rest of us, it's experiment time, self-discovery time—or simple avoidance.

Food Processing by the Body vs. Commercial Machine
Q. Where does the GLD's extra energy come from?
Ans. Processing!—at every level of the gross physical body, starting with the mouth and jaws, the stomach and small intestine, and the large bowel. After being processed by the GI (gastrointestinal) system, the food goes to the liver for its processing. Then, it goes to all the other systems, organs, and tissues. They all play a role in food, even if it's just nutrient metabolism, nutrient uptake by its cells.

A huge amount of energy is expended chewing, digesting, absorbing, assimilating, and finally moving and eliminating food and its waste materials thru the alimentary canal, mouth to anus. And then there is the metabolizing of food particles, which occurs all thru the rest of the body, all the other organs, and tissues.

Therefore, much energy is saved for purification by foods that have had their fiber extracted (juices) or otherwise broken into tiny bits (blender liquids). Here, of course, we're talking about living foods, solid and liquefied. Regarding the blended foods, the fiber has been broken down to such an extent that it is far easier to process by the body than if it were chewed in the whole state. That blender-processed bulk and ruffage are still quite useful by the bowel—as "union-scale" wages for the bowel muscles.

Energy expense and the Insult of Commercially Processed Foods
This food processing energy that is expended by the body, has, of course, an analog in food commerce and industry. The food industry is the biggest in the world, bigger than drugs, bigger than oil, bigger than insurance and banking. The food processing industry began in the late 1800s, perhaps with the invention of trans fats in 1890 or so. It is costly to "process" food industrially, turning produce into packaged foods.

When you get into the details of commercially and industrially processed food, and consider all that involves over against the great desire of us rushed, stressed-out, frustrated consumers for convenience, you begin to realize why we settle for a Gag-In-The-Bag burger and fries over against the 20 minutes it takes to prepare a big glass of RMVJ. Within 10 minutes of stopping at the burger joint on the way home from work, you have your "meal."

The money you just spent on the burger and fries could have purchased five meal's worth of raw produce. Of course, more than the money are the health benefits. When you consider the cost differences, the prep time, the health differential, and any and all other factors, you're still ahead by buying the raw produce and making your own meals. Of course, if you're living with others where you share household duties, self-prep wins easily!

Raw foods are industry processed by cutting, slicing, dicing, boiling, frying, mashing, adding food coloring, baking, cooking, broiling, mincing, shredding, powdering, adding surfactants, coloring agents and other preservatives, etc., etc. In other words, industry processing means raw food has had its integrity taken from it. It is no longer integral, whole. It is broken down, as when you slice an apple, but profoundly more. What happens to it?

Losing its natural vitality and integrity, processed food is thus insulting to the body. It is, in general, insulting to our consciousness to abuse the body with anything other than pure foods. It is even insulting to those who sell processed foods to receive money for something less than pure for the body. The only way we can justify this kind of food is as emergency rations or as celebratory fare.

Seeing Around Corners to Aid the Vulnerable

The liquefying factor may also help isolate allergens, irritants, and other food / dietary / orally-taken substances that do not belong in the body. Perhaps more specifically, ruffage and bulk processing by the body may slow down or otherwise somehow interfere with our discerning of which orally taken substances need to be eliminated or minimized by the body. In other words, GLD foods are only pure, natural, and mostly raw—which excludes the foods that tend to make us sick.

This is especially important with folks in significantly compromised states of health—the very young, the very old, those in shock, those suffering from weather extremes and disaster trauma, and those with chronic degenerative diseases. All of these people are more vulnerable to the effects of drugs, parasites, and crap food—the LQFs. The GLD provides them with immune-boosting strength and efficiency.

27—Intake Quantity

An Ancient and Realistic Formula

How much liquid can we drink on the GLD?

There is no limit to the amount or number of liquids you may consume on your GLD. However, over the days, we notice that we are naturally drinking less and less, and choosing the fresh raw juices and smoothies over the cooked or pasteurized liquids (store-bot juices, etc.). We will thus be drinking purer liquids and getting higher nourishment, since the raw juices provide our body with more of the living nutrients it was genetically designed for.

With the Green Smoothie, which is generally our most important GLD liquid, those of us who are more "physically abundant" (200 lbs. or more) may take 32 oz. per day or more. An average-sized person might take 20 oz. per day, while smaller people may take 16-18 oz. daily. Also, note that the stomach shrinks on the GLD, and the appetite with it, so you'll wind up not taking in as much food volume as you usually do when eating solid foods.

Age and relative energy output are two more factors in the question of how much to drink. Young persons are usually more active than are elders. They need to take in more nutrition. When consuming raw liquids, the judgment call is easy. The body tells us when to stop. This doesn't happen with cooked liquids or cooked solids. This is our next consideration.

The question of how much to drink can be answered by considering the question of raw versus cooked. Raw freshly prepared juices will stimulate the brain center involved with satiety (the feeling of being food-satisfied). This center tells us when we have had enuf of a particular nutrient or nutrients. Unlike with cooked foods, raw foods set off this mechanism because the cells of the body are programmed to receive only raw living foods as nourishment.

Therefore, when higher percentages of cooked food enter the body, the body tends to call for more in volume in its attempt to discover any real nutrients (which come from living foods) that may be available—so it can know when to quit. Thus, the human physical body demonstrates **no instinct for cooked food**.

Human Instinct for Food

So, we do have an instinct for food. This is easily proven. Purchase a large pizza. Eat as many pieces as you like—or as you can! Get stuffed on it. On your way to the frig to put away the remaining pieces, notice how it still smells so good! Take another bite. It still tastes good! Next day, prepare a large bowl of fresh strawberries and dive in. At some point, the strawberries

will no longer taste good! What is happening? Try this with apples. Same result! How many apples can you eat before they no longer taste good?

Your body is telling you that it no longer needs the nutrients in the apple—or the strawberries, or other raw natural living food. Your body has had enuf of the nutrients in them, so it turns off the "tastes good" switch. It cannot do this with the pizza ***because there is no instinct for pizza*** <u>or for any cooked food</u>—which is why the pizza will always taste good, even when your stomach is full to bursting with it!

Thus, when we drink more of the raw juices and liquids, we will automatically know when to quit, when our body has had enuf. However, during a given day, we may have both raw juices and cooked liquids—like soups. The body will not have the same simple response. Why not? The answer is because of the presence of the cooked (home-cooked!) liquids. But, don't make a problem out of it. As long as the liquids are as pure as you can find, it still doesn't matter terribly how much you drink.

This is especially so during the first few weeks of your GLD. Over time, after a month or so, it becomes easier to judge how much to drink, mainly because the purity of the liquids will necessarily curb your appetite so that your liquid meals will gradually and increasingly become smaller. In this case, the principle is: "*Purity counts—and almost nothing else counts*." So, the basic rule is: *drink until you feel right and comfortable but not stuffed*. Also notice any tendency to drink just for pleasure—a habit that can be overcome. Pray about it (Appendix G).

28—Age and Longevity
What We Know and What We Don't

A Loose, Relaxed, Youthful Body

At the level of the gross physical body, raw diet and yoga are two primary practices that guarantee good health. The musculo-structural system of the human body will "loosen" with raw food and yoga, and "tighten" with cooked and processed food (and no yoga). This looseness and flexibility is associated with youthfulness and strength.

When we say "tite" in this regard, we're not talking about the taut muscles of a bodybuilder. We're talking about the tightness, stiffness, and hardness of so-called "arthritis" and general body tissue inflammation—that comes with a diet of mostly cooked food. On such a diet, this tightness may start in the lower back when you first get out of bed. You may feel it in your hands and feet, then your wrists, ankles, and knees—first as simple stiffness, then, as the mineral buildup impinges on nerves, as real pain. Your choice: loose or tite, flexible or stiff, health or disease?

This painful and degenerative health phenomenon resulting from excessive cooked and processed food intake involves hi acid wastes circulating thru the body. During muscle activity, minerals are drawn out of bones and then accumulate in joints where they eventually impinge on nerves (the pain). These minerals can't get back into the bones where they came from because of the acid condition of the blood. There is not enuf natural salt—sodium—as in raw celery. This is why two big sticks of celery daily are so often prescribed for arthritis by Natural Health practitioners.

On the other hand, the body efficiently uses the living nutrients in raw foods and easily eliminates their wastes, obviating the cooked food/pain syndrome. Minerals easily pass in and out of bones and muscles as needed. In some sense, it's a percentage game: the higher the percentage raw, the more loose, relaxed and youthful the body.

Digestion, Absorption, and Assimilation on the GLD

Most *digestion* of food takes place in the stomach. Our work at Grand Medicine has confirmed medical research findings that beyond age 45, the stomach's ability to digest food decreases. As we age, stomach <u>acids</u> weaken, their output or secretion diminishes, and the stomach's muscular <u>walls</u> lose strength as the whole process of stomach digestion lessens.

This suggests the importance of....

(1) ***thoroughly chewing*** all foods (liquid or solid) before swallowing, and...

(2) gradually ***increasing the % of pure raw liquids*** as we age

Our experience at Grand Medicine, both personal and clinical, bears this out.

Assimilation is another related factor. It's one thing to digest food well, and yet another for the small intestine to absorb and assimilate it. An expression in the Natural Health field is, *"We are what we assimilate!"* While the stomach handles most of the *digestion*, most *absorption and assimilation* take place in the small bowel. And this is the center of most allergic reactions in the body.

Various toxics from environmental and food chemicals and other outside sources, toxins from the body's reactions, and parasites, can substantially interfere with the passage of nutrients from the small intestine (absorption and assimilation) into the liver for processing. (From the liver, nutrient-laden blood goes to all the cells of the body.) The pure liquids of the GLD solve the problem of efficient absorption and assimilation nicely. Gradually, on the GLD—whether the 1st, the 2nd, or an extended GLD, the small intestine and the rest of the body will be purified.

A Humorous Encounter with an Attorney
Once, we were called to a luncheon meeting by a Malibu attorney. We wondered, *"What have we done wrong? Are we being sued?"* It turned out that the attorney was managing the estate of an elderly man (age 96) and his former secretary (age 87) whom we had been treating as patients. Earlier, in our office, the caregivers described the common diet they'd been preparing for this couple. These old folks were suffering from dementia and needed round-the-clock care.

So, these old-timers were dependent on their caregivers, and the caregivers, on orders from the estate manager, were now dependent on what we recommended. Knowing the power of pure foods, we wanted to see how far we could go in improving the health of these senior citizens. We suggested a diet consisting of mostly pure liquids: fresh raw juices and smoothies, and a little cooked veggie soup.

Enter the attorney! At the luncheon, we awaited the reason for the unusual appointment. *"What are you feeding these people?"* was his first question. The bewildered lawyer wondered by what process our elderly patients had developed such spunk that they were jumping into bed with each other!

Children and the GLD
There is no "best age" at which to engage the GLD. Altho children below the age of 16 should not fast (they will spontaneously avoid food when

"sick" or otherwise when they don't feel well), those with various diseases may safely do the GLD—and for as long as their adult guides deem necessary. This is due to the hi-density nutrient availability in GLD liquids. Notwithstanding, placing children on the GLD should be done under the care of a qualified practitioner.

Chronic degenerative diseases tend to increase in frequency as we age, mainly due to...

- the increasing results of negative-reactive emotions (the NREs, egoity)
- the progressive degeneration of simple aging
- years of past &/or continuing dietary insult
- life-negative lifestyle factors
- the stresses and strains of living in our crazy random culture
- the lesser ability of the lymphatic-immune to respond to challenges
- unfortunate life circumstances

Thus, the elderly most often need the GLD—for improving their health, dealing with pain, and even saving their very lives. The GLD is an advantage for everyone, from ages 3 to 103 and beyond. The older the body, the more help the GLD will provide—and the more likely it will be appropriate. The GLD's liquids make digestion and all other body functions easier, overall, than virtually any solid food diet—including all-raw diets. The "raw" and the "liquid" factors make the difference.

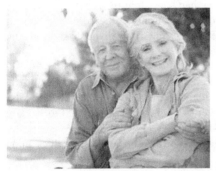

Unlike us adults, who eat vast amounts of cooked and processed foods (often just for fun, even when not hungry), infants and toddlers tend to stop when full. We adults, when getting into hi-raw or all-raw, also tend to stop when full. This is normal, since the body as a whole and in its parts—especially the satiety center of the brain—is satisfied genuinely on eating pure raw produce. The brain's automatic mechanism within the satiety center, sends this signal to the stomach saying, "*Hey, that's all you need; you can stop eating now.*" This occurs with raw foods but not with cooked foods.

So, toddlers fed a diet of all raw vegetal food—which is all they ever really need to be healthy—can have as much as they'll accept, and that includes the raw liquids. They'll naturally stop when they've had enuf. And while fresh liquids need to be diluted to some degree for infants, not so much or even at all for 1-yr-olds and above. Just make sure you're using untainted natural produce and staying with the three primary food groups.

Longevity

Can the GLD extend life? Yes! By how much involves several factors. How well are you applying your GLD? What is the general health of your body on initiating the GLD? For how long would it be best and most effective for you to continue on the GLD? What is your attitude about life and your use of the GLD? Do you understand the physical, mental, and emotional qualities that affect your immune response—big factors in health and longevity? Are you engaged in either religious or Real Spiritual practice?

As Avatar Adi Da says, "*The constantly changing body is really the product of a process of patterning that began at birth. Our current body isn't the same body as when we were a child. There is a complete change every 7-10 years in the elementals or material aspects of the body. It is a constantly self-replicating pattern that itself keeps shifting and changing, a process. The ego wants it to be an unchanging continuous person. But, it's not the same body even one moment to the next. Death is built in, intended.*"

Altho physical immortality is not the design of the human body, it seems to your author that, given our current technology, we should be able to live 150 to 200 years and more. In general, we could accomplish this by:

1 – Taking pure raw diet
2 – Fortunate life circumstances
3 – Avoiding hi-stress situations and environments
4 – Skillfully dealing with the body in its associations
5 – Engaging in life-positive lifestyle practices—***The BIG 7***
6 – living in a human-scale (cooperative community) circumstance
7 – Carefully observing the body's qualities, cycles, timing, changes, and responses
8 – Recognition of the Divine Reality and responding accordingly via genuine devotional communion

It takes most of us 60-odd years just to realize the importance of caring for the body to where we actually begin a program of regular life-positive activities. By then, it's often too late! We're already gray, wrinkled, ugly, gnarly, diseased, worn out, grossly tired, burdened by life-negative patterns, chronically sick, struggling with a whole series of bad habits, and otherwise going downhill on a sled! But, what if we could have a significant extension of our bodily life? Consider these possibilities:

Four Possible Lengths of Physical Bodily Life (as of 2019)

Average Length of Life of the human body *in our current world culture* = 68 years

Estimated *Projected Length* of the average body's life *with reasonable care* = 115 years

Estimated *Probable Length* of the average body's life *with high maintenance care* = 155 years

Estimated *Possible Length* of the average body's life *under optimum circumstances* = 230 years

As suggested, the average person doesn't even provide the body with "reasonable care"—much less "high maintenance care." Of course, we must take into account factors of world culture. It doesn't take a great imagination to grasp what these terms involve. But, what about "optimum activity" or "optimum circumstances"? What is that all about?

Optimum Activity: Keys to Longevity

All chronic degenerative diseases seem to have certain qualities in common. One of these is *a triggering factor*, which most often is diet insult. The average number of trigger factors is 2, but there can be as many as 10. Lack of exercise or far too much exercise can be (and often is) another. With diet, people in general, even those of us who have enuf food to eat, just <u>don't know *how*</u> to eat—which is often why our life is cut short.

On interviewing patients over the years, we've noticed these "trigger factors" again and again. E.g., if a person has a genetic tendency to heart disease and diabetes (easily seen in the irises of the eyes), poor diet and lack of exercise can bring on both of these disorders. On the other hand, even while their parents may have had those and many other diseases, and even if they inherited these tendencies, pure diet and life-positive lifestyle can obviate the disorders completely—and they will never suffer them: like, "the buck stops here!"

Regarding *#2 (fortunate circumstances)*: karma (egoity, the failure to practice rite life, failure to turn to the Divine) can bring all manner of stress and trauma to one's life. Those of us living in Western countries, and certain wealthier people in other locales, can enjoy less physical, mental, and emotional stress, plus reasonable safety and security. "Fortunate circumstances" can also involve simply acting intelligently, consciously staying out of harm's way, not having traumatic accidents, not placing oneself into problematic situations, and also Divine Grace.

Item **#4** (*skillful body management*) means intelligently handling the body in these various circumstances—like avoiding reaction, remaining calm and heart-peaceful, having faith in the universe (in God), taking pure food and life-positive lifestyle, and (most of all) remembering and turning to the Beloved of the Heart in every moment of life. (This last one sounds easy, but it's actually at once the hardest <u>and most important</u> activity anyone can ever do!)

Item **#6** (*observing bodily qualities*) means noticing how the body changes in the midst of its cycles, observing the timing of rest and sleep—like how much rest and sleep the body needs under various circumstances, what happens when certain kinds of food are taken, and how it responds and reacts when in certain environments. This is not about spending endless hours merely watching the body in its play. This "observation" is done naturally amid Spiritual practice.

Item **#7** (*real Spiritual practice*) involves engaging in <u>genuine</u> Spiritual practice, which is extremely rare. It's exceedingly rare these days to even know what Real Spiritual practice is—much less to do it. Most people don't know what it really is—or only think they do. What usually passes for religious or Spiritual practice these days is anywhere from watching sunsets to following prescribed rituals, rules, laws, and legalisms (Big religion)— nothing esoteric, nothing about submitting to, surrendering to, combining with Spirit—or how to do these practices.

While They were Alive in a human Body The Great Saints, Sages and Yogis both Knew and Taught the free and immediate Real Spirituality. It was always about God-Love and love of our fellow man. After Their death, however, as has happened so often historically, Big religion (downtown silly religion), in relentless efforts to capture and control the masses (us), eliminated virtually all references to True, esoteric Spiritual practice. Love of God became ritual and lip service. Love of man became "behead for Allah" and "kill for Christ"—i.e., service to the State.

Actually doing Real Spiritual practice requires the Good Company of other practitioners, studying the Teachings of the Adept Spiritual Master, and sacrifice of "self" to The Liberating Principle, the Divine in the Form of the Awakener. It requires Divine Grace. As Adi Da says, it is turning to the Divine whole-bodily via the four basic functions or faculties of (1) bodily activity, (2) breath, (3) attention (the root of mind), and (4) emotional feeling. This will certainly serve to enhance and lengthen your bodily life!

Old-Age and Vulnerability

As the body ages, the various systems tend to "wind down," to lose some of their functional ability to withstand the stresses of normal life. There are, of course, cultural mechanisms that can lessen the impact of this process, but much more can be done in this regard (see Appendix G). Meanwhile, the aging process generally makes us increasingly vulnerable to weakening of our basic senses, to infectious organisms, and to slow healing of wounds.

It can be quite irritating to notice that you can't see as well as you used to, to need hearing aids, to lose teeth, and to be bumping into things, not as well aware of the position of your body in space. This is in addition to the gray hair, baldness, memory lapses, wrinkles, and saggy skin. *"Hey, I'm not supposed to look like this! What's happening to me? Something's not right."* It's called aging, and, like it or not, it's here to stay. Might as well get used to it!

It's important to note, tho, that ***aging can be slowed down*** by simple health practices—like the yearly 30-day GLD! Right oral care can save teeth. Right exercise can help slow or prevent much of the wrinkles and sagging skin. Altho pure raw liquids (and raw diet generally) can help strengthen the immune system against infections and inflammation in general, infections and wounds will take longer to resolve. The elderly will be more vulnerable.

That said, you can still function well, even into your 80s, 90s, 100s, and beyond. Yes! With reasonable care, so-called old age can be the most creative and productive time of your life. This has been proven over millennia. True, there are certain limits in these conditional realms (Earth), limits to which the body is vulnerable. However, we needn't *presume* more limits than are real or merited! The body can remain balanced, and the mind can remain sharp and highly functional, especially when Guided by Grace and clarified by Wisdom!

The Food Connection

Food, of course, is crucial to longevity. The way we eat food, its quality, and its quantity—these enter into the equation of bodily longevity. Our food must be purifying as well as nourishing. When foods are liquefied, they are easier on the teeth, not just the stomach. Less bodily energy is expended altogether on the GLD compared with other diets containing solid foods. Therefore, the GLD can be useful for longevity, for extending the life of the body.

The GLD may thus be taken for indefinite periods of time—6 months and longer, with or without solid food breaks. Moreover, "fasting" (for our purposes, read "liquid dieting") is more basic to us as humans in our long history on this Earth than is eating solid foods. In our pre-history, we actually spent more time *searching* for food (fasting) than we did *eating* it! So, that makes fasting more fundamental than eating. Eating comes <u>after</u> fasting.

Fasting is about purification, and purification—at every level of being—is the name of the game in bodily life. Fasting is known, both historically and scientifically, to lengthen life. Given our world's current highly toxic environments, periodic fasting is basically intelligent. An intelligently applied yearly 30-Day GLD can be used very well for this purpose. BTW, one can be extremely old and still be healthy!

On learning of certain scientific studies, some have gotten into strategic "under-eating." They've heard about the scientific experiments with animals in which less food was fed to them which made them live longer. They've heard about the scientific experiments with animals in which less food was fed to them, and they lived longer. So these people get into what they think will be similar in order to lengthen their life.

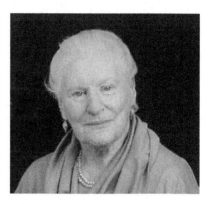

However, when taking *pure raw* food, whether as solids or as liquids, the life of the body will automatically tend to lengthen—without strategic under-eating—mainly because of the natural satiety factor signal from the brain.

As noted, the GLD is ***a food delivery system*** involving consuming *higher percentages* of pure raw foods—via the liquefication factor. The GLD won't make us happy, but if we pray while on it, engaging it <u>as conscious Divine Communion</u>, we sanctify it and are thereby Blessed—at all levels of being. This, plus the above practices, brings a life of equanimity, all serving the lengthening of life.

Certain herbs and SuperFoods have long been known to extend life. There are many ancient legends and tales, including in the Christian bible, of people living hundreds of years. More recently, it is said there are records of a man in China who lived for well over 200 years. He apparently used certain herbs such as ginseng, plus breathing exercises such as those described in <u>Conductivity Healing</u>, to gain and maintain longevity. He lived in the mountains and, of course, did not suffer the stresses of foreign chemicals, junk foods, and the threat of technological annihilation!

Intelligently making use of the Divine, we feed the heart with <u>true</u> Happiness (the hearts greatest desire). Happy, we will not merely live longer. Happiness can definitely <u>make</u> the body live longer. And, why would one want to live longer unless one could be happy in the process?

Enzymes, Health, and Aging

Enzymes are crucial to life. As already mentioned, there are basically three kinds of enzymes: *food*, *digestive*, and ***metabolic***. Food enzymes exist naturally in raw foods, digestive enzymes are produced essentially by the mouth and stomach, and metabolic enzymes are found all thru the body. Each type of enzyme has its role in the health and maintenance of the body.

Food enzymes mix with digestive enzymes to prepare the food as forms useful by the body. Digestive enzymes break the food down further for absorption and assimilation by the small intestine so it can go to the liver. From there, the food molecules are sent into the bloodstream for metabolic processing.

Metabolic enzymes are protein molecules that initiate and control almost every biochemical reaction in the body. They are needed to break down food particles into components our cells can use for energy, rebuild and repair all types of tissue, enable iron molecules to link with red blood cells so that they can carry oxygen throughout our bodies, detoxify blood and tissues, and help the immune system to function optimally.

Human digestive enzymes are present in a fixed ratio that is genetically determined in each individual—different for each of us. For some, the enzyme quotient runs out more rapidly than in others. But, it can be lengthened and maximized. So, in a real sense, the human body has a limited supply of digestive enzymes, which are at their peak between ages 16 to 23. For every ten years of life after age 23, we lose an average of 9% of our digestive enzyme "potential."

Digestive enzyme deficiencies show as gas, bloating, various bowel problems, fatigue after eating, abdominal cramping, and food allergies. This loss of enzymes (via *enzyme potential*) is apparently inexorable, continuing to the end of bodily life. As we age, enzyme potential slows, and digestive ability weakens. Most don't notice this as a "problem" until around age 45. Suddenly, we can't eat the food items as fast, as much, or at all, as we could when we were younger. At least, not without problems. The food just doesn't break down in the tummy like it used to.

However, there are ways to manage what could otherwise be a problem. For one, your digestive enzyme potential can be made to last longer by taking digestive enzyme supplements. For another, you can make the move to raw foods. Raw food intake allows our enzyme potential to be maximized, regardless of who we are or what that potential is. Careful and thoro chewing of all foods—and juices—is an even better way to avoid digestive problems.

Food enzymes are destroyed by cooking. Eating cooked food places more stress on our body by requiring it to produce more digestive enzymes.

Our body cannot naturally produce enuf <u>digestive</u> enzymes to keep up with the typical Western diet, with its enzyme-depleted cooked and processed foods. The result: digestive-dysfunction-related diseases—of which there are many.

But, there's another potential problem that arises with age: even with the <u>food</u> enzymes in raw foods, older digestive systems have trouble breaking down whole foods. Chewing is more difficult, often due to the loss of natural teeth. The use of dentures obviates eating many raw natural foods—including some favorites. Also, <u>digestive</u> enzymes have diminished in older stomachs.

Enter raw <u>liquids</u>—via the GLD! These raw liquids reduce the number of digestive enzymes needed and provided by older stomachs. The natural and intelligent way to prevent digestive dysfunction and disturbances, maximize body longevity, and enhance enzyme potential—and thus lengthen life—is to take pure raw liquids. At least, if the diet isn't all that great most of the year, an annual 30-day GLD can provide a huge boost in overall health.

Death as a Welcome Rest

It is in so-called "older age" (which in most world cultures starts at age 70) that we often notice we are no longer as afraid of death as we once were. In some sense, some of us even *welcome* it—as a "rest" from all the trials we've suffered and continue to suffer from "life's fitful fever." We notice how we're lucky if <u>anything</u> in life "works out" for our loved ones and us. Even if it does, it never grants the Perfect Happiness every heart truly craves.

For us as egos, life seems a perpetual struggle to survive in our endless attempts to become happy. So, why would one want to live longer if life isn't <u>already</u> happy? For the promise to *become* happy at some point, somewhere "down the line"? Yes, that's it exactly, and the ego actually believes this nonsense. Every culture encourages it. The problem is that it is just not going to happen. Ever!

What does it take, after all, to become happy? "Become?" Why not "already?" Any happiness we can gain, <u>we will *necessarily* lose</u>—at least via death. So, if one can't <u>become</u> happy, what's left? Without knowledge of and submission to the Divine, we live like a trapped rat, only suffering the essentially painful psychophysical life.

One has to be crazy or silly to avoid what is Higher in life. The only way for a sane person to tolerate life in this Earth realm is to submit utterly, to surrender completely, and in every moment, to the Great Consciousness of Radiant Light and Energy, the Very Context in which we appear.

Consider an average current length of bodily life (currently about 68 years). Now consider a possible *extended* or projected length based on better care. Let's imagine a person's *design* (or genetic) body length as 85 years. No one knows exactly what his or her *design* length is, of course, but just hypothetically, let's say 85. With current technology (2019), we can only make educated guesses based on our lineage.

However, with reasonable care (which most people rarely if ever provide their body), the body's length of life can be extended by another 45-50 years (Grand Medicine's estimate). So, our person would be living 135 years—with just reasonable care (see consideration above). What could you accomplish with that extra gift of time? What further purification, creativity, loving energy and opportunity for increased Spiritual practice could you bring that would help serve others and the Divine?

Aging and the Structural System

As the body ages, all systems, organs, tissues, and cells become more vulnerable. The body is programmed to do this, to wind down to the point of its death. Perhaps in some future time, much more will be known about this process, so that the life of the body can be much more extended—maybe to 1200 years or so—enuf time for just about anyone to figure out what life is really all about!

For now, we can do what we know best—be creative in the most positive sense, bring love, cooperation, tolerance, and good energy to everyone. Since the gross physical body is a "food" body, we can at least be creative with diet and lifestyle. And, since we know that conservation of energy has an impact on longevity, we can endeavor to avoid hi-stress situations.

An Age-based Diet Plan

Consider the structural system of the body, the bones, and teeth. We clearly know from skeletal remains of our ancient ancestors, their teeth were worn down by doing so much grinding of ruff vegetal foods. As we age, we can avoid this by taking in higher percentages of (especially fresh raw) liquids. What percentages? Let's see if we can use years of age as a guide. At age 60, we'd be taking in 60% of our diet as liquids; at 70, 70%, and so on.

How would this plan impact the health of teeth? With far less stress on the teeth from not doing all that extra chewing and grinding of solids, they'd last longer and be healthier—especially with hi-quality liquids. Of course, if we're regularly consuming colas, coffee, alcohol, and refined and chemical sugar liquids, we'll be undermining the teeth and bones from within. We can also stop brushing our teeth with sugary, gummy pastes, instead using harmless, cleansing, and far more effective Dr. Bronner's© liquid soap diluted 7:1 with pure water.

And, we can continue exercising the muscles and bones. In older age, this is accomplished simply by walking or swimming and perhaps some easy calisthenics such as Da Namaskars (video available thru *GLDLifestyle*). Da Namaskar, from "Surya Namaskar," or sun salutation, is an ancient rapid-movement in-place exercise practice from India that uses all the muscles of the body briefly and adequately without stressing them excessively.

Eventually, our technology will allow us to use stem cells to protect against premature aging, renew and strengthen tissues, organs, and systems, and help the body defend against various disease organisms. DNA tests will help us understand the body's potential for the length of bodily life. Various other more sophisticated technological means can be brot to bear in order to stretch our years. For the wise, *the longer we live in the body, the greater the opportunity to Awaken to the Divine, our highest purpose*.

An Attitude of Certain Elderly

We all know those "senior citizens" who act "old"—even at age 55! Are they seeking sympathy? Or are they actually mentally incompetent? There's a difference. In the past, we looked up to our elders for their wisdom, inner strength, and knowledge of the world, their understanding of life in the universe, and their respect for and honoring of the Divine. Nowadays, so many older people are just old punks, simply not worthy of looking up to.

Of course, they—like every other human being—are worthy of our basic respect and honor as living beings. But on another level, they're just old farts, silly characters, unwilling to give up their coffee, cigarettes, beer, indolence, sheer ignorance, insensitivity, and other bad habits and attitudes. They have no discipline to speak of, and want others to wait on them hand and foot. They are grumpy because they haven't dealt with what is inside: their unhappiness, their constant attention to worldly silliness. They haven't overcome much egoity.

These people figure they've gotten this far in life and so they're owed the rest, gratis. They have the appearance of lumpy, bumpy, withered old potatoes. Their wisdom is vanished. They talk only of themselves, the weather, or others, in gossiping tones. Their minds are narrow or closed to new ideas. They've learned nothing of real value from their lives. How can they be looked up to? They have achieved mediocrity—a common attainment! Their lives reflect our current society.

This points to our great need of a true Wisdom Culture (Appendix G), so we may once again enjoy the knowledge and understanding that <u>can</u> come with age, experience, careful observation, sensitivity to the feelings and real needs of all others and the world, and especially appreciation and practice of God-Communion.

Raw food alone will not necessarily bring longer life. It may, but it may not. There are many factors in longevity. But raw diet (as solids and/or as liquids) can definitely help bring balance and good health to the body. Add *The BIG 7* and the seven numbered items above and you are creating the foundation that allows you the best chance of living a long life.

Sexuality and Longevity

Yet another item we can consider for longevity is sex. Studies show that when the body is capable of sex play, people tend to live longer when they engage it. Many male bodies naturally lose the sense of sexual response and urgency between the ages of 55 and 60—some, a lot earlier, as a result of various forms of stress, toxicity (especially chemical toxicity), microwaves, RF, and other radiation, or disease.

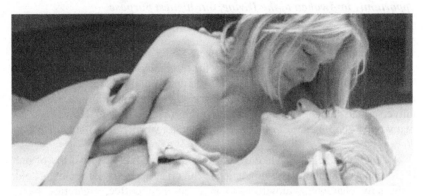

In older age, being free of the sex urge can be a distinct relief, a welcome freeing of energy for Spiritual practice. But, while that sense is there, it's best to use it correctly and regularly. This is best done in a socially acknowledged and positive monogamous relationship. The couple must have a happy and at least an acknowledged physical attraction for each other.

And it's clearly helpful for longevity to learn right practice of sexuality, including appropriate use (the withholding) of the vital fluids during sexual climax. This process and practice is described in wonderful detail in Sutras 40 and 41 of *The Dawn Horse Testament of The Ruchira Avatar* and also in the much smaller book, *The Complete Yoga of Human Emotional-Sexual Life* (both at www.adidam.org).

In other words, besides the simple pleasures of it, sex can be used as a means of health and longevity and as Communion with the Divine. Clearly, this is one possible beneficial and very positive future of human sexuality. The ancients knew of right use of sexuality for these purposes. Instead of casually throwing away sexual energy, it's time we used this great resource for its higher purpose and function in human life.

Toward a Flexible and Youthful Body

Basically, there are these two things to do to get and keep the gross physical body youthful and flexible: *Hatha yoga* and *raw foods*—preferably liquids…especially liquids in older age. Most people above age 60 are either flabby or hard—not hard as in strong muscles, but hard as in tissue hardness from toxicity and inflammation. How does this happen? Simply thru diet insult and life-negative lifestyle. It's from a combination of too much rich / cooked foods and a lack of adequate exercise.

Now, we're not suggesting that those over 60 should be doing hi-impact aerobics, running marathons, or otherwise engaging excessive wear-and-tear activities inappropriate to that age group. A simple Power (brisk) Walk of 15-20 minutes around the neighborhood would work for many over 60. Combine this with a 15-20-minute Hatha yoga routine and a diet of at least mostly raw liquids, and you'll see the improvement within 14 days.

Bad weather? You can do an indoor routine of several Da Namaskars, the extremely simple ancient exercise routine which requires a tiny space, no devices, and tones virtually every muscle in the body. The *GLDLifestyle* Yoga DVD shows a 66-year-old man doing Da Namaskars plus the full 20-posture Hatha yoga routine. Generally speaking, there's really no reason the body can't be relatively youthful and flexible right up to the last days of life.

Cultural and Other Longevity Factors

Some studies have shown that slower metabolic rates can help us live longer. As already mentioned, reduction in food intake (strategic under-eating) is another known factor—but that rightly involves cutting back on cooked food. Calm, peaceful, happy, clean, and orderly environments clearly help us live longer. Yes, genetics can play a role, but not the most important one. Environment is crucial—meaning what we *do* with what we *have*.

Bernard Jensen's "desk" analogy is an example of what we can do with what we have, what we've been given: When a pine desk (i.e., a genetically weaker body) and an oak desk (a genetically stronger one) are used and abused similarly, the pine desk deteriorates more rapidly. However, with care, the pine desk can outlast the oak! This is also an argument for carefully observing the body as it goes thru life, how it responds and reacts in various situations.

Insulin and IGF-1 have been shown to regulate longevity in all species tested. Altho most humans begin to develop degenerative diseases perhaps between ages 50 and 60, this needn't be the case. The most common age-related diseases include heart disease, cancer, stroke, emphysema, pneumonia, diabetes, kidney disease and Alzheimer's—all preventable. If you've reached "senior citizen" age (55) and your body suffers any of these disorders, the GLD can help you. Even in old age (70+), unless your situation is truly terminal, you still have room.

Emotional longevity factors include such qualities as:

- our expectations about the future
- how we explain past events
- our friendships and social ties
- how we feel about our education and income
- traumatic experiences that we <u>never disclosed</u> to anyone (ouch! Not good!)
- our ability to find meaning following adversity
- how all of the above influence our feelings and biology

Taking all of these into account, we can see how important *The BIG 7* really are to longevity and how the GLD can help. They can, at the very least, help us stay clear of drugs and doctors—and that's saying a lot!

Various organizations are currently working to develop both theories and practices that will extend the life of human beings. One of these is the *Life Extension Foundation* (www.lef.org). They discuss the strategic uses of various vitamins, minerals, herbs, and other nutrients, and also strategic calorie restriction, a proven way of extending life in both animals and humans. They also point to future uses of stem cell therapy to protect us from disease organisms and premature aging. (We just have to get past greedy corporate minds for this to work!)

Eventually, we should see therapeutic uses of gene therapy, nanobots (nano robots), and neuro-stimulatory therapies used to regenerate organs and body parts, improve vision, hearing, strength, intelligence, sexual powers, and other attributes. Meanwhile, we can intelligently use our GLD in the context of *The BIG 7*. The real biggie for us humans, of course, is growth in *moral* terms—which is where real Spiritual practice comes in.

Old Folks Homes Don't Cut It

Talk about "institutional nourishment" being a mutual contradiction in terms! What kind of food do they serve our elderly in these "retirement homes," "rest homes, "nursing homes," "old folk's homes," or "assisted living centers"? (All these euphemisms are given to the places we have to shuffle off our old folks these days!) Junk, plain and simple. Pretty much the same as in hospitals—and jails!

Yes, there is the argument that they're old and going to die anyway, so why not just give them what they want, or otherwise what they're used to— or, in some cases, what they couldn't afford in their youth. However, these are specious arguments. People deserve pure foods at any age, especially where (young or old) they can't prepare foods for themselves. Besides, crap foods will only hasten their death (which, in some cases, is what their families want!).

Where is the human dignity in all of this? Look at the circumstances we put these people in, separated from us, from their children and grandchildren. We visit them only occasionally. Yes, there are good reasons for that—as long as we have these current so-called "communities" of Western Civilization almost all of us live in. Which are actually "divide-and-conquer" moral prisons designed and encouraged by Big Corporate.

Do you really think our elders, those who lack the financial wherewithal to care for themselves, those who need help mentally, emotionally, physically, want to be shuffled off to some strange location with other suffering old characters, away from their loved-ones? How many of our seniors really want to live their last days with strangers, feeling outcast and like they are a financial burden on their children?

In most world cultures, our cherished old ones are surrounded by family—right to the end. In Western cultures like the USA, given the divided-and-conquered so-called communities, the single-family home designs, with children placed in day-care centers while both parents must work to cover expenses for a half-way-decent life, with no one around to check up with dad to be sure he's OK, what are the alternatives?

We need to get back to the cohesiveness and true intimacy of the human-scale genuine cooperative community (CoopCom—Appendix G), where our elders are kept close by, properly cared for, where they can interact with younger people in loving environments. Every human being needs to feel they are loved, safe, secure in their person, supported by loved ones, and able and encouraged to participate in life circumstances—birth to death.

PLEASE NOTE: a well-designed and executed CoOpCom is *not* idealistic. Nor is it expensive. Compared to what is currently called "communities" and what is now happening in our family lives, it is far less expensive and entirely realistic. A more careful and detailed comparison of these ways of living is presented thru *GLDLifestyle*.

In our current divide-and-conquer every-family-in-their-own-castle society, our elders—and even in some real sense, our children—are felt to be an imposition in our lives. True CoopCom pre-solves this and so much more. Instead of us struggling alone against the health problems and difficulties our old folks these days so often have, we could have our real and intimate community to help us. We don't have to depend on the imposition of expensive insurance plans and medical "care-giver" strangers infringing on our lives.

We hear these statistics lately about how our population is growing older by the day, how an ever-increasing percentage of the population in the USA is elderly. *We need to know how to treat our elders rightly, how to make their lives successfully and effectively integrated with ours, with younger people, with children and infants*. We can do this—thru creative human-scale arrangements that include real cooperative community.

The GLD can be part of this process—even used in the context of the current scheme of these facilities for the old and infirm—by insisting that the proprietors of these "homes" comply. Otherwise, whenever we do have any manner of control over their health and their diet, we can at least feed our elders pure liquids so they'll have whatever degree of honorable and noble ending to their physical lives that is possible, given their specific circumstance.

The so-called "elderly" of any society will tell you, almost without exception, that, while, yes, they value their privacy, peace, and quiet, they'd also enjoy access to the company of young people, children, and infants rather than to be stuck with only folks their age. They want to be with family, with people they've known all their lives, with kin and with those they know and love, those with whom they have been intimate, feel valued, and close.

The Hand That Rocks The Cradle
The society that we can and must create starts with the education of children. This is most beautifully and precisely described in the book, *The First Three Stages of Life*. Children raised with the principles described in that book will naturally know how to care for their elders—and all of life—with intimacy and love. *"The hand that rocks the cradle rules the world."* What are mothers teaching their children? What are their guidelines for how to live life?

As long as we have no accountability for dietary purity within our culture, from our government leaders, our institutions, and among ourselves as adults, we can expect to have our "senior citizens," our elders, suffering chronic degenerative diseases and prolonged illnesses in hospitals and nursing homes—instead of being active and strong thru-out life, until one day suddenly getting very tired, and then passing in their sleep, shortly thereafter.

Once, I had a friend whose very old mother lived in "the old country"—Europe. Wishing to have her near, she brot mother home to the USA. She built a little cottage for her behind her home. Mother would join her and her husband for breakfast each morning. One day, mother announced,

"Daughter, I've lived a long healthy life, and now it's time for me to die, to leave this place." "Oh, no, mother!" her daughter exclaimed. *"We love you. Stay with us."*

The next morning, she and hubby were enjoying breakfast when she noticed her mother's absence. *"Where's mom?"* she asked. Then, suddenly remembering what mother had said the day before, she jumped up and ran to mom's cottage. There, she found mom, silently, softly and pleasantly lying in her final sleep.

There are noble and ignoble ways to die. While bodily death is a certainty, no one knows for sure when or how it will come. It is possible that, thru fortunate life circumstances and consciously bringing sufficient care to the body-mind, it can enjoy a relatively healthy normal number of years, or even somewhat extended years, in disease-free comfort. Unfortunately, for most people these days, this is not the case—for both personal and cultural reasons.

You can have your hi-tech death, with machines pumping drugs thru tubes running in and protruding out of your body, lying there as a motionless lump, unable to speak or respond to anyone, with nurses and doctors hovering over you, blood-thirsty insurance agents and money-hungry relatives in the waiting room. For my passing, I'll take a quiet afternoon at home with loved-ones, thank you—every time!

29—The GLD and Restaurants

Right Use to Avoid Health Destruction

Restaurants are fun to go to, especially because (1) we are waited on, served food by others, and (2) we can choose food we don't normally eat at home. However, except for a very few Natural Food types, restaurants are in business to make money—not to make us healthy! At Grand Medicine, we urged all our patients to generally avoid regular use of restaurants—especially when on solid foods. We used the phrase, *"If you want to get sick, eat at restaurants often!"*

Opening the restaurant menu, it never says, *"Tonight's Dead Animals!"* But, there they are on the menu. And most of the rest is cooked, degenerated by chemicals, and otherwise unwholesome. Even the salad bar is likely GMO and sprayed with preserving chemicals! And, notice how restaurant food is rarely the quality and taste as its advertising photos seem to suggest—even in those beautiful ads that are often found rite there on the restaurant menu.

Of course, there are those times when restaurant eating is next to impossible to avoid. Like when traveling to foreign countries—especially by air. On the GLD, restaurants can be particularly challenging, since we will be drinking tea while watching as others consume foods that we savor but must avoid. The aromas of various dishes can tax our restraint to the limit. At these times, recall why you are doing your GLD, and visualize a resulting slim, strong, and radiantly healthy body.

If unavoidable, it's usually best to order fruit juice, tomato juice, or even V8©. If they have a homemade veggy soup, ask them to blend it for you. They usually will. Herb tea is fine, if they have it (sometimes they have only caffeinated tea, which you should reject). Resist using refined or chemical sugar substitutes to sweeten tea. Stay with purity, even if relative! Bottom line: if you can do so, avoid going to restaurants whenever possible.

Beware of Microwaved Food

Another thing about restaurants and the food we eat: AVOID microwaved food! It may <u>look</u> like food, <u>smell</u> like food, and even <u>taste</u> like food. But, nuked, it is no longer fit for human consumption. Its nourishment has almost entirely been destroyed in the microwaving process. Infants in hospitals have died when nurses, trying to cut corners by microwaving bottled milk, innocently feed this to them.

A major study (available on the Net) was done in Switzerland some decades ago by a renowned physicist, proving conclusively that microwaving food destroys its nutritional value. Two groups were fed the same food, the first without the microwaving and the second with. Those receiving the microwaved food had blood workups matching those with cancer. Therefore, avoid eating microwave food while on (or even off) your GLD!

The Restaurant Exception

There are times when it's appropriate to visit a restaurant. Certain celebrations, like one's birthday, anniversary, etc., emergency, a break from some very hi-stress situation, or other such time when you've just gotta cut loose from an otherwise very strait hi-raw or all-raw practice, take your buddies, and go get some ordinary, common food! This, of course, should be rare. Use your good judgment.

30—Sweets, Salts, and Spices

Satisfying Natural and Basic Taste Qualities

Sweets Allowed on Your GLD

There are basically three kinds of sugars: (1) *natural sugar* found in most raw natural foods, (2) *refined sugars*, and (3) *chemical sweeteners*. Natural sugar is needed by the body to perform many critical functions. Most natural foods contain sugar, some—like dates, pineapples, beets, and bananas—in big doses. Refined sugar robs the natural plant source of its natural nutrients to one or another degree. Chemical sugar is human-made, contrived junk.

Natural sugar is necessary for the functions of the living body. Most living raw foods contain this sugar. This is the source we recommend first and foremost. Some reports suggest that common white granulated sugar has been refined 62 times. In any case, we consider it an addictive poison, the worst non-food you can eat, and thus to be at least minimized (celebratory occasions) or avoided altogether. The same for the chemicalized sugars or sugar substitutes (see Appendix D).

If you wish to use any refined sugar, the only one we recommend is pure raw coconut sugar. Coconut sugar is slowly drained by hand in the tree from coconut flowers, heated once in a vat, allowed to dry, then broken up into small crystals—thus, it is minimally refined. Perhaps even better is homemade date sugar, which you can make by drying organic dates in a food dryer and then crumbling the resulting dried dates—which can then be called sugar.

Stevia (a natural herb-derived sugar) is also OK as a sweetener. Avoid most other sweeteners (see Appendix D), especially regular granulated cane sugar and the chemical sugars (Equal®, Sweet-n-Low®, aspartame, etc.). Whole dates can be blended into smoothies. Pure raw coconut sugar can be used in teas and cocoa drinks. Real unrefined cane sugar and juice may be available in certain countries (Brazil, Mexico, e.g.), but not in the USA.

Dates are among the very best sweeteners because of their hi natural sugar content, the kind our body needs—especially the brain—which doesn't do well at all on the unnatural, refined, and chemicalized sugars. That's why your head and thinking often go weird after eating it. Pure raw coconut sugar (foto image) is our choice for a sugar-type sweetener, but dates are the number one whole natural sweetener we recommend.

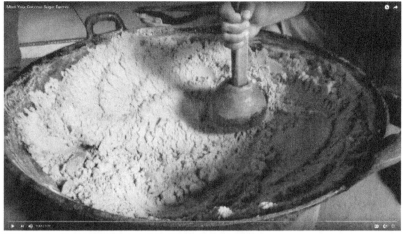

Minerals, Salty Foods, and Salting Agents

Minerals are nutrients crucially needed by the body to function. There are *organic* minerals and *inorganic* ones. Plants have <u>roots</u> to process *inorganic* minerals from the earth and turn them *organic*; we don't have roots, so we can't do that. We rely on plants to do that for us. Essentially, we can only use <u>natural</u> *organic* minerals—as found in plants. "Essentially," but our bodies <u>can</u> process a small amount of *inorganic* mineral. Salt is perhaps the best example of this.

Salt (sodium chloride) is a mineral necessary for good health. Raw foods provide all the salt and rest of the minerals the body needs. However, over millennia, we've developed a real and abiding <u>taste</u> for it—mainly because of our ever-increasing intake of cooked and processed foods! While on your GLD, you may notice a need something salty—usually from a lifetime of eating mostly cooked foods. Blended veggy soups, broths, or a sip of liquid from a jar of pure olives, dill pickles, or sauerkraut can suffice.

Any number of veggies can be used to make these salty soups and broths (see Appendix A). If you are allergic to any of these ingredients, your pulse will race right after their consumption. If you make soup on your GLD, be sure to blend it before consuming it.

For broths, you may simply pour the liquid off the cooked veggy soup and drink it as-is or add a pinch of pure salt or a natural salting agent. The best salting agents include the various untainted broth powders and untreated natural sea and earth salts like <u>Pink Himalaya Salt</u>© and <u>Celtic Salt</u>®, or other natural solar evaporated salt. These can be added just before the blending process or simply placed on the tongue.

Important: Do not use common table salt (Leslie's© Salt, Morton's© Salt), which have been heated or processed, causing loss of vital energies. They usually contain added anti-caking agents (calcium silicate), stabilizers (dextrose), and perhaps other unnecessary or otherwise toxic materials. Also avoid any broth powders containing hydrolyzed or texturized vegetable protein, MSG, or other chemicals. Broth powders should contain only powdered dried veggies.

Spicy Foods

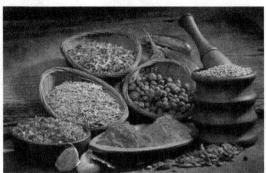

As suggested, it can be fun during your GLD to take a sip of the liquid from a jar of natural style dill pickles, sauerkraut, or even jalapenos—if you can handle the heat! You may also wish to add a few Tbsp. of these liquids (or a few chopped fresh jalapenos themselves) to soups for a very special hot and spicy flavor (remember to blend before consuming). You will also note that with time and bodily purity on your GLD, you'll feel far less desire to use spicy foods. You will naturally choose the simple purity of fresh raw fruits, veggies, nuts, and seeds.

31—Fruits

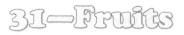

Liquefying the More Purifying Foods

The category called "fruits" includes berries and melons. Always try for fresh, ripe, natural, local-grown, and in-season fruits. Fruits will be going into the blender to make smoothies, and also into the juicer to make single or combination juices—like RMVJ. It's best to use fruits that grow in your local area. However, there may be little or even no fruits that grow in your area of the world—unless there are proper greenhouses—in which (rightly made) any fruit, nut, herb or veggie can be grown (Appendix G). On the GLD, fruits are used mostly to sweeten green smoothies.

Therefore, short of the greenhouse, it's OK to use fruits from far away areas, including tropical, like pineapple, papaya, banana, mango, guava, and more—the fresher, the better. The possibilities and possible combinations, especially when mixing fruits and nuts/seeds, seem endless. You will never run out of ideas for combinations of fruits, nuts, and seeds to make delicious smoothies. Of the three essential food groups, fruits are the more <u>purifying</u>. They are also the seed-bearing parts of certain plants. Most fruits grow in trees.

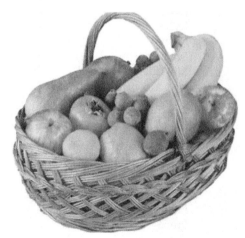

Everything in the conditional or cosmic realm (where we bodily beings currently live) is vibrations, hi and low. Higher vibrations make religious and Spiritual practice easier. In terms of food, red meat has the lowest vibration. Fruits, as food, have a fine, hi, lite vibration. Noticing this, some people have tried living exclusively on fruits. Altho this can be done, it takes time and preparation. You have to be ready for it—so you don't "drift off into the etheric."

It's best to begin at the dietary beginning: where you are currently. If that involves a disease process, do not go immediately to fruit—especially whole fruit—unless directed to do so by your Natural Health Practitioner. It can be a shock to the body to suddenly move into such a powerfully purifying diet—which will happen on all fruits. It's best to begin slowly and gently. The GLD is excellent for this. On the other hand, some people, with good strong direction from the experienced healer, are well-advised to go onto an exclusively fruit regime for a time.

Preparing Fruits

Unless you have your own natural garden and orchard, purchase your fruits at local natural grocers to be reasonably assured of relative purity. Wash them in hot soapy water, removing any dirt or accumulated dust or attached bugs. Rinse in cold clear water. Certain peels are essentially inedible, as in bananas, melons, oranges, and pomegranates, and so these should be removed. Other peel coverings, like those of apples, pears, cherries, peaches, and nectarines, e.g., can and should be eaten, because this is where much of the nutritive value is found.

Lemon peels can be used with the fruit of the lemon in the RMVJ recipe. Lemon is perhaps the only citrus fruit in which the peel is rite to use this way. *Note*: If at any time any certain fruit doesn't taste good to you, don't eat it. Your body probably doesn't need the nutrients of that particular fruit at that time. Or, you may be allergic to it.

A few of the more popularly grown fruits

Apple	Loquat
Apricot	Lychee
Banana	Mango
Blackberry	Mulberry
Blueberry	Muskmelon
Cantaloupe	Nectarine
Cherimoya	Orange
Cherry	Papaya
Currant	Peach
Date	Pear
Elderberry	Persian melon
Fig	Pineapple
Gooseberry	Plum
Grapefruit	Pomegranate
Grapes	Prune
Guava	Raisin
Honeydew	Raspberry
Huckleberry	Sapote
Kiwi	Strawberry
Kumquat	Tangelo
Lemon	Tangerine
Lime	Watermelon

Combining Fruits—and Other Foods

We have noted three food groups as essential in human nutrition: fruits, vegetables, and nuts/seeds. In certain persons, due to genetic inheritance or developed weaknesses, certain food combinations need to be avoided in order to prevent digestive problems. Each has his and her particular stomach / digestive strength. Because of some folk's lesser digestive capability, food combinations thus need to be taken into account. Of course, some peoples' stomachs seem to be able to handle any and all food combinations without the slightest complaint.

Elaborate designs of pure produce food combinations have been proposed so as to minimize irritation to the body and manage problems of digestion, absorption, and assimilation. Foods from different groups are more easily combined in most bodies thru using one or more of the following:

(1) liquefying

(2) careful and thoro chewing

(3) having an average strength digestive system

(4) including digestive enzyme tablets in the diet

(5) staying within one food group

(6) taking pure natural produce

(7) eating in calm, peaceful and altogether happy environments

(8) dining alone or with the "good company" of friends &/or peaceful, happy people

(9) praying over your food, asking for Divine Blessing on your meal—and thus remaining happy while eating

There are other theoretical factors involved in food combining. If you seem to or tend to have difficulty digesting food, the best rules are to liquefy, pray over your food, chew everything exceptionally well, don't be in a hurry when you have a meal, and keep simple any recipe involving different types or groups of food.

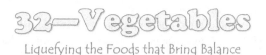

32—Vegetables

Liquefying the Foods that Bring Balance

While fruits are referred to as <u>purifying</u>, vegetables are <u>balancing</u>. During our clinic years at Grand Medicine, we came across many examples of patients with chronic diseases—especially bowel-related—who suggested that they couldn't eat raw vegetables. They knew this from experience, they claimed, and balked at the very idea of eating a salad. However, we pointed out to them that they could *drink* a salad! Enter the Green Smoothie and the GLD. Not only did this solve the problem of eating salads, it cured their bowel problems altogether.

A wide variety of raw veggy juices and liquids are possible on the GLD. The Green Smoothie (Appendix A) is the one most essential drink on your GLD and should be emphasized. In fact, ***it is recommended that the Green Smoothie be taken @ a minimum of 16 ounces daily (average person), and even a quart or a liter or more in chronic degenerative situations***. With cancer, at least a quart of RMVJ is usually appropriate.

One may wish to experiment with veggy drinks, both as blender (smoothie) and juicer (juice) drinks, including the use of carrot, celery, beet, cucumber, cauliflower, cabbage, zucchini, broccoli, and so on. Carrot, celery, and beet, is the most frequently used combo (see RMVJ). Other combinations can include mixing with various nuts or fruits, like carrot-coconut or carrot-apple, depending on your digestive capacity as well as your taste buds.

Remember to use enuf fruit along with the raw greens so that your drink tastes good to you—or you won't want to drink it. Fresh mint leaves can also be added. Fresh mint, orange juice, and coconut make a great combo goes excellent with orange juice and coconut. Yes, apple and lemon with peel may be juiced with the veggies—they are compatible with most digestive tracts and add significantly to the nourishment of the drink.

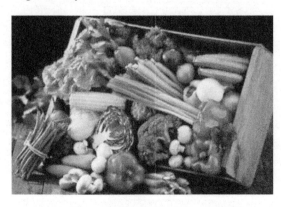

Always prefer <u>fresh, natural produce</u> to bottled juices, and try to consume whatever you make <u>the same day made</u>—or at least the very next day. GLD liquids always taste best the day they are made. If drinking them the day they're made is not possible (e.g., when you must leave very early for work), make your juices as late as possible before bedtime, refrigerate them, and take to work the next day.

Grasses and Sprouts

Various grasses and sprouts can also be juiced. Among the more popular grasses are wheatgrass and barley grass. Other grasses are possible, too, and many still need to be experimented with as to their nutritive and therapeutic value for human beings. To our present knowledge, *wheatgrass is, along with aloe vera, certainly among the very most powerful and nourishing substances currently available in this world*.

Growing Wheatgrass

Wheatgrass can be made in about two weeks per batch by soaking wheat seed (often called "wheat berries," "winter wheat," etc.) for 15 hours, rinsing and draining them twice daily, and allowing them to sprout in a dark place (like a cupboard) for another 15 hours. Special sprouting jars for this purpose are available in Natural Food stores. Then, fill a plastic "flat" or garden tray (available at nurseries) with about 2 inches of the following mixture: 1/3rd soil, 1/3rd peat moss, and 1/3rd planter's mix.

Apply water to the mix and spread the new sprouts over the surface. Cover the flat with newspaper or dark plastic to simulate the underground environment. Remove this daily and sprinkle with water. On the 3rd day, remove the covering permanently but keep the tray out of direct sunlight. Water the grass daily or as needed, allowing the grass to grow to about 7 inches tall. It is now ready to harvest.

Wheatgrass can be taken orally as nourishing drinks and also injected rectally and vaginally as a therapy against diseases of the bowel and urogenital system. As a drink, wheatgrass can be combined with pineapple juice for an improved taste—the so-called "Green Cocktail" (see Appendix A). It is made by combining chopped wheatgrass and several chunks of fresh pineapple in the blender, blending, straining, and drinking. Here is a list of only some of the more commonly used vegetables:

Arame	Kelp
Artichokes	Kombu
Asparagus	Leek
Barley grass	Lettuce
Beets	Mushroom
Bell Peppers	Mustard greens
Broccoli	Nori
Brussels sprouts	Okra
Cabbage	Onion
Carrots	Parsley
Cauliflower	Parsnips
Celery	Peppers
Chard	Persimmon
Chili Peppers	Potato
Chives	Pumpkin
Cucumber	Radish
Dandelion greens	Rutabaga
Dulse	Shallot
Durian	Spinach
Eggplant	Sprouts
Endive	Squash
Garlic	Tomato
Hiziki	Turnip
Jicama	Watercress
Kale	Wheatgrass

33—Nuts and Seeds
Liquefying the Sustaining Foods

While fruits are <u>purifying</u>, and vegetables are <u>balancing</u>, nuts and seeds are <u>sustaining</u>. True, green veggies are our most important food, but…nuts and seeds have their place, too. Nuts and seeds contain a wide variety of minerals, which are more important than vitamins as nutritional substances for us humans. Perhaps equally nutritionally important, nuts and seeds contain fatty oils, which sustain us for more extended periods than the other nutrients such as vitamins, minerals, and enzymes.

Once again, it is best, in general, to *emphasize green veggies* over fruits and nuts. The chlorophyll, which is the blood of plants, and other nutritional ingredients within the living greens, are more important than the nutrients found in the fruits and nuts. And yet, all three groups are necessary for human health. Try to get all three daily. It's easy on your GLD.

On the GLD, nuts, and seeds are used in smoothies and nut-seed milks as bases for smoothies and other drinks. Currently, at GranMed, we make up and use both thinner and thicker (Extra Rich) nut-seed milks. A wide variety is possible. Five ounces of Extra Rich Nutmilk plus 5 ounces of pure water, plus a peach, a big handful of mixed greens, and maybe a date, blend, and you've got a delicious, health-bringing green smoothie.

Among our favorites nuts is coconut—and its oil. Coconut is a nut (coco "nut"). Coconut is a true SuperFood. We use two tsp. of coconut oil in our Extra Rich Nutmilk (Appendix A). Purchase all your fresh, raw nuts and seeds from your local brick-and-mortar store or online. Best is in-the-shell, but next is in coolers at the market. Keep nuts and seeds refrigerated because their oils are volatile and will go rancid at varying times and in different environmental conditions.

Avoid salted or roasted nuts or seeds except for special occasions. If a raw nut and/or seed tastes hot at the back of your tongue, it's rancid, so throw it into the compost bin. Any nut or seed you are not allergic to is OK to use in smoothies. Peanuts are legumes, not nuts. Typical seeds include sunflower, pumpkin, sesame, flax, and hemp seed. The nuts that are most commonly allergens include English walnuts, cashews, and macadamias.

Typical nuts used these days as food include (especially) almond, walnut, avocado, coconut, brazil, macadamia, filbert, hazelnut, pecan, and pine. Many people are allergic to peanuts (which are legumes), so it's usually best for most people to avoid peanuts—and peanut butter. On making smoothies with the nuts and seeds, the soft nuts may be placed directly into the blender—altho a VitaMix© will easily blend the hardest nuts and seeds.

Typically, almonds and pumpkin seeds are the harder ones used by vegetarians. Almonds, the king of nuts, are packed with protein, fiber, and omega-3 and -6 fatty acids. It's best to soak almonds and pumpkin seeds in a bowl of pure water for at least 3 hours or overnight to release enzyme inhibitors, free up more nutrients, and make them easier to blend. Then, rinse them three times, the last time (at least) in pure water before placing them in the blender.

Enzyme Inhibitors
A certain controversy has developed regarding the propriety of taking nuts and seeds directly from the shell as opposed to soaking them overnite. The argument centers around enzyme inhibitors found within the membrane surrounding the flesh of the nut or seed. The presumption is that these enzyme inhibitors need to be eliminated by soaking for the nut or seed to be nutritionally available to one or another degree.

Theoretically, the enzyme inhibitors are eliminated by either 3-hour or overnite soaking in pure water. The water would then be poured off, then do a rinse, and the nuts or seeds consumed. We at GM feel that altho this soaking process is not crucial to obtaining the nutritive value of the nut or seed, it does improve digestion and assimilation, and, of course, it also helps make the nuts or seeds more easily chewed and blended.

Allergic to Nuts on The GLD?
You may be allergic to certain nuts, as many people are. The ones that are typically allergy-reactive are peanuts (which, as legumes, tend to more rapidly attract mold), English walnuts, and macadamias. You can do a pulse test to determine allergy and then act accordingly. Check your pulse directly after eating a mouthful of any nut and see if your pulse races. Check your pulse at your wrist before you eat the specific food and then within seconds afterward. If it's faster after eating that food, you're likely allergic to it.

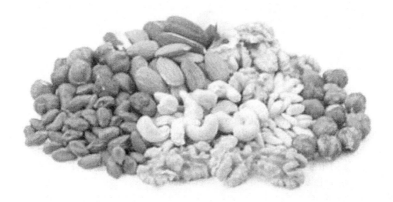

If nuts are rancid, you'll be more likely to be allergic to them, and your body will react. At the least, they'll cause a burning sensation on the back of your tongue. This is how you can tell they're rancid—if not by smell. It's best to keep all hulled (shelled) nuts and seeds refrigerated—especially if you are not planning to use them within a few days of purchase.

Some people have allergies to many nuts. You can use seeds as excellent alternatives to nuts. Among the best seeds are ***sesame*** (which can be taken as "tahini," a raw butter), ***sunflower***, and ***pumpkin***. Avoid packaged powdered nuts/seeds, since, even if they are "natural," they've lost a lot of their nutritional value in being ground. Whole is best. Grind them up yourself in your nut-seed grinder, blender, or juicer.

For those needing to gain weight on the GLD, oils, nuts, and nut butters are excellent. Some delicious nut and seed preparations are possible, both for those needing weight gain and those looking for snacks. Nut and seed butters can be mixed. For those losing weight, just a teaspoon daily can taste like heaven itself! Several spoonfuls daily plus nut and seed smoothies will put on the pounds (or kilos) for thin-body and fast metabolism types.

34—Food Combining on the GLD

Helping the Stomach with some of the More Delicious GLD Meals

Nut and Fruit Liquids

Some delicious drinks can be made by mixing certain fruits with nuts and seeds. This includes both blended and juiced combinations. For example, grape and coconut: wash and rinse a large bunch of grapes, leaving them on the stem (and it's even better if they have seeds in them!). Place into the blender with a few chunks of fresh coconut (or a few lge Tbsp. of dried raw shredded coconut). You may need an ounce or two of raw apple juice to get the blender started. Blend well, and then strain through a wire mesh veggy strainer.

Another great drink is apple-coconut, and yet another is carrot-coconut. These last two are <u>juicer</u> drinks, however, and it doesn't take much imagination to figure how to make them! In their case, it's fun to use mature coconut fresh from the shell, poking the holes and draining out and drinking the coconut water (assuming it's sweet), then prying out the nutmeat with a soupspoon or butter knife. Brief Net videos show this being done.

One of our favorite drinks is made with fresh orange juice, shredded or whole coconut, and fresh mint. Just placed these in the blender, blend well, strain, and drink.

Smoothies

A typical smoothie is a blender drink that consists of fresh fruits (try to avoid using frozen fruits and/or berries—altho blueberries are an exception), fresh greens, and pure raw nuts or seeds. Into the blender, place a freshly peeled banana, six strawberries (frozen strawberries if fresh ones aren't in season or otherwise available), 4-6 ounces of nutmilk, a handful of greens, a few almonds, and blend. You can change the amounts to suit your taste.

An ***avocado smoothie*** can be made by placing half an avocado into the blender with a banana, two big Tbsp. of shredded coconut, a small handful of almonds (or nutmilk), 3-5 pitted dates, and 4-6 ounces of pure water. For an exceptional taste, add half a non-GMO papaya.

Carob powder may also be combined with banana, walnuts, perhaps dates, and rich nutmilk to create that chocolate taste and effect. Some of the more common smoothies include strawberry and pineapple. A simple strawberry smoothie combines a handful of fresh strawberries with a banana and a small handful of soaked nuts or rich nutmilk. Greens can be added or not (see Appendix A).

A pineapple smoothie can use the same recipe, but substituting fresh (or, if not available, frozen) pineapple chunks for the strawberries. Beware of using canned so-called fresh pineapple or other fruit that contains refined sugar.

Fruits can be mixed in a wide variety of combinations. Berries can also be used, preferably raw and in-season. Be sure to try different nut and seed combinations. Bananas are frequently used in smoothies as a kind of thickener. The most common base for smoothies is either homemade almond or other nut or seed milk, pure water, or raw apple juice.

One of our favorite nutmilks is made from fresh coconut: place the chopped (or shredded no-sugar) coconut into the blender, add pure water, blend very well, strain thru a wire-mesh veggy strainer, and you're done. You can add a few dates as a sweetener to this already rich milk, but it will not last as long in the frig as without the sweetener. An excellent tropical smoothie uses shredded dried coconut, papaya, mango, banana, and pineapple, with rich nut milk as your base. Mint or other greens may be added to make it a green smoothie.

Recently, we've been making a rich nutmilk for general purposes on or off the GLD. Place a handful of raw almonds, another of raw cashews, ten raw macadamias, + ½ handful of pecans into a bowl to soak in pure water for 3 hours. Pour off the water, rinse 3x in pure water, blend with 2 cups of pure water, 2 Tbsp. virgin coconut oil, 5 Tbsp. shredded coconut + 1 Tbsp. sesame seeds for two full minutes and pour into a half-gallon bottle. Fill the rest of the bottle with pure water, and you have an excellent rich white milk that will stay fresh in a cold frig for about five days.

35—Sauces, Pastes, and Pates

Spicy Entertainment While Staying Liquid

Fruit Sauces

Applesauce can be used on your GLD. It should be homemade to assure maximum nutritional value—which is easy. Place 2 oz. raw apple juice into the blender with four cored unpeeled raw natural apples, and blend. Other such fruit sauces can be made similarly, such as pear, apricot, peach, and combinations of fruits blended together. Thus combined, these sauces can, for some folks, have a Tbsp. of plain yogurt added as a topping or barely stirred (swirled) in. Bee pollen can then be sprinkled on top for a unique added flavor—and added nutrition.

Guacamole

Salsas and guacamole can also be made at home, using all raw ingredients. Homemade natural style crackers and/or food dryer veggie chips can be used with these, or you can simply spoon them up plain, without the crackers or chips. Guacamole can be made with a ripe avocado, ½ onion, 1 garlic bud, ¼ fresh lemon with peel, 1 raw jalapeno (optional), 2 Tbsp. chopped cilantro leaves, ½ tsp. Cumin powder, perhaps a tsp. of natural-style broth powder, and one tomato. Place these into the blender, add an ounce or so of water, and blend.

As you progress along your GLD, maybe not the first one or the second one, but at some point over the years, your desire for crackers and other snacks, soups, and broths, will lessen, and you will choose the pure raw liquids pretty much exclusively. Your body will demand it.

There are several pastes and pates available in Natural Food Markets that can be used as a base for guacamole or other such sauces. These may include various pestos (ex. sun-dried tomatoes, basil, garlic, pine nuts, etc.), hummus (made from garbanzo beans), and tahini (made from sesame seeds).

It is very important to your health that you make sure that there are no chemical preservatives or other foreign ingredients in these packaged sauces. If the only "preservatives" are the natural kind (citric acid), you're OK. Better still, make your own such sauces. They could wind up tasting better, and they'll certainly be healthier.

Possible Sauces and Associated Items on the GLD
(preferably homemade)

- Fruit sauces (apple sauce, pear sauce, etc.)
- Certain natural snack crackers (temporary, perhaps three once per day max—if that)
- Salsas and guacamole (@ a few Tbsp./day)
- Nut and seed butters (almond butter, sesame tahini, etc., taken @ 1-2 Tbsp. per day max.)
- Pesto sauces (use discretion)
- Humus (use discretion)

Nut Butters

We've mentioned that we don't recommend consuming either peanuts or peanut butter. The main reason is that, somehow, peanuts more readily attract mold. As such, it causes many people who eat it to suffer allergic reactions to it. The mold is responsible for this reactivity. And, BTW, a heavy mold infestation can wreak havoc on your body, causing great pain and even death. If you smell mold anywhere in your home, eliminate it immediately. Peanuts are miss-named, anyway. They are legumes, not nuts. We suggest avoiding peanuts and peanut butter entirely.

Nut butters are easily made, using the rite juicer. Among the better juicers for making nut butters is the Champion© and the Omega©. Because almonds are comparatively dry when compared to other nuts, you may need to add coconut oil during the almond butter manufacturing process. Virtually all other nuts can be used to make nut butters. Mixing certain nuts during the nut-butter-making process, we can create some rather tasty combinations. Consider cashew-pecan, walnut pecan, almond-hazelnut, and so on.

36—Water

It's Everywhere, but Which is Right to Drink?

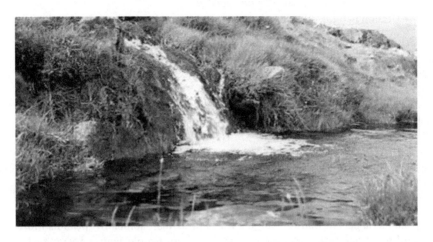

Crucial for health and life, water is subtly and profoundly connected to everything on Earth. It covers some 70% of our planet and comprises about 12% of the approximately 60% liquids of the human body. In general, we cannot live gross bodily life without it. Those of us who live where it is plentiful tend to take water for granted. It is not only the <u>fact</u> of the water itself, but the <u>quality</u> of it that is important.

For most of us, the days are long gone when we could simply dip into a local stream or river and get pure water to drink. We humans have a lot of self-purifying and Earth-purifying to do to get back to that level of water quality—if, indeed, that can happen at all, at this point, given the amount of pollution that we have thus far created.

Water comes from our tap at home, at work, and in public. Why not just drink that? As we all know—despite what we're "officially" told—most municipal tap water is not safe to drink. That is, it is not of a quality that our body can easily process and remain healthy. In many cases, with the chlorine or fluoride, it doesn't even taste good. So, what should we do about getting pure water? Go to water bottled in plastic? How safe is that? Install a water filtration system? How do we know what water is best for us, healthiest, most free of contaminants?

The Contaminants

Our on-the-go convenience lifestyles plus the overwhelming greed and sheer inhumanity of Big Corporate have created environmentally untenable circumstances for us and the other life forms on our planet. There are so many contaminants in water these days that we cannot reasonably list them all. We can create categories of these water contaminants, such as (1) plastics, (2) heavy metals, (3) chemicals, and (4) parasites.

Plastics debris in the marine environment, including resin pellets, fragments, and microscopic plastic balls, contain organic contaminants, including polychlorinated biphenyls (PCBs), polycyclic aromatic hydrocarbons, petroleum hydrocarbons, organochlorine pesticides (2,2'-bis(p-chlorophenyl)-1,1,1-trichloroethane, hexachlorinated hexanes), and so many more.

The chemical contaminants include such as the municipal water additives like chlorine and DBPs, and then fluoride, various other VOCs, THMs, and MTBEs. The heavy metals include lead, arsenic, cadmium, and mercury. This list just scratches the surface. *Warning!* Do NOT trust bottled water! So much of it is contaminated these days. Better to steam-distill it and let the sun purify it (see Appendix B) and add its own magic.

According to Dr. Edward Group, DC, many municipal water supplies in the USA are contaminated with a varied mix of chemicals. These can include such as fluoride, chlorine, lead, mercury, PCBs, arsenic, perchlorate, dioxins, DDT, HCB, dacthal, and MtBE. There are more possible chems in our waters coming from the city or county, but "they" are not significantly concerned for our health to take the necessary measures to clean this up.

Parasites commonly include e. coli, Cryptosporidium parvum, Entamoeba histolytica, the Copepods, and Giardia lamblia in cysts and other forms. There are the various protozoans, helminths, and flatworms. Giardia intestinalis is also a common parasite found in drinking water.

Water Purification and Filtration Systems
There is "water *filtration*," and then there is "water *purification*." Filtering water is not necessarily the same as purifying it. Water can be filtered without rendering it potable, or fit for human consumption. Perhaps the best way to go for preparing drinking water in these times (best price, effectiveness, and value overall) is to purchase a good steam distiller unit and allow the sun to purify the water after the steam-distilling process (see below).

Alternatively, you may consider getting a high quality six-stage home filtering/purification system and follow up with a good steam distiller. There is plenty of information (maybe even too much!) currently available on water filtration and purification systems on the Net. How does one choose among them? In our best understanding, this listing shows the various generic types of systems, from best to least effective:

Estimated Relative Effectiveness of Water
Purification and Filtration Methods

1-Steam Distillation (then placed into the sun in glass)

2-Multiple Stage Selective Filtration

3-Ozone Filtration (best for municipal use)

4-Reverse Osmosis

5-Charcoal Filtration

6-Backwashing

7-Ultraviolet Exposure (alone)

8-Water Softening

9-Deionization

10-Chemical Exposure

Literature from the local municipal water company tells us that if we leave an open container of tap water in the frig, we can expect the chlorine taste to be eliminated, since, they say, the chlorine dissipates into the air when the water is chilled. This may be so with perhaps up to 60% of the chlorine, but do we want to go to that length to drink that kind of water? If this is all you've got, it's worth the effort, but there is usually much more you can do to make the water drinkable.

Our first choice of pure water to drink and use for other personal purposes is steam distilled that has been exposed to the sun for at least 3 hours in glass containers (see notes on sun exposure below). Among the overall better family and personal systems we've studied, our first choice is the *Pure Water© Mini Classic II* (about $575USD, www.purewaterinc.com). Yes, companies come and go, everything in the conditional realms change, but if you can get this quality or better, go for it.

Second on our list of home filtration systems (just below steam distilling with sun exposure) is multiple-stage selective filtration. There are many brands of home multi-stage filtration systems currently available. In past editions of *The GREAT Liquid Diet*, we listed a few. Since then, more good ones have appeared, varying in price from $100USD on up. Multiple Stage Selective Filtration leaves important natural minerals in the water.

Perhaps third on our list of quality filtration of water (mostly for municipal water systems, and not so much for personal and home use) is ozone types. Ozone is said to kill bacteria 3000 times faster than chlorine, making it excellent for municipal water filtering. Ozone municipal water filtration is used in European countries extensively. Why not in the USA?

Why are our town and city water systems still poisoning us with toxic chemicals? You might ask our wonderful government servants who were long since tricked and paid off by the phosphate mining industry. It has long been known that there are "probable carcinogens" lurking in virtually every municipal water supply in the USA—including chlorination byproducts such as trihalomethanes, volatile organic compounds, and haloacetic acids. The worst is hydrofluocilicic acid.

It is hard to go wrong with steam distiller water processing units. Add a little carbon filter at the end (which the *Pure Water©* distiller system does), and they remove virtually all that is currently present in water, including minerals, leaving pretty much only H$_2$O. Minerals useful for the body <u>are already present in raw foods anyway</u>, so we need not be concerned about them being missing from steam distilling.

Water and Sunlight

The best possible water yet remaining on planet Earth may well be found in high altitude streams where it is exposed to the sun. Optimally, water should have such sun exposure, a natural physical course as its path (instead of running thru right angle pipes), and be without toxics and bacteria—which "without" is virtually impossible in most places in the world these days.

Rainwater has usually been good for drinking when found in clean, remote, natural, non-industrial locations. But in recent times, winds have carried airborne industrial pollution to even isolated areas where rainfall now brings it to earth as "acid rain."

Even worse, we now have "chemtrails" to contend with. This involves the seeding of clouds and otherwise aerial spraying of atmospheric powdered metals such as aluminum and other chemical substances for who knows what purposes. These toxics and toxins have been detected in soils and on produce, on trees, in soils and in rivers in many and varied world locations.

Water bears energy. How water is stored makes a difference. Water takes on qualities of its environment—because water, like everything else, has consciousness. Sunlight purifies and revitalizes water. We should use water that is sunlight-purified for drinking and other internal uses. Whenever possible, we should also use such water to wash the body.

Within the Third Century Aramaic manuscript called the **Dead Sea Scrolls** (translated by Dr. Edmond Bordeaux Szekely), the One reputed to be Jesus admonished those seeking health advice from Him to *"Drink the water that bubbles over the rocks in the sunlight."* Today, Avatar Adi Da Samraj Gives us similar instructions regarding water. Probably **the very best water to drink** in these polluted times **is steam distilled that has been exposed to sunlight in glass jars for at least 3 hours**.

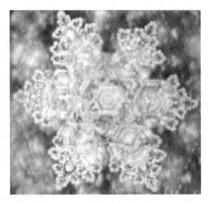

Water Temperature

Regarding a healthful water temperature for drinking, one argument suggests room temperature to avoid irritating the stomach. Sounds logical, except that water occurring in nature is rarely "room temperature." Spring waters, river and stream waters, ice melts—these are almost always cold—and refreshing. Room temp water may be fine for many occasions and stomachs, but on hot days, a nice cold drink is far more useful and natural—as well as satisfying.

Environmental Influences on Water

There are many other properties of water that we're now discovering that are nothing short of astonishing. Like food, the taking of water (and all liquids) is rightly a sacred act. Therefore, prayer is always appropriate when drinking water. Another exciting discovery along the lines of prayer, affirmation, and the rite use of mind and emotions, was that of the creative and visionary Japanese researcher Masaru Emoto.

In his book, _The Message From Water_, Emoto provides factual evidence that human vibrational energy—emotions, thots, ideas, and music—affect the molecular structure of water. He has photographed the crystalline structures of water that has been frozen. Water taken from pure lakes high in the mountains shows beautifully-formed crystalline patterns (*see upper foto, right, showing spring water from Saijo, Japan*), while water from polluted streams and industrial areas shows randomly distorted and ugly crystal patterns.

Emoto also noted that photos of various personalities can affect these crystalline structures. Images of saints attached to glasses of water were frozen, and their structures examined—and found to be beautiful. When photos of murderers and other criminals were applied, the results were the opposite. Prayer over bodies of water also changed these structural patterns.

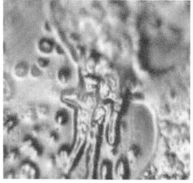

All of this points strongly to the way we so effectively influence our environments—and how they influence us—by our very thots and feelings. Dark emotions and thots such as "*You make me sick; I will kill you*" brot ugly patterns (*see lower foto, right*). Emotions such as gratitude, joy, love, and compassion produce beautiful patterns—and therefore enhance not only water quality but the quality of our very lives.

In the book, *Conductivity Healing*, Adi Da mentions water as a means of strengthening and conducting the flow of etheric energy in the human body. He describes the healing properties of water accordingly, and how it can be used by us intelligently. Water is not just something for us to drink and to bathe in. It is conscious Earth energy—and, as such, to be honored and cherished.

37—Ending your GLD

Transitioning Back to Solids

In this chapter, we are concerned with bringing your GLD to an end and returning to a hi-raw essentially solid food diet. Part of the process of breaking a fast includes taking special precautions such as *gradually phasing onto* certain solid foods so the stomach is not shocked. This is also the case with the GLD but essentially with less caution. The richness of the nutrition and the viscosity of the liquids obviate the need for exaggerated "breaking the fast" measures.

So, there is a certain caution when transitioning from your GLD to solid foods. Having learned the importance of diet purity while on your GLD (to the degree you practiced such purity), your body will complain if you break your GLD on junk food—like a hamburger and fries. This shows us that while the body can be trained to accept a wide variety of "foods," it likes and actually thrives on pure vegetal foods.

Therefore, this transition will be made easier by starting with a bowl of fresh chopped fruit or whole fruit or melon, for example—especially after a GLD of 30 days or more. A veggy salad, a baked yam, or even a bowl of hot veggy soup can be your next meal. **IMPORTANT!** *Try to keep the percentage of raw food at or above 80% while on solid foods.* This will keep your overall health relatively strong and stable, and make it easier for you to transition back into your GLD when needed.

Cereal for Breakfast or Any Solid Food Meal

Nut and seed milks are great on cereals with fresh chopped fruit on top. They're terrific with a little natural-style non-sugared flake cereal or home-made granola placed in the bottom of a bowl, then adding fresh berries &/or otherwise chopped fresh fruit on top. Coconut or almond milk are excellent. Some like to add a dollop of plain yogurt and sweeten with sprinkles of pure coconut sugar or chopped dates.

A few pre-soaked almonds could be added. Or, sprinkle with shredded coconut and drizzle with a little raw almond butter. It's beautiful to look at, delicious to taste, and very healthy! What more can one ask of a meal—after asking God's Blessing? Add a mixed veggie salad (greens, cherry tomatoes, avocado) topped with your favorite natural dressing, plus your green smoothie or RMVJ, and your set for the day.

On solids foods as with liquids, try to get the three basic food groups in daily. Meanwhile, we will continue to help you in health and life practices with ongoing tips and suggestions from our clinical work (since 1972) and from a lifetime (since 1940) of experience via *GLDLifestyle* (go to www.GLDiet.co). We welcome your energy and your feedback. It is our sincere desire to serve you.

As you proceed on your health program of doing more and more GLDs, you will notice how the body adapts to increasing levels of purity. This continues until a place of genuine balanced health is achieved—which is relatively rare in human life, especially in these crazy times. Your GLD will help you maintain this balance, this equanimity in health. Use it as appropriate in disease and health, and always as your return gift to The Divine Reality, the Most Beloved of every heart.

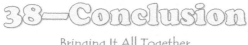

38—Conclusion

Bringing It All Together

Creating the Circumstance for Superior Health—and Everything Else

OK, fine, this is what we need to do to get and stay healthy. So, how can we do it? Who has the time to live this way of life?

Who can spend time in the sun, do skin brushing, prepare juices and other liquids, take an exercise walk, get to bed early, and do yoga—much less do Spiritual study, meditation, and other real Spiritual practices? Let's get real about this! Otherwise, it's just pipe dreams, fantasy, idealism, wishful thinking, an exercise in frustration. These days, for most of us by far, that's precisely what life is: frustration.

Childcare, shopping, paying bills, keeping up with technology, keeping the house in repair and orderly, cleaning, maintaining the family car, keeping up with friendships, family harmony, business relationships—in this increasingly complicated society, the list of responsibilities is endless. The hardest part is just starting. Do a little at a time. Add a bit each day until you've got a strong, stable routine.

It's maddening to live this modern life. You have to be crazy to think it's all going to work out for you. And yet...there is a way to do it that "pre-solves" managing health and most other current problems and situations simultaneously. It's not something we tend to think of at all. And yet, it's our roots, where we came from, what we were doing long before we even developed the current civilization, cities, large gatherings of people. It's about cooperation, tolerance, and love—only *human scale*.

In real cooperation, people join together to accomplish what the divide-and-conquer "every man in his own castle" principle cannot: namely, time and energy freed up to do real human things—to walk out at nite and watch the stars, to have a face-to-face family conversation at dinner—and, mainly, engage in that which is truly exceptional in life: real Spiritual practice. Who, tell me, these days, has that kind of time?

Our ancient ancestors, and even the remaining few indigenous tribes, worked 2-3 hours per day to sustain themselves. How many hours per day do we need to work—just to survive? And who is happier? We used to live cooperatively. We had to—in order to make it!

We need that kind of time, that cooperation—to be human. We need that kind of luxury, that kind of what now seems like an extravagance, to be truly elegant in life. And, we're not talking about just money here, or about destroying civilization to get what we are told to want, but instead creating a strong and authentic foundation for our real needs.

We all, at some time or other, have expressed the desire to have a nice big home to live in. We also want safety and security all around us. Today (2019), we don't have safety or security, no matter how big our house. The MSM suggests to us we shouldn't trust our naybors, and should rely on the government and the police for protection. Our government has proven itself a pack of unruly self-serving thugs, while the police look and act increasingly like the military—and treat ordinary citizens like potential enemies.

In a Wisdom Culture with authentic human-scale communities, we have the relative comfort, security, and support of others around us whom we know intimately and are similarly disposed in belief and feelings. Working with them, we can have beautiful homes and live close together—in peace and privacy but with them as community plus whatever happiness we can enjoy. Most importantly, we can have an environment in which to grow Spiritually according to our heart feeling.

The Politics of Living in the Modern World

Lewis Mumford, in his 1969 introduction to a book by Ian McHarg, wrote, *"[regarding] man's relation to his environment as whole… …man's life, in sickness and in health, is bound up with the forces of Nature, and that Nature, so far from being opposed and conquered, must rather be treated as an ally and friend, whose ways must be understood, and whose counsel must be respected.*

He goes on, *"…ignorant violations of Nature are so quickly penalized by physical disorders. Despite Nature's many earlier warnings, the pollution and destruction of the natural environment have gone on, intensively and extensively, for the last 300 years, without awakening a sufficient reaction."*

These days, the word "green" means more than a color. It's a whole way of life that we humans must embrace, or we will soon lose our beautiful planet. Greenhouse gasses—the results of waste products of fossil fuel production, burning, commercial animal factory processes, and the dumping of various other chemicals into the atmosphere and oceans—are destroying our living host Earth's thin layer of breath.

We cannot wait for our government to see this and mandate the needed changes. They are apparently owned and controlled by a global-money/business-oriented Big Corporate. We must require our elected officials to be responsible, yes, but meanwhile, we can and must act locally and personally to initiate the positive changes and live them ourselves as individuals. Each day, we can do little positive changes.

In terms of pollution, the USA is the biggest offender, the most destructive to this blue envelope of life. Therefore, Americans must take the lead. But, wherever in the world we live, we all can help. We must break away from our dependence on fossil fuel for energy and move swiftly into renewable resources: sun power, wind power, fusion power, tidal power, and so on. We must break away from abuse of animals.

We can start by walking and riding bicycles, purchasing hybrid automobiles, using mass rapid transit, eating natural vegetal foods, using non-chemicalized hygiene products, etc.—all of this as our conscious gift to each other, the planet, and the Divine Reality. We can do the GLD and tell others about it. We can learn and practice higher ways of life described in detail via *GLDLifestyle*.

We do not have to give up our machines, our computers, our washers and dryers and refrigerators and all. We need only change the way we think and act about them, how they work, the kind of energy needed to power them. We can find and practice ways of sharing our wealth and our skills and abilities, and to educate our children in ways of kindness, cooperation, tolerance, and love.

There is so much fear in the world now, and so many wars, people being told they must shake their fists at each other. Adi Da says, "***When you open your hand, what happens to your fist?***" (In other words, what happens to your hate or your fear?) Children have to be taught to hate (the "fist"). Otherwise, when they're very small, they naturally love and play with each other, regardless of color, culture, or ethnicity.

Everything we do is a political act—even brushing our teeth—affecting everyone and everything. If we make these changes now, our children will have a safe home on this Earth. And, speaking of children, the most wise, insightful and loving instruction we know of is in the book, ***The First Three Stages of Life***.

A New Culture, a New Civilization
The earliest human inhabitants of USA America are now (as of 2019) estimated to have entered the continent and lived here some 32,000 years ago, possibly having come from Europe. In those ancient times, we knew everyone in our group, our local community—for our whole life. We grew up with them, watched them give birth, get born, be sad, cry, laff, get injured, get well, be strong, be weak, grow old, and die.

It wasn't too very long ago, only a few decades, that we shared and borrowed food from our naybors, and let young children wander around the local nayborhood without fear. Our doors were never locked. As children, would lie down in grassy fields and ponder the shapes of clouds. Rivers and streams ran clear. There were frogs in local ponds in summer, and we'd watch tadpoles hatch and grow.

What is happening to us, to our culture, to the cultures of this world? Can we reclaim these parts of life—and still have our computers, and continue to maintain the more life-positive aspects of hi-culture and technological sophistication? Of course, we can! We can live peacefully, cooperatively, tolerantly. The Net is how we have best seen these changes—and it is our means of connecting with each other worldwide.

Human Civilization has been breaking down for the past 60-or-so years now, and this trend is continuing today. The major cracks began with WWI and then WWII. War as a means of settling human disputes *must be outlawed!* This current civilization has to be replaced by something…but, what? The increasing trend toward cultural globalization has its positives and negatives.

On the *plus* side: worldwide Internet communication, connecting people, and encouraging education in ways and at distances previously unimagined. The *minus* side: global Westernization spreading modern forms of military imperialism, crass scientific materialism that denies our full human sensorium, and a junk food restaurant on every corner. We can do a lot better than this!

Many of us who can buy food don't know what or how to eat to be healthy, while most of the rest of us starve. Our untrustworthy governments and corporate interests serve the enrichment of the wealthiest and most powerful. Earth is a conscious living being. It will inevitably react with natural violence to the random and reckless pollution we've laid on it—and the results will be excruciating, if not (eventually) catastrophic. ***We need a whole new paradigm for living. We need it now!***

"If you go deeply into the physical dimension, you see it is simply energies. It is mainly space. When you get down to the atomic level, there is a lot of space in between so-called 'particles'. It is a field of energy. The particles are not particles—when seen truly, they are energy-fields. Everything is energy-fields—everything! There is no 'matter'. There is only energy-fields. Everything is an apparition of energy-fields.

"Everything cosmic, everything conditional, is energy only. There is no matter otherwise. What appears to be matter is a mode of energy. If you get close enough to it, you find matter to be energy. If you get more of a distant view, you feel it as 'stuff'. But, in truth there is no 'stuff'"—there are only

fields of energy. Functioning on the basis of this understanding is fundamental human responsibility. Right-life practice is energy-practice relative to the life-domain." —Adi Da Samraj

We need a new way of life, a new basis for Civilization as a whole. We can no longer build our cultures on cold, shallow, scientific materialism (phony science) or on cockamamie downtown religion. It has to be based on something truly strong, steady, entirely self-authenticating, and thoroly acceptable by everyone: ***Consciousness***.

Looking at the world situation positively and realistically, we can use Adi Da's term, *"positive disillusionment"*—meaning while we must remain positive about life, we have no illusion about egoity in ourselves and in others. No need to be idealistic and imagine wishing away the darkness. Instead, we can act intelligently and in positive, caring, sharing, tolerant, and cooperating ways.

"We are a binary or bipolar form, with only two options: (1) contraction or (2) radiation, either being (a) a closed fist, or (b) an open hand, a "no" or a "yes", a "zero" or a "one", a "minus" or a "plus, a "negative" or a "positive." We can contradict each other or we can cooperate with each other. We must be positively, responsively, and cooperatively purified and transformed as an integrated whole thru our surrender to the Unbroken Light of The Beloved Divine Person." —Avatar Adi Da Samraj

Reality-Humanity
In an amazing and revolutionary essay in the book, <u>*Not-Two Is Peace*</u>, Adi Da describes why the present world situation seems so intractable, and how we can turn things around. He suggests creating a "Global Cooperative Forum" and speaking with one unified voice—basically acting "everybody-all-at-once." The Net allows this to happen.

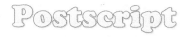

Earth Mandala

Our Earth is a beautiful world, gorgeous in so many ways and places, with wonders that a thousand lifetimes couldn't embrace. Bodily life here is a paradox of opposites: plus and minus, good and evil, high and low, mother-force and father-force. You must grow, but not without adversity. The lover devours you. The young and graceful gazelle is killed and eaten by the cheetah. So, where is the justice? What is the point? Neither going outward nor going inward grants true freedom. There is no such escape.

As delightful as this Earth-place appears, everything we love here dies here. As realms go, ours is in the gross area, the outermost band of The Cosmic Mandala (illustration ©ASA). All the universes, planes, and realms of being, are within the Conditional domain, each participating in a general level of vibration or energy that is lower (grosser, more difficult) or higher (more refined and pleasant). Each of us can participate in the various levels of this Mandala, and often go thru a range of these levels on any given day.

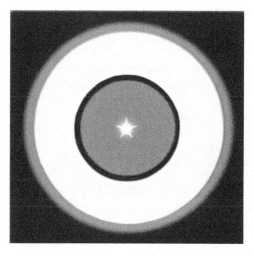

The lowest realms within the Mandala are the so-called "hell realms," within the red band or circle. Our best understanding suggests that, overall, Earth is just inside the red band. Some worlds are further down in the red realm than our Earth. Life in those realms is shorter and more brutish. The yellow band represents the etheric, pranic, universal life energy of conditional experience. The soft white band represents the ordinary sense-based or ego-mind. The black band is a transitional space where mental activity is suspended.

The **blue** band is the domain of higher mind, the mind beyond the brain. The brilliant white 5-pointed star is the doorway to the Divine Domain—which some think of as the God-Man, the Spiritual Master, the Threshold Personality. The significance of The Cosmic Mandala is described in precise detail in the book, *__Conductivity Healing__*.

We picture it here to illustrate the various planes of being that have been described perennially thru our human Great Tradition of Spiritual literature. Every heart longs for the Great Happiness, the kind that never goes away. Some are told (and become convinced) that such is found in the "heavens" of the blue realms, so-called "cosmic consciousness," the Disneyland-like realms of higher mind.

But, it's just another trap—granted with many lovely places, where beings live much longer, and war has long-since been abolished. And, yes, everyone does Spiritual practice, and folks are much happier, but it's not the capital "H" Happiness every heart longs for—The Divine Reality, the Place of Eternity.

Consider how we might move our world up out of the hell (red) realms and into the etheric (yellow) realms. How could we do that? One way could be to get together on the Net and insist our leaders outlaw war as a means of solving human disputes. Remember John Lennon's song, "*Imagine*"? It can happen. Believe it. The process is described in the book, <u>*Not-Two Is Peace*</u>. We can do this.

I tell you true, there would be a cry of happiness and delight like this world has never known. As suggested in that amazing book, there would likely be a call for a whole month of world-wide celebration! And it would be justified. This is cooperation on a grand scale. Let's do it!

Oh, and one last thing! If you feel moved by what you have read here, I urge you to get a copy of four audio talks by Adi Da Samraj:

(1) *A Birthday Message From Jesus and Me*
(2) *Submission to The Self*
(3) *The Secret of Suddenness*
(4) *Renunciation and the Gift of Community*

They will teach you much more about how life and afterlife work. If you listen to them 100 times, you will learn something new each time— something wise and even critically important.

How do I know? I've done it!

May you enjoy your GLD into the future.
May you pass your gifts on to everyone.
May you be Blessed!

Appendix A — Recipes

Preparing Liquid Meals that Both Nourish and Please

Introduction

IMPORTANT: For many more recipes, go to www.GLDiet.co and click on **GLDLifestyle**.

First, check Appendix B to decide which Helpful Kitchen Devices you want. After purchasing them (at least the blender—if not also the juicer), note that for most health purposes, blender liquids are more vital than juicer liquids because of the bulk and ruffage retained for good bowel health. However, for fasting and juice dieting, the variously diluted and undiluted juicer drinks are essential. On your GLD, as well as with fasting and juice dieting, the green drinks are the most important of all.

Remember, always use pure water for internal body nourishment. Most tap waters contain the poisons chlorine and/or fluoride, and therefore are unhealthy and should be avoided. Also avoid water stored in plastic bottles. Store your liquids in the frig, using glass, stainless steel, or ceramic containers. Whenever possible, consume fresh-made liquids directly after making them.

Avoid keeping home-prepared smoothies and fresh-squeezed juices overnite as they are volatile and will lose their nutritive power over certain hours. Veggy juices tend to last a bit longer than do fruit juices. If liquids can't be drunk right away, store them overnite in a cold frig. Some juices store better than others—including apple and pineapple. A covered container helps, and refrigerating them will make them last longer.

If you have to go to work, OK, make your liquids that day, put them into a thermos (chilled or heated, as appropriate) and take them along, but if at all possible, consume them that same day. Otherwise, a day later, they may still taste good but, remember, you'll be getting less nutrition from them.

Avoid purchasing pasteurized drinks in bottles. Commercially bottled drinks have lost their food enzymes from the Pasteurizing (heating) process, and also some of the vitamins, but other vitamins will remain, and at least some of the minerals will remain intact. Altho commercial vacuum sealing helps preserve the nutrients, under most circumstances by far, *fresh is best!*

SPECIAL NOTE:

The USA is still behind the curve with metric measurements. We still use the old British Imperial system, where oz. = ounce, Tbsp. = tablespoon, tsp. = teaspoon, qt. = quart, and c = cup. Also, it is assumed that all recommended recipes use the purest **water** available (see Chapter 36). Our Rx is steam-distilled that has been in the sun in a glass jar for 3 hours. See Appendix B for our juicer and blender suggestions.

Always use only the purest untainted fresh raw fruits, veggies, nuts, seeds, and spices. Sweeteners could be dates, date sugar or coconut sugar. For salt, use Himalayan or other untainted earth salt or sea salt. Let's start with some smoothies!

Blender Recipes

Basic Instructions

Smoothies are often the tastiest and most important of all the liquids you'll be drinking on your GLD. You need a sturdy blender (e.g., VitaMix® or Blendtech©) for making smoothies. The blender must be strong and capable of making the widest variety of drinks, from simple nutmilks to complex green smoothies to hot raw and cooked veggy soups. Other more common blenders are usually weaker, slower, and less capable of the quick results and fine blending (with fewer chunks).

Base Smoothie Blender Liquids

Introduction

Included here, besides milk for people of all ages, are some ideas on making milk for infants and babies that are not being breastfed. Please note that it's best to breastfeed babies until they are at least two years of age—if not three! Breastfeeding boosts a child's immunity, creates a special bond of intimacy between mother and child, and brings many other positive qualities to the infant.

If breastfeeding can't happen, your first choice is the water inside young coconuts (see below). After eight months, many of the other following milks may work for them—in other words, after children have been weaned. Let's start with some GLD blender foundation or "base" liquids, the first thing you put into your blender. Typically, you will be using about 10 ounces of some liquid, which could be…

(1) pure water
(2) a nutmilk (or seedmilk, or combination milk made from nuts <u>and</u> seeds), or
(3) a fruit juice

After the base smoothie liquid, you add your solids to the blender. These are typically a handful of greens (if making a green smoothie), one or more pieces of fruit, and (if not using nut-seed milk as your base smoothie liquid) a few nuts or seeds.

At Grand Medicine, some of us like our smoothies rich, so we use about 5 oz. of the Rich Nutmilk formula, then add about 5 oz. pure water. Then, we add the other ingredients, depending on the desired smoothie. This process can be used for almost any kind of smoothie—except for such very simple smoothies as the Orange-Coconut-Mint Green Smoothie (recipe below).

Some people like rich, thick smoothies. Others—including those in more of a hurry—prefer quick and thin smoothies. You can avoid making the nut-seed milk by simply adding a few nuts or seeds to a water base. Whichever way or viscosity you like—thick or thin—you can add more or less water, or more or fewer nuts / seeds, for the desired consistency or viscosity.

Pure Water Smoothie Base
Ingredients
- 10 oz. pure water (prefer steam distilled)
- (fruits, veggies, nuts/seeds)

Procedure

You place the water into the blender, then add the other desired ingredients, blend, and serve.

Simple Nutmilk (smoothie base)
Ingredients
- 10 oz. pure water
- One handful nuts

Procedure

Pour the water into your blender. Add the nuts (preferably almonds, but whichever you choose, they are best soaked for 3 hours in a bowl of pure water before placing into the blender; such seeds and raw sunflower, pumpkin, or sesame may also be used instead of the nuts; sesame seeds, if used, do not need to be soaked). Blend well on hi-speed. Pour into a quart-size bottle and store in a cool frig to use as needed.

Simple Almond Milk
Ingredients
- 1 handful raw almonds
- 2c pure water
- 1 tsp. raw sesame seeds (optional)

Instructions

Soak almonds in a bowl of pure water for 3 hours or overnight in the frig. Rinse this well with pure water and place into your blender with water (prefer steam-distilled). Add the sesame seeds now if using them (for added calcium). Blend for a minute or so. For a rich and more healthful milk, add a Tbsp. of virgin coconut oil per quart. Pour into a quart container and fill the rest of the container with pure water.

When kids get funny about wanting it sweeter (usually around teenage), you can add 1 or 2 dates or a tablespoon or so of pure coconut sugar. Strain thru a white hemp cloth if the milk is being presented to an infant (to eliminate any chunks or particles that could irritate a tiny throat). This same formula can be used with just about any other nut or seed, especially the hard nuts and seeds (almonds, pumpkin seeds, filberts, and hazelnuts). This milk stays white and will remain fresh for 4-5 days in a cool frig.

Almond-Cashew Milk

Ingredients

- 1 lge handful raw almonds
- 1 lge handful raw cashews
- 2 cups pure water
- 1 big Tbsp. pure coconut oil
- 1 Tbsp. raw sesame seeds (optional)

Instructions

Blend ingredients for 1-2 minutes on hi-speed. Coconut oil must be unrefined raw expeller-pressed (cold-pressed). Pour into a half-gallon container and add pure water to the top. Place in the frig.

Coconut Milk (intro)

Coconut milk is made from the white flesh of the nut. It is among the most nourishing of all possible milks, and can be drunk by everyone over nine months of age. It's best to use fresh young or mature coconuts for this, or, if these are not available, at least raw natural shredded or flaked unsweetened coconut. *Caution:* avoid commercial shredded coconut containing refined sugar and/or preservatives. Mature coconuts are lite brown to white in color. First, break off the goatee at the bottom of the nut and note its color. If black, it's probably moldy. If lite brown, it's likely OK.

To open and prepare it: use a sharp-pointed knife to poke a hole in the "monkey's mouth," which is the larger of the three markings on its top. Once you get a good hole, invert it and drain out the liquid inside. Taste it. It must be sweet. If it's not sweet, take it back to the store for a replacement or break it into pieces and place it into the compost pile.

The Net describes several ways of opening a coconut. One way is by placing it into 2 or 3 plastic shopping bags and swinging it down hard to crack it on the concrete outside. Then CAREFULLY pry out the nutmeat with a butter knife. Either drink the sweet coconut water or place it in the blender to use for making your nut milk. (It may also be placed into a nipple bottle for an infant to supplement or replace or augment missing mother's milk.)

Coconut Milk

Ingredients
- Several chunks of freshly cut coconut or 4-6 heaping Tbsp. raw shredded or flaked coconut
- 10 oz. pure water
- 1-2 tsp. coconut sugar or 2-3 dates (optional)

Instructions

After draining and breaking open the nut, cut the nutmeat into manageable chunks and place them in the blender. Blend them with half of the water for 2-3 minutes. Strain this thru a wire mesh food strainer, stirring with a spoon. Save the liquid to one side and place the pulp back into the blender with the rest of the water and repeat the procedure. Throw the remaining pulp into the kitchen waste container for composting.

The resulting liquid makes a delicious and very nutritious milk. OK to add a little pure coconut sugar or a few dates for those who like their milk sweeter.

Coconut Milk for Infants and Children

Ingredients
- Gel-like nutmeat of a young coconut
- 5-6 oz. pure water
- 2-4 dates (optional sweetener)

Procedure

Find an unhusked young coconut. At one end, cut away the lite-colored husk with a sharp knife to expose the end of the nut. Puncture a whole and drain out the liquid, which is excellent **for infants**. Then, break a large hole in the end of the nut, and, using a large spoon, scoop out the soft gel-like nutmeat, place this into the blender, add 2-4 dates for sweetness to taste, blend and you have your milk **for children**.

Smoothie Foundation Liquids

Among the better bases or foundation liquids to use to mix your smoothie's solid ingredients is simple nut &/or seed milk, like almond-cashew milk, most often made with raw almonds, raw cashews, and perhaps a Tbsp. or so of coconut oil blended with pure water. Alternatively, you may wish to use just pure water, or raw, unfiltered apple juice, or fresh-made coconut milk (recipe below).

Home-made almond-cashew milk stays white and keeps in a cool frig for 4-5 days. Coconut milk keeps safely in the frig for about four days. Using a combination of nuts and seed, plus a cold frig, your milk could last a week. Commercially available almond milk is a poor substitute for your own nut and seed milks. Avoid soymilk, dairy milk, and rice milk. The only ingredient in Aroy-D© 100% coconut milk (in a box) is coconut—acceptable for the GLD and currently available at "Asian Food" stores.

Smoothies—Almost Infinite Possibilities

Feel free to experiment with different kinds of fruits, veggies, nuts, and seeds, remembering that a smoothie almost always has "the basics": fruits, veggies, and nuts/seeds. Change the base liquid now and then; use different nuts or seeds in your mix, switch veggies, and also your fruits. Our favorite base is some kind of nut-seed milk, but you may prefer apple juice, pineapple juice, or plain water. Use your creativity and imagination.

Tips

- Share your recipes with others.
- Avoid blending melons with any other foods, even fruits (somehow, they don't combine well)
- Melons can be used by themselves (without nuts or seeds) to make delicious liquids
- Use virtually any nut or seed or combo thereof (besides almonds and coconut) to make nut-seed milk
- The sweet water inside a fresh young or mature coconut will nourish an infant unable to take mother's milk. On removing it from the coconut, always taste it first to be sure it's sweet.
- A heaping Tbsp. or so of plain yogurt can be added to smoothies to enrich them, if desired and appropriate.
- Smoothie recipes are made with a blender, not a juicer.
- Altho there are a variety of blenders available for purchase, only a few (like VitaMix and Blendtech) have the real power and ability to quickly support efficient, effective smoothie production.

For Green Smoothie recipes, we simply place the greens into the blender, add some water (or nut-seed milk), and the amount of fresh fruit needed to make the drink palatable and blend on medium-to-hi speed. Slower speed may leave some (usually undesirable) chunks. Hi-speed makes the smoothie viscosity and consistency smoother and finer. Thicker or thinner, you decide what is just right.

BTW, with the Vitamix and other power blenders, always start at the lowest speed and gradually raise the speed, **never** on higher speeds. Starting them on hi-speed settings can harm the Mechanisms. It's like starting a car in the wrong gear.

Many different fruits and berries could be used as sweeteners, besides dates. You may use only one vegetable and one type of fruit or mix and match. More likely, you'll use two veggies and perhaps 2 or 3 different fruits. It's best to switch veggies and fruits at least weekly for a variety of nutrients. The amount of water used depends on the amount of smoothie needed and viscosity (thickness) desired.

Coconut Milk (smoothie base)
Introduction

      Coconut Milk is made in any number of ways. One is made by blending the grated flesh of a fresh mature coconut with pure hot water. The result is a rich white liquid that looks very much like cow's milk. When refrigerated, coconut milk (fresh or canned), if not shaken, separates into two layers, the thick (upper) cream layer and the thinner (bottom) milk layer. The top layer can be skimmed off with a spoon and used for recipes requiring cream (usually desserts) with the bottom layer reserved for coconut milk recipes.

      Canned, frozen and powdered coconut milk are widely available, convenient to use, and generally of good quality. (Just be sure to check the container for excipients. If anything but coconut and water, avoid it). However, they do not usually achieve quite the quality of coconut milk prepared at home from good fresh or desiccated coconut. Never buy shredded (desiccated) coconut containing refined sugar or chemicals!

Procedure: Preparing Coconut Milk from Fresh Coconut

      Pierce the larger of the three eyes of a fresh coconut with a sharp-pointed knife. Drain the liquid inside it into a glass. Taste it to see if it's sweet. If moldy, break up the nut and put it into the garbage for compost. If sweet, place the coconut into a doubled ordinary plastic shopping bag, take it into the garage or outside and swing it onto the pavement, breaking the shell into several pieces.

      Carefully remove all the coconut meat from the shell using a butter knife. Leave the brown skin on the nutmeat and cut the meat into small cubes. Place these into a glass container and keep in the frig if using them within three days or into the freezer for use a week or more later. (Other means of opening whole coconut shells—whether young or mature—are available on the Net.)

      For one quart of coconut milk, place a small handful of the nutmeat pieces into a blender, add 2 cups of very hot water and blend on the highest speed for two full minutes. Place a fine-mesh sieve or strainer over a bowl and pour the blended nutmeat into the bowl thru the strainer and stir with a spoon until most of the milk is in the bowl.

      Discard the resultant coconut meat into the compost, pour the milk into a quart container, fill with pure water, and refrigerate. You can blend in 2-4 dates to make it sweet to your taste. Be sure to use this white milk within four days max. Use these recipes as milk for cereals, granolas, and other preparations.

Procedure: Alternative Desiccated Coconut Milk Recipe

Unsweetened desiccated coconut can be prepared in the same way as with the fresh chunks of coconut. Empty an 8 oz. package of unsweetened desiccated coconut into a blender and add 1 cup boiling water. Blend for two full minutes and allow the mixture to cool a bit.

Place a sieve over a bowl lined with cheesecloth. Ladle the mixture into the cheesecloth, fold the edges over the coconut meat, and twist the ends to extract as much milk as you can into the bowl. Compost the squeezed coconut meat and refrigerate the coconut milk you've extracted into the bowl. Refrigerate the milk and use it within 3-4 days.

Raw Almond-Cashew Milk (smoothie base)

Ingredients
- Gel-like nutmeat of a young coconut
- 1 handful raw almonds (36 or so)
- 1 handful raw cashews (36 or so)
- 1 Tbsp. pure unrefined virgin coconut oil
- 1 Tbsp. sesame seeds (optional—for added calcium)

Procedure

Soak nuts in pure water for 3 hours or overnite; rinse well in pure water, place in your blender with 15 oz. pure water, 1 Tbsp. pure virgin coconut oil, and, if you like, the sesame seeds. Blend very well (1 minute), pour into a half-gallon glass container, add pure water to fill the container, refrigerate. This white milk will remain tasty and viable for 5-6 days in a cold frig. For sweeter milk, add a few dates or pure coconut sugar to taste. (Ex. www.CoconutSecret.com)

Extra Rich Nutmilk (smoothie base and more)
Ingredients
- 1 handful almonds
- 1 handful cashews
- 8 raw macadamia nuts (or other raw nuts)
- 10 pecans (or other raw nuts)
- 1 Tbsp. raw sesame seeds (for high calcium)
- 1-2 Tbsp. coconut oil (raw, cold or "expeller"-pressed, unrefined, chemical-free)
- (optional) two 250 mL boxes Aroy-D© 100% coconut milk* (see *Procedure*)
- 15 or so oz. ounces of pure water (see *Procedure*)

Procedure

Place the nuts (not the sesame seeds, tho) into a bowl of pure water and allow to soak for at least 3 hours or overnite. Rinse at least three times with pure water. Place into your blender, add about 15 oz. pure water, and the sesame seeds and coconut oil. Blend on hi-speed for a full minute. Pour into a half-gallon bottle and fill the rest of the bottle with pure water. Shake to mix, and place in the coldest part of the frig (NOT the freezer) for maximum life.

This very rich, creamy white milk should keep for about six days—IF sweeteners are not added to it. It can be used as a base (instead of water) in virtually any smoothie AND for cereals, granola, hot cacao, etc. Excellent for those thin-body types wishing to avoid too much weight loss. Otherwise, yes, if you like, you can thin it down by adding more water.

*This boxed coconut milk is available in so-called "Asian" stores. Four Tbsp. of raw untreated unsweetened shredded coconut or several chunks of fresh coconut may be substituted.

Sweet Basic Nut Milk (a good smoothie base)
Ingredients:
- 1 cup of pure water
- 1 handful (about 30) raw almonds
- 3 Tbsp. pure coconut sugar or 4-5 dates

Instructions:

The almonds should be fresh-ground or (preferably) soaked priorly overnight. Blend very well (for about 90 seconds on hi-speed), pour into a quart container, add more water to fill quart container, blend in a few pure-water ice cubes if instant cold milk is desired. Experiment with pumpkin seeds, sunflower seeds, and various other nuts as your base, especially including coconut.

Hot Cacao (cocoa)

Ingredients

- 1 level tsp. cacao powder
- 1 level tsp. carob powder
- ½ tsp. whey powder
- 3-4 tsp. coconut sugar
- 5 oz. (±) pure water
- 3 oz. Extra Rich NutMilk

Procedure

"Cacao" and "cocoa" are the same thing. Just be sure to buy <u>only</u> raw <u>un</u>processed fair-trade cacao powder (NOT "alkaline processed," "alkali processed," "Dutched," or "Dutch-processed"). The carob must also be raw unprocessed. The best whey powder (I think) is <u>Capra Mineral Whey</u>©. Insist on genuine pure coconut sugar as your only sugar—which amount you adjust to your taste. Put the powders and the sugar into your cup, pour on about 5 oz. boiling water, stir, add about 3 oz. of the Extra Rich NutMilk (see recipe in these pages) and enjoy a delicious and nutritious hot beverage!

Green Smoothies

Basic Green Smoothie
Ingredients
- 5 oz. Extra Rich Nutmilk
- 5 oz. pure water
- One large handful of fresh raw greens, either as a single veggie or various mixed veggies (ex: baby spinach, chard, kale, beet greens, cilantro), or use some broccoli, a few asparagus spears, celery sticks, etc.
- 1 peach
- 1 organic date

Procedure

  Add nutmilk to blender, then water, then the other ingredients. Blend, pour, serve, and drink!

Orange-Banana Green Smoothie
Ingredients
- One large handful of fresh raw greens
- One peeled orange
- One peeled banana
- 1-2 cups pure water

Procedure

  Blend, pour, serve, and drink!

Kale Orange Mango Smoothie
Ingredients
- 1 medium handful Cilantro
- 2 large leaves kale
- 1 peeled Orange
- 8 large Strawberries
- 1 mango
- 1 date
- 1-2 cups pure water

Procedure

  Blend, pour, serve, and drink

Banana Berry Green Smoothie
Ingredients
- 10 oz. raw, unfiltered apple juice
- 1 banana
- 1 handful berries
- 1 Tbsp. shredded coconut
- 1/3c (or small handful) raw nuts or seeds
- Several sprigs of fresh mint leaves

Procedure

   Place apple juice in your blender. Add banana, nuts, or seeds (or a combination thereof), then the shredded coconut. Add the berries (OK frozen if they are blueberries). Blend, serve.

Pineapple-Coconut Smoothie
Ingredients:
- 10 oz. fresh-squeezed pineapple juice
- 3 heaping Tbsp. plain yogurt (optional only)
- 2 large medjool dates (or 4 smaller dates)
- a few chunks of fresh coconut (or 2 big Tbsp. shredded coconut)
- 1 banana

Instructions:

   Use fresh-squeezed pineapple juice (via your juicer) whenever possible because of its far higher nutritional qualities. If not, use a high quality non-adulterated bottled or canned pineapple juice. Place into blender, add the other ingredients, and blend until smooth. Note that the yogurt is not a necessary item. However, for chronically toxic bowel systems and with dysbiosis (full of unfriendly organisms), the yogurt can be very helpful. (Yes, yogurt can also be helpful by injecting it rectally. See Chapter 9.)

Orange-Coconut Drink

Ingredients:

- 8 or so oz. fresh orange juice
- 1 big Tbsp. grated raw unsweetened coconut
- 1 or 2 pitted dates

Instructions:

The orange juice should be fresh-squeezed. Make sure the dried coconut does not contain refined sugar or any other ingredient. Alternative to the dried coconut, you can use a chunk of fresh coconut from the shell. The date or dates can be dried (commonly the way they're sold) or fresh. Blend well. This is a delicious and powerfully nourishing breakfast drink—orange with a taste of coconut.

Carob Smoothie

Ingredients

- 1 banana
- 2 Tbsp. raw carob powder
- 1 big Tbsp. coconut flakes, shreds or chunk
- 2 lge medjool dates
- 2c pure water
- 2-3 heaping Tbsp. plain yogurt (optional)
- 12-16 almonds (or use almond milk or Extra Rich Nutmilk)

Instructions

Blend well. Note that for a hot carob drink, the water may alternatively be boiled, then poured into the blender, then the other ingredients added.

Strawberry Smoothie

Ingredients:

- A handful of fresh strawberries
- 4 oz. pure raw apple juice
- 4 oz. almond milk (or coconut milk)
- A small handful of fresh raw pecans or walnuts
- one banana

Instructions:

Blend. (Add 2-3 pure-water ice cubes if a cold drink is desired.)

Pineapple Smoothie

Ingredients:

- 1 cup fresh chopped pineapple
- 1 cup of pure water
- 1 cup almond milk
- 1 banana
- ½ apple

Instructions:

Blend ingredients, adding 2-3 pure-water ice cubes if a cold drink is desired. Other nut or seed milks can replace almond milk if desired. ALWAYS make your own nut and seed milks!

Avocado-Coconut Smoothie

Ingredients:

- ½ avocado
- 1 banana
- 2 heaping Tbsp. plain yogurt (only if appropriate)
- 1/3 cup shredded coconut (not sugar-sweetened)
- 1½ cups almond milk, coconut milk, or Extra Rich Nutmilk
- 5-7 pitted dates (for sweetness to your taste)

Instructions:

Add 2-3 pure-water ice cubes if a chilled drink is desired. Add 1 or more Tbsp. pure coconut sugar or more dates if more sweetness is desired. Blend well; add more water if a thinner liquid is desired. We like it thick enuf to hold up a spoon! It's green, it's Martian, and it's delicious!

Blueberry Smoothie

Ingredients:

- ½ cup blueberries (fresh or frozen)
- 2 large dates
- 1 Tbsp. pure coconut sugar
- 2 cups pure water

Instructions:

Two lge Tbsp. plain yogurt may be used if appropriate. Blend well. Check before serving to see if it's sweet enuf; then add coconut sugar to taste as desired.

Hot Raw Soup

Ingredients:

- 3c pure water
- 1 garlic bud
- 1 slice of onion
- 1 ear corn (cut from the cob)
- 1 slice cabbage
- 1/3rd bell pepper
- ½ carrot
- 1 small bunch fresh cilantro (or parsley)
- ½c natural style corn chips
- Veggy broth powder (or sea salt) to taste

Instructions:

Boil water and let stand until still hot but no longer boiling. Place in blender with other ingredients and blend well. Be sure broth powder has no TVP or HVP (texturized or hydrolyzed vegetable protein).

Basic Juicer and Other Thinner Liquid Drinks

RMVJ—Raw Mixed Vegetable Juice
Ingredients

- 1 handful raw almonds (36 or so)
- 3 large carrots
- 3 stalks celery
- 1/3rd beet
- 1 garlic bud
- ½ zucchini or cucumber
- 2 large apples with peel (prefer Granny Smith green apples)
- 1/3rd fresh lemon with peel
- Optional (for the stomach) add 1 small slice fresh ginger

Procedure

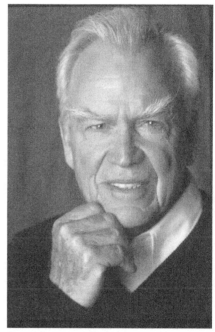

Scrub and rinse ingredients in cold clear water, leaving their peels on as it is in the peels that most of the nutrition is found. Cut ingredients into sizes that fit easily into juicer. ***Note***: carrots, beet, garlic, lemon, and apple should always be included. Other veggies, especially greens, can be substituted for the celery and zucchini—such as asparagus, kale, broccoli, chard, spinach, parsley, cabbage, etc. It's good to do such substitutions now and then to bring other nutrients into the recipe. Yield: about 20 oz.

Story

We first came across Jay Kordich, "The Juiceman," in the 1960s. One of the heroes of Natural Health, a true pioneer in this field, later referred to as "The Father of Juicing," Kordich lived to age 93 in good health. He introduced us to his Juiceman, Jr., juicer, and to the RMVJ recipe. Over the decades, we would make this recipe from time to time. Currently (September 2019), we drink it almost every day.

While teaching Eyology in Australia, three nice ladies in one of our classes secretly purchased leprechaun-like tall green hats. Whenever we would mention RMVJ, they would all stand up together, wave those hats, and say, "*RMVJ—all the way!*" Years later, on hearing this story, a friend had manufactured for us our own RMVJ caps to wear!

317

Alternative (and powerful) **RMVJ Recipe**
Ingredients
- 4 large carrots
- 2 sticks celery
- 1/3rd beet
- 1 garlic bud
- ½ zucchini
- 2 large green apples
- 1 lemon with peel
- A few buds of broccoli
- 2-4 sticks of large asparagus
- A small handful of fresh spinach
- A few large chunks of fresh pineapple (possibly including the core)
- 1 thumb-size chunk fresh ginger root

Holly's Mini-RMVJ
Ingredients
- 1 small beet
- 1 beet leaf
- 3 carrots
- ½ cucumber
- ½ c distilled water

Procedure
Process these thru the juicer, serve!

Salty Sipping Beverages
Ingredients
- 2 oz. juice from a jar of pure dill pickles, or…
- 2 oz. juice from a jar of pure sauerkraut, or…
- 2 oz. liquid from a jar of pure jalapenos

Instructions

The pickle juice (from a jar of pickles) must have nothing more than (possibly) water, cucumbers, red bell peppers, carrots, salt, distilled vinegar, and dill weed. The sauerkraut juice must have nothing more than water, cabbage, sea salt, and maybe organic garlic (Costco has this). The liquid from a jar of jalapenos must have nothing more than jalapeno peppers, water, vinegar, sea salt, and spices (La Costeña© Nachos).

Absolutely no chemicals! If you like, you can use any of these deliciously salty liquids separately or mix them together, place in a jar, and keep refrigerated. When feeling the need for something salty (and you <u>will</u> on your rightly done GLD!), pour some of this mix into a small cup and take an occasional sip.

Coconut Nectar
Ingredients
- Several chunks of fresh coconut

Procedure

Coconut nectar is made by running the chunks of mature coconut meat thru your juicer. Altho centrifugal juicers will work in this case, the masticating juicers (<u>Omega 8006</u>, <u>Oscar</u>, <u>Champion</u>) will do best. The resulting liquid is thick, rich, and delicious—all of which you may wish to drink immediately! Great for cereal, granola and as dessert toppings. Otherwise, add water and perhaps a few dates, blend, and you have coconut milk.

Note also that blending fresh chunks of coconut involves adding water, blending, and straining, whereas juicing the chunks produces more immediate results. However, with juicing, the result is thicker and leaves far less product. Juice or blend, then, according to your needs and desires.

Pineapple Nectar
Ingredient and *Procedure*

Prepare a fresh whole pineapple by twisting off the top. With a sawing motion, cut away the skin in strips. Lay it down and cut long strips of the pineapple thin enuf to fit thru the hopper of your juicer. Be sure to include the core, which has strong anti-parasite properties. Bottle and place in the frig to chill.

REAL Orange Juice
Ingredients and **Procedure**

Peel 4 or 5 oranges (preferably navel type) with your hands or a citrus or potato peeler. Quarter the resulting white balls with a knife, then blend well to produce "real" orange juice. This yields 100% of the nutritional value of the oranges—instead of the usual 4-10%, you get when purchasing commercial orange juice!

In order to make this "Real OJ" palatable, you may wish to add the juice of 2 or 3 oranges squeezed the usual way. (What people normally think of as "orange juice" is really more like "orange water"!) OK to use Real OJ as a base for certain smoothies. Approximately 92% of human-useable nutrients are derived from the whole juice of fresh raw ripe oranges, with about 8% sacrificed in the pulp (the orange-colored outer peeling has few human-useable nutrients).

Snacks

Raw Hummus
Ingredients
- 1 cup chickpea sprouts (sprouted overnight)
- Juice of 1 lemon or lime
- 2 Tbsp. fresh orange juice
- 1 clove garlic
- 2 Tbsp. raw sesame tahini

Procedure

Optional seasonings: ground cumin, sea salt, chives, paprika, cayenne pepper, dried onion powder, or dried garlic powder—to taste. Blend all ingredients. Add water in order to thin to the desired consistency. You can add sun-dried tomatoes, roasted bell pepper, cilantro, and jalapeno to achieve different flavors. Delicious when spread on leafy greens, red bell pepper strips, or even celery. Enjoy!

Veggie Chips and Hummus Dip

There are several currently available veggy-based "chips" made from carrots, beets, tomatoes, and other vegetables that can be used as snacks while on your GLD. There is almost an equal variety of dips, many made from hummus, which is made from garbanzo beans, or other dips made from other beans or vegetable materials.

Any of several fresh veggies can be fine-chopped and mixed into dips purchased for GLD snacking. Our choice includes onions, garlic, celery, parsley, jalapenos, tomatoes, and cilantro. Avoid any chips or dips that contain chemical preservatives, coloring agents, or foreign chemicals of any kind other than citric acid from lemons. Limit the number of chips to a few while on GLD *Level 2* and *Level 3*, none on *Level 1*.

Figs, Apricots, and Soaked Nuts

Ripe and whole, figs and apricots are magnificent foods. When properly dried, figs (Calimyrna golden or black) have a white coating of natural sugar from the fig itself. They are sweet and delicious. Avoid the stupid companies that still process figs and other dried fruit with sulfur dioxide or other chemicals. Carefully processed, dried fruits do not need the chemicals and are devoid of moth eggs.

Dried fruits including figs, grapes (raisins), apricots, pears, apples, and peaches of many kinds have been used perennially by school students in Europe and other countries as a primary snack in delightful combination with nuts to create a nutrition packed, hi-calorie, delicious, energy-rich and powerful snack combination. Limit this combo to a handful on GLD *Levels 2* and *3*, none on *Level 1*.

Crackers and Guacamole

Open a ripe avocado by slicing it lengthwise and twisting it apart, as shown in our Lifestyle DVD. Using a fork, mash it into a bowl. Add finely chopped onion, garlic, cilantro, jalapeno (optional—because it's hot!), and tomato. Stir and either eat with a spoon or with a few natural style chips or crackers—a favorite evening snack.

Solid Food Meals
Salads, Granola, and Desserts

Raw Coconut-Vanilla Granola
Ingredients
- 1 cup sprouted buckwheat
- 1 cup sprouted sunflower seeds
- 1 cup sprouted pumpkin seeds
- 1 cup chopped soak almonds or other nuts like pecans, walnuts, etc.
- 1 cup raw coconut flakes
- 1 cup of coconut crystals
- ½ cup raisins
- ¼ cup of coconut oil
- 2 Tbsp. vanilla extract
- A dash of sea salt

Procedure

    Sprout buckwheat, sunflower, and pumpkin seeds in large jars for two nites with water. Mix all ingredients together with your hands in a big steel mixing bowl. Spread on a dehydrator sheet and dehydrate at 115 degrees for 8-12 hours or until crunchy. Serve with Nut milk and dried or fresh fruit. Enjoy! (Note: this private recipe is an original creation of Nenita Sarmiento-Mehlmauer)

Creamy Cashew Dressing
Ingredients
- 1½ cups cashews
- 1 cup peeled cucumber *(or water)*
- 3 Tbsp. lemon juice
- 1/4 cup apple cider vinegar
- 1 Tbsp. honey
- 2 cloves garlic
- 3 tsp. onion powder
- 1 tsp. sea salt
- 1/3 cup extra virgin olive oil
- 1 tsp. dried dill

Procedure

    Blend everything but the dill and olive oil in a blender. Then, gently blend in the dill and olive oil.

Crisp Green Salad with Vinaigrette Dressing
Ingredients
Salad

- 1 head butter lettuce
- 1 whole avocado, chopped into chunks
- 1 cup sunflower seed sprouts
- 1 medium tomato, chopped into small pieces
- 1 medium cucumber
- ¼ cup raw pine nuts

Dressing

- ¼ cup olive oil
- 1 cup balsamic vinegar
- 1 clove garlic, crushed
- 1 teaspoon Dijon mustard

Procedure

Rip or cut the lettuce leaves and place them in a big bowl. Cut the remaining vegetables and place them in the bowl with lettuce. Apply the pine nuts. Whisk together the olive oil and vinegar, then add the crushed garlic. Pour over salad and serve immediately.

Zucchini Linguine with Basil Pesto
Ingredients
Basil Pesto

- 2 cups tightly packed basil
- 1/2 cup pine nuts
- 1/4 cup walnut or pumpkin seeds
- 1 Tbs lemon juice
- 1 clove garlic
- 1/2 tsp. Himalayan or Celtic sea salt
- 1/4 cup cold-pressed olive oil

Spring or Filtered Water
Procedure

Soak the pine nuts and walnut/pumpkin seeds for at least 4 hours. Drain and rinse.

Zucchini Linguini
Ingredients
- 3 large zucchini
- 2 medium tomatoes
- 8-10 dried olives
- 1/2 red capsicum (cayenne)
- 2 Tbs pine nuts
- 1/2 cup basil pesto

Procedure

Using a julienne peeler or a spiralizer, slice the zucchini lengthways into long noodles and place them in a large bowl. Place all ingredients (except water) into the food processor and process until almost smooth (you still want a little texture to it). Add a little water at a time if it seems too dry. Store in a glass jar in the fridge for up to a week. Chop the tomatoes and capsicum, de-stone and chop the olives, and add these with the pine nuts to the zucchini. Add the pesto and mix thoroughly to combine. If you would like the noodles to soften a bit, leave the mix sit for 1 hour before serving.

Mock Salmon Pate
Ingredients
- 2 cups almonds, soaked overnight
- 1 cup celery, finely chopped
- 1/2 cup green onions, chopped
- 1/4 cup pure water
- 2 medium or large carrots
- 3 tsp. lemon juice
- Dulse flakes, rinsed
- 1 head romaine lettuce
- Parsley

Procedure

Run almonds and carrots through your juicer, using the "blank" or nut butter plate to make a smooth pâté. Mix all ingredients except lettuce in a bowl, adding the dulse to taste. Form the mixture into a rounded (or other shape) loaf and garnish with the parsley. Spoon onto the lettuce leaves and eat like a sandwich, or spread onto celery sticks. *Note*: this pate can also be used as a snack (as appropriate) on your GLD!

Raw Raspberry Cheesecake
Ingredients
<u>Crust</u>

- 2 cups raw macadamia nuts
- ½ cup pitted dates
- ¼ cup dried shredded coconut

Procedure

     Prepare macadamias and dates in your food processor. Sprinkle dried coconut onto the bottom of 8" or 9" spring-form pan. Press crust onto the coconut to prevent it from sticking.

<u>Cake</u>
Ingredients

- 3 cups chopped raw cashews (or 1½c cashews & 1½c macadamias) soaked for at least 1 hour
- ¾ cup lemon juice
- ¾ cup honey
- ¾ cup of coconut oil
- 1 tsp. vanilla
- ½ tsp. sea salt

Procedure

     Blend cashews, lemon, honey, gently warmed coconut oil, vanilla, sea salt, & 1/2 cup water. Blend until smooth and adjust to taste. Pour the mixture on the crust. Remove air bubbles by tapping the pan on a table. Place in the freezer until firm. Remove the whole cake from the pan while frozen and place it on a serving platter. Defrost in frig

<u>Raspberry Sauce</u>
Ingredients

- 1 bag frozen raspberries
- ½ cup pitted dates

Procedure

     Prepare raspberries and dates in a food processor until well blended. *Note*: Do NOT use a blender for this, or the raspberry seeds will become like sand.

Raw Mango Pie

Crust Ingredients
- 2 cups raw almonds (or walnuts or pecans; I use mainly pecans with a few almonds)
- 1 cup unsweetened shredded coconut
- ½ cup pitted dates (adjust so that mixture becomes slightly sticky)

Procedure

In a food processor, process the nuts and coconut together until the lumps are gone. Do not over process. Add the dates, then process until the mixture resembles coarse crumbs that stick together. Press into a pie plate.

Filling Ingredients
- 2 fresh mangos
- ½ cup organic dried mangos

Procedure

Peeled and cut up the fresh mangos. Cut or tear into small pieces the unsweetened dried mango, then soak it for about 10 minutes and drain. Optional: other fruit that can be used as topping includes kiwis, strawberries, or blackberries. In a blender, process the fresh and soaked dried mangos until the mixture has a pudding-like consistency. Pour into the crust and decorate with other fruit.

Delicious!

Fresh Blueberry Pie

<u>Crust</u>

Ingredients

- 2 cups almonds
- ½ cup pitted dates
- pinch of sea salt

Procedure

Grind almonds in your food processor until fine. Add dates and salt. Blend 'til mixture binds together between your fingers when pinched. Press into 9" glass pie pan and set to one side.

<u>Filling</u>

Ingredients

- 5 cups fresh blueberries
- 2 bananas
- 1½ T honey

Procedure

Combine four cups of the berries, bananas, and honey in your food processor. Blend 'til smooth. Remove from the processor bowl and stir in remaining berries. Pour into the prepared crust. Refrigerate for at least three hours. Serve and enjoy.

Chocolate Bliss Pudding with Coconut Cream

<u>Coconut Cream</u>

Ingredients

- meat from 2 young coconuts
- water from 1 young coconut
- 1 vanilla bean or ¼ tsp. vanilla liquid
- 1 chopped raw date

Procedure

Blend until smooth and creamy. Chill thoroughly for the best flavor.

<u>Coconut Bliss Pudding</u>

Ingredients

- 1 ripe avocado
- 10 pitted dates, soaked
- 1/3rd cup filtered water
- 2 Tbsp. raw cacao or carob powder
- 1 Tbsp. raw cacao nibs
- 1 vanilla bean or ¼ tsp. vanilla
- 1/8th tsp. sea salt

Procedure

Blend everything until smooth and creamy. Chill thoroughly for the best flavor. Serve topped with coconut cream.

Banana Cream Pie with Sweet Walnut Crust

Sweet Walnut Crust:

Ingredients

- 1 cup walnuts
- ¾ cup chopped dried apricots
- ¼ cup chopped dates, or raisins
- 1/3rd cup 100% pure coconut sugar

Procedure

Place the first three ingredients in the food procedure and process them into a moist meal. While the processor is running slowly pour in the coconut sugar until the mixture turns into a ball. Press sweet crust into a 9-inch pie dish to form piecrust. Set aside.

Cream Filling:

Ingredients

- 1 cup cashews
- 2 bananas
- ½ vanilla bean or 1 teaspoon vanilla extract
- 1 tablespoon psyllium husk powder, optional

Procedure

Place all ingredients into a blender and blend until smooth.

Topping:

Ingredients

- 2 - 3 bananas

Procedure

Cut bananas into ½-inch rounds.

Assembly

Pour the cream filling into the sweet piecrust. Top with sliced bananas in a circular pattern for a pretty presentation. Serve at room temperature or chilled.

Peanut Butter Chocolate Cups

Ingredients

- ¼ cup coconut oil
- ¼ cup natural peanut butter
- 1 Tbsp. honey
- ¼ cup cacao
- ¼ cup pure maple syrup (also taste great with real agave syrup)
- 1 tsp vanilla

Procedure

Melt the oil, butter, and honey together on the stove, then add the rest. Let simmer for 5 mins or so. Pour into containers you can pop them out of, or into small cupcake type wrappers and place in the freezer. Enjoy! *Note*: The last time I added shredded coconut and dried cranberries. Instead of pouring the mixture tediously into little molds, I just poured it onto parchment paper in a baking or casserole dish and cut it into pieces once they are hardened. Leonard greatly enjoys them! They are delicious, to die for, and definitely addictive!

Almond-Date-Raisin Sweet Rolls

Ingredients

- 2 cups almonds, soaked overnight, blanched and dehydrated
- 2/3 cups pitted dates
- 2/3 cups dates
- 3-4 Tbsp. raw cacao powder
- 2 Tbsp. expeller pressed coconut oil
- 1 Tbsp. coconut sugar
- 1/3 cups pure water
- Wax paper
- Cinnamon powder

Procedure

Grind the almonds in a food processor using the S-blade until well chopped. Mix in dates, raisins. Process again until they stick together. Transfer into a bowl. In another bowl, mix together the raw cacao powder, coconut oil, coconut sugar, and water. Sprinkle cinnamon onto the wax paper (10"x10"). Using your hands, spread the almond-date-raisin mixture to form a thin square onto the wax paper with the cinnamon. Once spread evenly, add the cacao mixture as the next layer, then roll like a sushi roll and cut into pieces. Chill, serve.

Avocado Salad

Ingredients

- 1 cup wild rice, soaked 3 days (change the water daily)
- 2 Hass avocados, organic, mashed
- 1 small red onion, minced
- 1 small red bell pepper, minced
- juice of 1/4 lime
- ½ tsp. cilantro, dried
- ¾ tsp. kelp powder
- a few sprigs of oregano
- pinches of cayenne to taste

Procedure

Mix all ingredients; serve

Nourishing Popcorn

Ingredients

- 1/4th cup Organic (non-GMO) yellow popcorn kernels
- 1 stick pure raw unsalted butter
- Kelp powder
- Parsley flakes
- Dulse powder
- Granulated (or powdered) garlic
- Granulated (or powdered) onion
- Chives (dried, flaked)
- Nutritional Yeast flakes (or powder)
- Powdered (or shredded) Parmesan cheese (keep this refrigerated)
- Italian Organic Seasoning (marjoram, thyme, rosemary, savory, sage, oregano & sage)
- Kirkland Organic (Costco) No-salt Seasoning (onion, garlic, carrot, black pepper, red bell pepper, tomato, orange peel, parsley, bay leaves, thyme, basil, celery, lemon peel, oregano, savory, mustard seed, cumin, marjoram, coriander, cayenne, citric acid, rosemary)

Procedure

The preferred way to pop popcorn is in an electric hot-air popper, like the Rival© RV-932. IF YOU DON'T HAVE ONE: in a large stainless steel pot, set heat at medium or medium-to-hi. Apply 3 Tbsp. pure organic coconut oil (other oils can more quickly polymerize); place 3 or 4 popcorn kernels into the pot, cover it, wait until they pop, then add 1/4th cup popcorn kernels and replace the lid. Slide the pot around a bit on the burners until the popcorn stops popping; this makes about 3 quarts of popcorn. Meanwhile (while the popcorn in popping), allow the butter to melt <u>on very low heat</u> in a separate small covered saucepan.

Hot Air Popper or big steel pot, next, place the popped popcorn into a sturdy but light container (that has a lid of some kind) and pour on the melted butter, using a circular pouring motion so as to distribute it evenly. Then, generously sprinkle the rest of the ingredients, one at a time, onto the buttered popcorn. Place the lid onto the popcorn container and shake it in several directions to distribute the ingredients thru the popcorn. They will stick to most of the popcorn—wherever the butter went. *Note*: there's no need to add salt: dried veggies are already quite salty. The result is both tasty and wholesome.

VERY IMPORTANT: Make sure your ingredients do NOT contain MSG or any other excipients (chemicals, unknown factors)! If you can't pronounce it, it doesn't grow in the ground or in the trees! For the sake of your health, your food MUST BE PURE! For more recipes, go to www.GLDiet.co

Appendix B — Helpful Devices

Where to Get What You Need on Your GLD

The following products and materials are needed on your GLD. Some technical details are provided so you can make more informed decisions regarding these items. Prices and specific product references reflect the date of this printing (2019) and the Country in which it was written (USA).

- NATURAL FOOD SOURCES

  —Most urban areas of the world now have a sufficient number of Natural Food Stores. Increasingly, supermarkets carry organic produce because the people are demanding it. There are also many smaller, local Natural Food outlets, including farmer's markets and even local food stands that sell organic produce—whether they are required to pay expensive licenses for it or not.

- FRUITS/VEGGIES/JUICES

  —Use any fresh raw ripe in-season naturally-grown fruit or veggy that you are not allergic to. Small amounts of the extremely nourishing ocean veggies arame, wakame, and especially <u>dulse</u>, <u>hiziki</u>, and <u>kelp</u>, can and should be ground and sprinkled onto salads or very usefully added to soups and broths.

- LEGUMES/GRAINS

  —<u>Legumes</u> can all be used on the GLD cooked into veggy soups as appropriate to your health situation. <u>Grains</u> should be minimized or eliminated altogether. It's probably best to avoid or at least minimize peanuts and peanut butters since they quickly and easily attract fungi. **Also**: never blend killed (flesh) foods (animal flesh, red meats, fish, and poultry) into soups. This defeats the purpose of the GLD, which is purification toward balance, equanimity.

- NUTS/SEEDS/OILS

  —Most nuts or seeds are good to make into nut-seed milks as bases for smoothies or just to drink by themselves, singly, or in combination. The top nuts and seeds in nutritional terms are almonds, coconut, pumpkin seeds, sunflower seeds, and sesame seeds. When nuts or seeds are rancid, you'll feel a hot, burning sensation on the back of your tongue. Note that African shea butter and pure coconut oil are among the best skin products.

- WATER

—Our first choice is steam distilled water. Currently among the better personal household units is the *Pure Water© Mini-Classic II* (about $575USD). After steam-distilled in terms of quality water, we suggest multi-stage carbon filtering for household use, as a quality choice. We choose steam-distilled for many reasons and after decades of continuing research and ongoing study of all available water purifying and processing methods and equipment.

- JUICERS

—For a juicer, we recommend the *Omega® J8006HDS* (about $300USD). Overall, we find this to be the best juicer currently available. It's easy to clean, break down and put back together, extracts about 97% of the juice from the fruit or veggy, can juice grasses and leafy greens, and can make nut and seed butters. More expensive juicers are available, but—everything considered, including price—none does a better job. In Australia, the apparent equivalent is the *VitalMax® Oscar 900*.

—*Braun®* makes fairly good orange/citrus juicers for about $18-20. Many other companies make adequate products in this genre, but the best citrus juicer we've ever found is the *Breville 800CPXL* (about $200USD), which we use weekly at Grand Medicine.

- BLENDERS

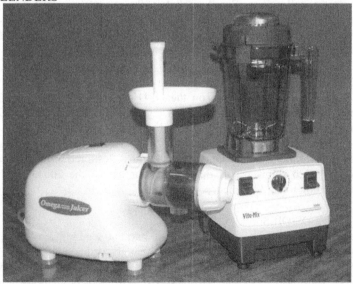

—Adi Da calls the power blender the most important machine humans have ever created regarding food. The best instrument in the USA and Canada for making virtually all liquids containing pulp (blended) is the power blender, of which the *VitaMix®* is an example. The older 5200

model shown here can be found at \$275USD; the S30 model is \$300 on sale, while the Ascent 3500 is \$600; see www.vitamix.com for all models. We can hardly say too much about the efficiency and utility of this item for use on the GLD and beyond.

Along with the Omega juicer, or even by itself, it does most (or all) of the liquids needed on your GLD. In Australia, the *VitaMix* is available but comparatively much higher priced than in the USA, so we recommend the *Breville® Optiva* in that country.

—We do not recommend the common blenders (usually priced at \$35-80) for your GLD. One can also purchase higher-end (and more expensive) so-called "commercial" or "professional" blenders, the kind used in bars and soda fountains or otherwise wherever smoothies and mixed drinks are sold to the public. These are available at Smart & Final Iris Company© (USA) and commercial/industrial restaurant supply outlets. Other, very effective big, strong blenders include such as the **Waring MX 1050 XT** 3.5 H.P. blender or the **Blendtech HP3A**. These are fine for your GLD. Other companies, including **Hamilton Beach**, are in the competition.

- NUT-SEED GRINDERS
    —**Braun®** and **Waring®** (usually about \$18-20) are only two of several companies that make good nut-seed grinders. It's hard to go wrong with these little machines. Nut-seed grinders (also called "coffee mill") are very useful for grinding the harder nuts and seeds (almonds and pumpkin seeds) needed for cereals and toppings when you are on solid foods.

- ENEMA BOTTLES

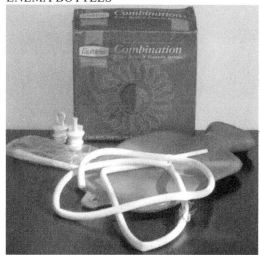

-

—The *Faultless*® enema bottle is among the best and well-priced on the market ($10-$17US) with its accessories, from any drug store or large department store (Wal-Mart). Other thick rubber bottles are available, often with trademarks of the store thru which they're sold (try www.optimalhealthnetwork.com and www.enemabag.com). Be sure the bottle is made of thick rubber and comes as a kit with hose, bottle holder, anal tip and vaginal douche tip included. *Note*: Do not purchase a "fleet enema" kit. These are made of thin rubber or plastic and are basically use-once-and-throw-away items.

- TEETH CARE PRODUCTS
  —***Dr. Bronner's Liquid Soap***©. www.drbronner.com; Of the six different "flavors" of these liquid soaps, almond and peppermint are our personal favorites for tooth brushing. These soaps are made from natural coconut, olive, hemp, and jojoba oils. A 32 oz. bottle sells for $12.99, and—if used only for tooth brushing—can last about four years when diluted 7:1 with pure water. We also use it at the same dilution for bathing, shaving, and as a shampoo. *Note*: Much more information on tooth care will be coming soon thru *GLDLifestyle*. Be sure to floss your teeth—at least nitely before bed!

- SPECIFIC DISEASE PROTOCOLS
  —For information on specific disease processes and what to do about them in terms of both standard allopathic and Natural Health practices and procedures, you can google your condition and otherwise see your Natural Health Practitioner or other qualified health professional. Information on how to become a Natural Health Practitioner is available on our website at www.eyology.com.

Appendix C — The SuperFoods

Certain foods and herbs have extraordinary qualities, such as much higher concentrations of certain nutrients, more potent anti-parasite activity, strong healing properties, combinations of these, and so on, placing their value for our health well above the average food—the "SuperFoods." At Grand Medicine, we recommend taking at least 2 SuperFoods in your daily diet. When suffering from chronic degenerative disease, or otherwise when feeling ill, we suggest you increase this to 4 or more on your GLD.

ALWAYS make sure your sources are "organic" and all-natural, no chemical fertilizers, unsprayed (non-pesticide) and non-GMO home-grown or otherwise locally-grown in-season produce. And stay on a hi-raw (80%+) or all-raw veggie diet as much and as often as possible. Try to start each day with a green smoothie. For many reasons, this is the most important meal of the day.

Acai	Goji Berries
Acerola Berries	Hemp Seed Oil
Almonds	Hempseed
Aloe Vera	Hiziki
Ashwagandha Root	Incan Berries
Asparagus	Kakadu plum
Bee pollen	Kale
Black Cumin Oil	Kelp
Black Currants	Krill Oil
Blue-green algae	Maca
Boku	Mangosteen
Cacao	Maqui Berries
Camu Berries	Matcha Green Tea
Cannabis	Monk Fruit
Cayenne	Moringa
CBD Oil	Mucuna
Chaga	Noni
Chia Seed	Pomegranate
Chlorella	Propolis
Coconut	Rose Hips
Comfrey	Royal jelly
Dates	Shiitake
Dulse	Spirulina
Flaxseed	Turmeric
Garlic	Watercress
Ginger root	Wheatgrass
Ginseng	Yacon

Leonard Mehlmauer, ND

Appendix D — The Many Names for Sugar

In this list, the five artificial sweeteners (*acesulfame K, aspartame, neotame, saccharin*, and *sucralose*) and their variants have been added. These chemically manufactured molecules do not exist in Nature. **Bolded** are the substances generally recognized by Natural Health authorities as among the least harmful of the common sweeteners.

Acesulfame K
Acid Saccharin
Aclame (or Alitame)
Advantame (aspartame / GMO)
Agave nectar
Alitame
AminoSweet (contains aspartame)
Aspartame
Aspartame-Acesulfame Salt
Barley malt
Beet sugar
Blackstrap molasses (sulfured)
Brown rice syrup
Brown sugar
Buttered sugar (buttercream)
Calcium Saccharin
Candarel (w/aspartame)
Cane juice crystals
Cane juice
Cane sugar
Caramel
Carob syrup
Caster sugar (superfine sugar)
Coconut sugar (crystallized coco-palm sap)
Cologran (w/saccharin and cyclamate)
Confectioner's sugar (powdered sugar, icing sugar)
Corn sweetener
Corn syrup
Corn syrup solids
Crystalline fructose
Cyclamate
Date sugar (crystallized dried dates)
Demerara sugar
Destran
Dextrose
Diastatic malt powder
Diastase
Dulcin (banned in the 1950s)
Equal (aspartame)
Ethyl maltol
Evaporated cane juice
Fructose
Fruit juice concentrates
Galactose
Glucose
Golden sugar

Golden syrup (refiner's syrup)
Heremesetas (w/saccharin)
High-fructose corn syrup
Honey (especially pasteurized)
Invert sugar
Lactose
Malt syrup
Maltodextrin
Maltose (malt sugar)
Maple syrup
Molasses syrup
Muscovado sugar
NatraTaste (w/aspartame)
Necta Sweet (saccharin)
Neotame
NutraSweet (aspartame)
Organic raw sugar
Oat syrup (Avena Sativa)
Panela (boiled, evaporated cane juice)
Panocha (penuche, brown sugar fudge candy)
Rice Bran Syrup
Rice syrup
Saccharin
Sodium Saccharin
Sorghum
Sorghum syrup
Splenda (w/sucralose and maltodextrin)
Stevia (a natural herb sweetener)
Sucaryl (w/saccharin and cyclamate)
Sucralose
Sucrose (table sugar)
Sugar
Sugar Twin (aspartame)
Sunett (acesulfame K)
Sweet and Safe (acesulfame K)
Sweet One (acesulfame K)
Sweet 'N Low (saccharin)
Sweet Twin (saccharin)
SweetyHi (inulin, herb extracts)
Syrup
Treacle
Tapioca syrup
Turbinado sugar (raw sugar)
TwinSweet (w/aspartame & acesulfame K)
Yellow sugar

Notes:

Some "honey" that comes from China has turned out not to be honey at all! If you use honey, it should be local-grown pure raw organic unrefined, and unprocessed. Maple syrup can occasionally be acceptable IF it is 100% pure top grade. Date sugar is excellent if you make it yourself in a food dryer from organic dates. Otherwise, it's OK to use pure raw coconut sugar as your primary sweetener—short of stevia.

Appendix E — The Devotional Prayer of Changes

A Prayer as Described by Avatar Adi Da Samraj

Some years ago, I was given an exceptional gift: a special way of praying. I'll never forget the first time I used it. My men friends were telling me that after many years as a bachelor, I was ready for a wife, for a life-friend, an intimate partner. I had been trying, dating all kinds and ages of women, but nothing was working. They suggested this prayer, and within nine days I heard her name! A Gift of Bhagavan Adi Da Samraj, this powerful prayer method is called "*The Devotional Prayer of Changes*."

The Devotional Prayer of Changes

The Devotional Prayer of Changes is a higher form of prayer. Unlike other forms of prayer, it does not separate the person praying from God, the Divine Source. It can be done at any time of day or night. The best location for this prayer is a Communion Hall or quiet place set aside for God-Communion, somewhere you are unlikely to be disturbed. There is no limit to the number of times you can do the Devotional Prayer of Changes (DPC). The only caution: with right use of the DPC, you should be careful what you pray for because you will very likely see it happen!

Since the DPC is not done from the "separate and separated" position of the ego-"I," it is therefore not a request for favors of a "separate deity"—as most prayers are. The DPC begins immediately with whole-bodily surrender to Real-God, or the Spiritual Master. In the "position" of non-separate heart-felt devotion, or love, or oneness-Communion with the Divine, the prayer is continued and engaged. This "adult disposition" is the reason it is so effective: no separation from God is presumed at any time during the prayer.

"*The Devotional Prayer of Changes is a participatory process that has a real basis in the psycho-physics of the universe. It is a means for participating in the real universe, and in Reality Itself, in such a manner as to release the characteristics in the human body-mind-complex which are holding certain conditions in place, and to animate the characteristics in place, and to animate the characteristics in the human body-mind-complex which can be exercised so as not to hold those conditions in place.*" —Avatar Adi Da Samraj

To prepare for your DPC, create a concise list of your specific desired positive changes. Bring it with you into the Hall. Sit comfortably on a cushion on the floor or in a chair. After full submission to The Divine Reality, you will be clearly stating your intention and *visualizing the details clearly with the mind's eye* while *feeling the desired changes*.

The prayer has five parts. The last part is the Faith presumption—"trust in the universe." The DPC is effective to the degree that you establish and maintain a "bridge to God" via your continuing intensity of attention and devotion to The Divine Person. You and God Are One! Be submersed, lost in God, thru-out the DPC. Always be turned to The Lord!

The Devotional Prayer of Changes (simple form)

—*Surrender*: While engaging breathing conductivity, *devotionally invoke and heart-surrender completely to Beloved Guru* (to the Spiritual Master or the Very Divine) from your heart. In feeling, surrender everything—body, mind, soul, material wealth, friends, relatives—until you feel this is done for real. (It's all "owned" by The Great One, anyway!) Affirm the Divine Self-Condition that always already transcends all conditions.

—*Intention*: Clearly and precisely *state the purpose of the prayer* to The Beloved Lord (Spiritual Master or God), out loud or quietly, with the tongue of the mind, focusing on the positive.

—*Visualization*: Remaining in God-Communion, on inhalation *receive with heart-feeling all particular and intended positive conditions &/or changes*, visualizing them, seeing them and feeling them actually happening—in detail.

—*Release*: Remaining in God-Communion, on exhalation *heart-relinquish all doubts*, negative thoughts, and identification with problems *and negative conditions*. Feel them fading away.

—*Have Faith*: Remaining in God-Communion, arise. Stay positive and change your action. Assume, live, and do all you can that is required to serve and bring into being the intended changes. (This is your part. The Divine Reality Does the rest!)

"This process is not magic—although it is magical in some general sense, you could say, or (otherwise) extraordinary. Rather, this process occurs based on a law of conditional existence—that all conditions arising are the product of deep-seated presumptions. If you can change those presumptions, and (likewise) change your behaviors (and so on), then conditions change. This is because the presumptions exist at the level of energy-modification that is the source of conditions, which can very directly affect the grosser, more peripheral aspect of 'experience.'"
—Avatar Adi Da Samraj

On p522 of the book, *The Aletheon*, Adi Da elucidates the DPC further: *"Therefore, if change is required (or would-be), do not <u>ask</u> for changes and then wait for the changes to 'happen' as a result. Instead, always intrinsically <u>be as</u> changed, and (thus and thereby) always priorly and actively <u>be</u> (and categorically presume) the would-be changes (<u>as</u> being in fact the case)—and, on that basis, always and only (or merely) <u>observe</u> (and do not seek or merely intend and look for) the 'experiential' evidence. This is how Reality Itself 'Works'. This is how Real God—Which <u>Is Only</u> Reality Itself—Is."* See www.adidam.org

And finally, *"The Devotional Prayer of Changes is simply an expression of the right disposition. It is the willingness to be changed in your disposition and your life altogether and to make changes in life."*
—Avatar Adi Da Samraj

Appendix F — How to Meditate

A Practice Based on the Teachings of Adi Da Samraj and Four Decades of Direct Experience

Introduction

Meditation is a traditional means devotional communion with The Divine Person that has the secondary effects of calming the body-mind, focusing attention, and finally transcending attention toward Divine Self-Realization. The intensity of one's application of these principles, combined with Divine Grace, determines one's results. (In some real sense, meditation IS the "result"!) When real, even brief meditation is helpful. Most important is <u>what</u> you meditate on. There are a few principles or factors to manage:

Location

Find the quietest place, somewhere you will be least likely to be disturbed by noise or other intrusion. If at home, a dedicated Meditation Hall is best. For most Westerners, a part of one's bedroom may suffice. Lock the door! Perhaps hang a sign on the doorknob: "**Meditating. Do not disturb!**" The room should be as quiet as possible. Use earplugs if needed to avoid sound distraction. Darken the room against all visual distractions except on the focus of your attention (see below).

Bodily position

Best is a sitting position on the floor, rug, or mat, in which you hold yourself upright. The body should be relaxed and yet alert, able to focus attention. If in a chair or couch, there can be a tendency to fall asleep, so use only if you have a problem that requires them. A small cushion under the backside provides a little lift, allowing comfortable sitting. Sitting cross-legged is fine until lotus positions become comfortable. Sit upright, back in a straight line, but without forced or otherwise uncomfortable rigidity. This can take some weeks to get used to but is entirely worthwhile.

Focus

You are what you give your attention to! This is a Great Law. Whatever we consistently give our attention to (person, place, or thing), we "become," or take on qualities of. Focusing on a candle flame, e.g., makes us like the flame: simple, quiet, serene, and consuming oxygen. However, if all you want to do with your life is to be quiet and calm, go for it. On the other hand, **the desire of every heart** is for far more.

If real human growth beyond all stress interests you, if transcending everything in Absolute Happiness, Eternal Peace and Perfect Freedom seem more important—as displayed in the lives of Jesus, Krishna, Gautama, and (historically most recently) Avatar Adi Da Samraj—then there is something better for you than candle flame meditation.

Traditionally, the Adept Spiritual Master, The Divine Realizer of any degree, is the best focus for your attention—simply because you will, thru your steady attention on the Master, take on His Qualities. If you are Christian, get a large murti (image) of Beloved Jesus, one that you relate to in feeling. If you are Hindu, Buddhist, Muslim, Jain, or of other religious or Spiritual tradition that has a specific one or several possible Spiritual Masters, you may wish to use an image of Him or Her, accordingly. Place your murti a few feet before you and elevated a bit such that your gaze is slightly upward.

If you have no specific tradition, see the book, *The Gift of Truth Itself* (Amazon) or go to www.adidam.org and copy or purchase a murti image of Avatar Adi Da Samraj. Full, large murti image fotos may be purchased from Adidam.org. It will not be long before you begin to feel or otherwise notice the Grace of Real Meditation (see below).

Submission
The four principle human faculties—body, mind, feeling, and breath—are to be submitted or "surrendered" to the Spiritual Master or Divine Condition during meditation. This submission—giving yourself over, surrendering—comes naturally over time. As you sit for meditation, the body becomes progressively relaxed and ready to submit.

The mind will wander, usually a lot at first. Just gently and consistently notice this and bring it back (thru your attention) to the image of the Master. Do not be disturbed by that wandering—no matter how much. The feeling part is whatever degree of devotion for or feeling-connection you have with the Beloved.

The breath is relaxed, slow, and deep (see *Conductivity Healing*, p168-169), breathing the in-breath down the frontal line of the body to the abdomen, allowing the etheric energy to cross under the perineum while briefly holding the in-breath. Then, on the out-breath, allow the etheric energy to move up the spinal line to the heart, then the rest of the body, then outward in all directions to infinity.

Over time, this process will deepen, eventually with the breath even stopping for long moments, as the faculties focus ever more intensely on the Master. (This process is enhanced by regular Spiritual study of books in your religious tradition and/or those mentioned in this document. Audio of Adi Da is available at www.adidam.org, and video clips of the Spiritual Master can be viewed on YouTube. These will significantly assist your meditation.)

Timing

Before even attempting to meditate, it is best to have done some Spiritual study. If already practicing within a religious or Spiritual tradition, with daily scriptural study, you can start meditating. If there has not been such a tradition for you, there are many study options. You may wish to begin with the book, *The Gift of Truth Itself* ($12.95US paperback, Amazon). Other books include *The Knee of Listening* (by Adi Da Samraj), or *The Avatar of What Is* (by Carolyn Lee).

Begin meditating for no more than 15 minutes at a time. Your mind will not be prepared for more than that. Gradually, over time, you can increase to 20, then 30 minutes, eventually moving to a full hour, as Divine Grace enters the body-mind, allowing for deeper and more effective meditation. If the mind wanders—which it will—no problem, just bring attention back to The Master. On some days, meditations will seem not to work at all, while at other times they will be blissful.

The best time to meditate is first thing in the morning and last thing at nite. On awakening, go to the bathroom, then immediately go to the Meditation Hall to sit before the murti and begin meditation. This sets the right tone for the day, grounding you in Happiness—and preparing you to deal with the world.

BLESSINGS!

Appendix G — Espheria

Human Scale Living for a Higher Way of Life

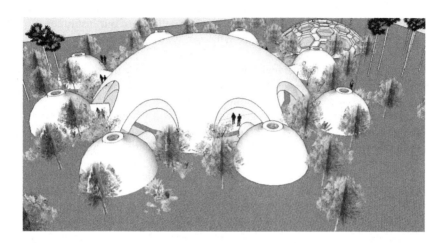

The Perennial Cooperative Life

Introduction

Def. *"Espheria,"* from the Spanish—*"sphere."*

Espheria is an original cooperative community design for disaster-proof spherical structures for optimizing living that is simple, low-cost, safe, secure, efficient, effective, and peaceful, and with a potential for higher human life.

Quick View

Espheria is a housing and living design for extended families and small groups of 16-25 persons. With both *privacy* <u>and</u> close-proximity (*community*) living—and therefore the necessary human sharing of energies—**Espheria** provides occupants with instructions in this currently different but ages-old and time-honored way of life.

The peripheral *Satellite Domes* are your private housing, the *CentralDome* is for community life, and the attached *GardenDome* provides your food. Off-the-grid, self-sustaining, virtually disaster-proof, very low maintenance, largely autonomous, safe, and secure low-cost living frees up time, money, energy, and creativity. Designed for any extended family or group of optimally 16-25 persons, folks *with values and beliefs that are similar or otherwise compatible.*

Motivation

Let's get real. It doesn't take a genius to see that our current world is ego-mad. Constant wars, the occasional random threat of nuclear annihilation, ongoing environmental pollution, and destruction, massive starvation, poor leadership, enormously exaggerated economic inequality, the breakdown of civilization, the corruption of virtually all of our institutions—the list of insanities goes on and on. What can we do in this midst?

As individuals, we feel helpless, and yet we sense that if we can only somehow join together—we ordinary people who love peace—we can turn this picture around. Strength in numbers. But what numbers? One? Two? What if we got together a small group of those with whom we enjoy certain sympathies—like religious beliefs or social concepts or general philosophies? Could that work? It has in the past—and is working in the world right now.

Nenita (my intimate partner) and I traveled to many countries while teaching science classes. Among the perceptions that stood out—almost everyone we met was kind and decent. They wanted peace. Including the Russian people, who we had been told (at various times—even recently) were our "enemies." They were fine. So, what enemies? If at least most of the ordinary people of the world are like this, why don't we have peace? Are we being played by our so-called leaders? Is our world condition essentially about egoic control, maintaining wealth and power for a few psychopaths?

However that may be, there are various things we can do to help ourselves to a better world, at least on a local level—perhaps on a VERY local level! Yes, we can email our members of congress, join environmental groups, pitch in to help at local community events, etc. Good! But, amid these gestures, we can do something we haven't done in a long time—at least since the Industrial Revolution, since around the mid-1700s.

Even tho towns and cities have existed for thousands of years, most of us lived in small villages where we knew everyone. We knew who could be counted on, who had integrity, and who didn't. We could make agreements and hold each other accountable. We didn't need tens of thousands of laws, rules, and regulations created by bureaucrats in order to live our daily lives sensibly. (That's for big cities, for huge numbers of people, and it doesn't work in the present world model, anyway.) Life was much simpler back then, and it can be again—even with (rightly used) technology.

Espheria is an entirely realistic design that is based on (1) evidence of peaceful and effective human interaction during most of human history, (2) the author's personal experience in many countries, plus (3) the Wisdom of the Divine Adept Realizer, Adi Da Samraj.

348

An Optimum Human Living Circumstance

What kind of future do you want to make? What would be optimum for happy, heart-fulfilling, and self-transcending lives? Let's think of one. Imagine a gathering of 16-25 intelligent people, folks you know and feel good about, living cooperatively and privately in a small graceful community. The idea is based on principles of (1) strength in numbers, and (2) the perennially proven fact that small groups can cooperate responsibly, accountably and peacefully.

The 16-25 persons "optimum number" comes from (1) the fact that this was the approximate size of successful human Hunger-Gatherer cultural groups for perhaps over 100,000 years, and (2) the Divine Wisdom of Avatar Adi Da Samraj in describing "human-scale" living and working groups. Less than this number tends to bring out a single dominating character. More than 25 people is difficult for most of us, personally, to keep up intimate communication day-to-day.

This group size, while much smaller than most communities, provides many advantages over the current "divided-and-conquered" family home, everyone needing their own same things as everyone else, each struggling alone for survival in their own little separate castle kingdom. The sharing we used to do, way back then, essentially happens now only in emergencies. We knew the value of strength-in-numbers, and that "teamwork makes the dream work." So, we stuck together.

CoOpCom and the Psychopathology of Everyday Life

So, if it's so great, why isn't "democracy," working in the world? The answer is simpler than our so-called leaders and top thinkers would let us believe—if, indeed, any of them knows, him or herself. It's egoity! The sense of separation, of separateness, of separativeness. It is a lie that virtually everyone has accepted and is living by. And yet, there is not one jot of separation anywhere in the universe. Never was. Never will be. Everything is wonderfully, intimately connected!

Everything is one "Thing," one Reality, called The Great Consciousness, God, Allah, and all the other names we dream up for "It." Despite all the names we've come up with, and all the sometimes bizarre attributes we have assigned to "It" (some bearded guy in the clouds!), "It" is beyond anything the human mind can comprehend. But the Divine Realizers have consistently told us it is Beautiful beyond anything we can possibly imagine. It is capital "L" Love—in Person!

Need I say it? Our current world culture is not based on appreciation of, or connectedness with, The Divine Reality. **And this is the whole trouble!** It has, from time to time in this world's past history, but it certainly isn't now. It is now based on pseudo-scientific materialism. Our current world culture, altogether, can be considered an ego-mad "crazy-random" culture, not at all a Wisdom Culture. It is generally based on personal self-*fulfillment*. If truly religious ("re-lig", meaning re-join with The Divine Reality), it would be based on self-*Transcendence*. not self-Transcendence—which is what they'd be based on if they were truly "religious" ("re-lig" = re-join with The Divine Reality).

Yes, we've all been beaten over the head by self-righteous silly down-town religion followers, those whose institutions have caused the destruction of whole cultures, enormous suffering, and even death in the world—in the name of the Great Saints they purportedly espoused. And we've been approached by well-intentioned and more peaceful religious adherents who asked us to merely *believe* in this or that Saint and by doing so we'd be immediately absolved of our "sins" and have access to some "heaven." (No Saint ever asked for our mere belief. They wanted us 100%.)

In my studies of many Saints, Sages, yogis, and wise men and women of our Great Tradition of Spiritual Literature, it was always the same with them. They were about real love of the Divine—love to the point of us actually *becoming* Love (capital "L"), whereupon we could then truly love all others. And they all said Spirituality was going to be hard work, not about our mere belief. Belief is of the mind, and the mind—I'm sure you've noticed—is capable of all manner of craziness.

These Great Ones wanted it all—full submission, surrender, self-sacrifice to The Divine—in order for us to Transcend "self," "world," and everything else—in Awakening to Divine Happiness, Eternal Peace, and Perfect Freedom. They weren't saying we were to have no fun at all in the world. No. You can still do that, but in the knowledge that fun isn't the point of your life.

The Great Ones say that if we're not up for this "turning," we waste our lives, die, and keep recycling back to the same thing—indefinitely. They describe how they themselves had to "earn" Realization, Awakening, thru this real sacrifice of "self" into The Divine Reality. It wasn't just given to them thru their mere belief in someone, something, or anything—or thru someone else's death or sacrifice.

Personally, Spiritual life has been the very hardest thing I've ever attempted—but at the same time, the most deeply rewarding—heart-rewarding. It is all about a personal relationship—THE personal Relationship, the one with The Divine Master. I bring this up not just in the context of the world (why the world is in such bad shape), but also because religion and community have always been together, have always been intimately associated. Religion isn't just something one does alone, in private —it's something one does together with others.

350

Obviously, then, the current world is not about the Divine. Unlike certain civilizations have in the past, it is not truly about honoring the sacred—including this most sacred relationship, that with the Divine Guru. We have lost our sympathy with the truly sacred. Our world is steeped in self-*fulfillment*—not self-*transcendence*. There's an old expression, *"Power corrupts!"* The more the **power**, the more the **corruption**. As before, this seems to be the rule of the day.

An important aspect of this (necessarily egoic) lust for power, money, and control is that it invariably involves the **psychopathic** character. Look up the definition and the characteristics of **the psychopath**. Only a very small percentage of people in the world, perhaps 1%, develop this way. They are intent on gaining positions of power over people. They are capable of doing awful things to get that power. Finally, they cannot *empathize* with others. They can't feel others' suffering.

If this sounds like the attitude and activities of most government officials, heads of corporations, and the so-called "elite" or shadow government, CIA, NSA, FBI, DARPA, and the big militarists, could this be a major reason why we see so much suffering in the world? Are people born this way—or is this developed thru their individual experiences? If it is not *nature,* but *nurture,* then it's true that *"the hand that rocks the cradle rules the world!"* It's about our earliest education—by mothers immersed in God-Love!

Enter Espheria

While we can and certainly should (even must!) do all kinds of little things every day, in each of our ways, to make our world a better place for everyone to live, meanwhile we have this design called Espheria. It's about getting together in small groups to live a simpler, less expensive, more creative, and generally higher way of life.

Some Advantages of Espheria CoopCom Living
—Simpler, less expensive lifestyle
—Safe, secure living environment
—Low-stress natural surroundings
—Year-round built-in childcare
—Year-round built-in senior care
—Low or no insurance rates/payments
—Low food expenses: most food grown onsite
—Companionship / fellowship on-demand
—Spiritual practice of your choice, unhindered
—Low cost, lovely, disaster-proof housing
—Increased human growth potential
—Hi potential for Spiritual growth
—No outside HOA (homeowner assn.)
—No need for outside nursing homes
—Trees and flowers outside &/or inside
—3-4 generations living only steps away
—Truly healthful living birth-to-death
—Self-owned off-the-grid water & power
—Inhabitants share your religion
—Greater peace of mind potential
—More free time for creativity
—Privacy and community as desired
—Responsibility and accountability
—Home safety covered when traveling

An Espheria community "Unit" is a design for both a series of inter-connected disaster-proof structures of various sizes. While many different shapes, sizes, colors, and configurations of the live-in structures are possible, the original design calls for a series of connected Monolithic Domes. In general, there is the large (3-story) community CentralDome surrounded by and connected to eight or more private Satellite Domes. A large GardenDome is connected to the CentralDome.

All of these structures are disaster-proof (fire, hurricane, earthquake, and flood). Of course, they should not be built on a floodplain or on the primary dune (directly on the beach). Among other qualities, they are:

—Beautiful, elegant, pleasing to the eye—not angular, weirdly colored, and painful to look at
—Human scale (basically 16-25 persons)—within the size needed for comfortable associations
—Blending with nature, in shape and color, with decorative trees, flowers, hedges, and shrubs
—Off-the-grid, self-sustaining in food, water, and power terms

Monolithic domes, for example, are relatively inexpensive to build, cheap to maintain, sustainable, very low or no insurance (because they're disaster-proof), using no wood in their superstructure (thus not requiring the destruction of forests), lasting many centuries, and employing rounded natural shapes (www.monolithic.com). A monolithic dome home on the Florida coast survived a hurricane intact while all the homes around it were totally destroyed—one of many examples.

With nothing to catch hold of, hurricane or typhoon winds benignly swirl around a dome. Fires can't do more than superficial damage. Built on this principle, we would not be hearing of all this property destruction from natural disasters on the evening news. Build these lovely homes in clusters of Units, using true CoopCom principles, and you have communities with the opportunity for a safe, secure, intelligent, simple, more permanent, less expensive, and higher way of life.

The three-part climate-controlled GardenDome, where most of the community's food is grown, is maintained by experienced gardeners who live within your group. The garden's soil contains ground glacial rock and other factors to help support enzyme action. Kitchen scrap-recycle-produced compost complements companion planting and other natural pest control. Those in your group who enjoy gardening maintain the GardenDome, for pay or voluntarily as community service.

While we work out the various possible financials, we know how people live together in close conjunction successfully. We continue to study the many current and historical models. We have experienced CoOpCom directly by living it in various ways over decades. And, we have been Given guidelines from our Beloved World-Friend, Adi Da Samraj. For more details on the Espheria project, contact us at gm@grandmedicine.com.

Last Word

The word "sacrifice" usually elicits thots of negative events of the past, even savage ones, like wantonly killing humans or animals, or destroying things or throwing away something we like. But on the plus side, sacrifice is Love, Real Love, releasing "ownership" of people and things. Sacrifice is also letting go of fixed habit patterns of the body, brain-mind and sub-conscious mind (or "soul"). These are necessary for our Real human growth.

We are always free to see and drop these negative patterns. We can do so a little at a time or wholesale. In any case, whichever way determines our destiny. Make few or no changes and your next incarnation will be very much like this one. It's the Law. Grow or not. The process, described in a Talk by Adi Da Samraj called, "*Attention Is Destiny*", involves contemplation of the Divine Reality and tapas. It's about devotion, service and self-discipline.

If and when we consistently grant attention to something higher than our current worldly (generally gross-level) patterns, a higher destiny awaits. This is sadhana, Real Spiritual practice, and the path and gate are narrow (Matthew 7:13-14). In these Dark Times, few are interested. Most only want self-*fulfillment*, not self-*transcendence*. Consistent devotion, service and self-discipline involve purification, change of habits, self-sacrifice.

We define the results in our life, the limits we place on this sacrifice. Attention is destiny. How are you using your attention? Is it consistently going to the same things, the same patterns? This defines the state of your existence. You can change it. Find this out. Mere belief doesn't determine destiny. It's what you do with attention. You must change your act. What attention associates with has dimensions in space and time. This is destiny.

We tend not to think of, or be aware of, this process. We allow attention to wander into dark places—without realizing that this establishes and perpetuates a dark destiny accordingly. If we are not moved to go beyond these patterns of gross possibility, they will simply continue. Even the subtler planes of existence are limited. They can be gone beyond, too. Attention is like a wild pony, jumping into this and that pasture, finding fixed places.

Only when attention's location becomes unsatisfactory do we move it elsewhere. But where we move it is up to us. Everywhere in the grand matrix of the universes and planes of existence we find limitation. The wise discover this and decide to go beyond all limitation to Realize What Is Great. That requires great sacrifice. Grace is Given. The Sadhana is Given. But we must then do it. Is purification happening only in your imagination?

Where are you now in your life? Age doesn't matter. How are you motivated? For a major change of destiny there must be an extraordinary sacrifice of self. Even for a *moderate* change, you have to do something different. Don't wait 'til you're on your deathbed, then look back on your life, saying, "*I could have done this purification!*" Grace is here. The process is here. Help is here. You can do this!

The usual life is a self-perpetuating cycle of mediocrity and suffering, with occasional pleasure and pain, while seeking permanent happiness and self-fulfillment via minimal self-discipline and more than occasional self-indulgence. **Get better results via the GLD and GLDLifestyle**. Do them as your heart-felt return gift to the Spiritual, the Eternal Divine Presence, the Person of Love.

Leonard Mehlmauer
Lake San Marcos California
20 November 2019

Bibliography

Below are listed only a sampling of the books we've used in the creation of the fifth edition of *The GREAT Liquid Diet* book. The titles are in *bold italics*.

Adidam Radical Healing; by Avatar Adi Da Samraj; some material found in ***Conductivity Healing*** (see below).

At The Feet Of The Spiritual Master*, by Gerald Sheinfeld; go to: www.storiesofthespiritualmaster.com

Conductivity Healing, from teachings on the subject by His Divine Presence, Avatar Adi Da Samraj; Dawn Horse Press

Death is a Living Process, based on the Wisdom-Teaching of Avatar Adi Da Samraj; Dawn Horse Press; www.adidam.org.

Design with Nature, by Ian L. McHarg; paperback edition 1971; Doubleday/Natural History Press; NY

Dining in the Raw, by Rita Romano; 222 pages; 1992.

Disease Prevention and Treatment, expanded 4th edition; Life Extension Media, 2003; Life Extension, P.O. Box 229120, Hollywood FL 33022-9120

Easy Death; by Avatar Adi Da Samraj; Dawn Horse Press; USA; www.adidam.org

Fasting for Regeneration: The Short Cut, by Julia Seton; 84 pages; 1929; http://www.healthresearchbooks.com/index.php

Green Gorilla, by Adi Da; 184pps; $16.95 from Dawn Horse Press, www.adidam.org; also available from Amazon

Juice Therapy Remedies A to Z, by Jay Kordich—The Juiceman

Natural Annie's Fresh Tastes for Breakfast; by Ann Miller-Cohen, Green Gourmet Cookbook, Vol. 1; July 2005; Earth Angel Publishing, Manlius NY 13104; gg_naturalannie@yahoo.com

Not-Two Is Peace, by The World-Friend, Adi Da; 4th edition, August 2019, Dawn Horse Press

Raw Food Made Easy, for One or Two People, by Jennifer Cornbleet; 187 pages; 2005.

Raw Foods for Busy People, by Jordan Maerin; 88 pages; 2004.

Raw Vegetable Juices; by N. W. Walker, D.Sc., Norwalk Press, 1970; Phoenix AZ 85002

Rebuild Your Health with High Energy Enzyme Nourishment, by Ann Wigmore; 93 pages; 1991.

Santosha Adidam; by Avatar Adi Da Samraj; Dawn Horse Press; USA; www.adidam.org

Take Control of Your Health; by Elaine Hollingsworth, Hippocrates Health Centre of Australia; 617-5530-2939; 9th edition; www.doctorsaredangerous.com.

The Aletheon, by Avatar Adi Da Samraj (Dawn Horse Press)

The Basket of Tolerance, by Avatar Adi Da Samraj (publication forthcoming from Dawn Horse Press)

The Complete Yoga of Human Emotional-Sexual Life, by Avatar Adi Da Samraj

The Dawn Horse Testament of the Ruchira Avatar, by Avatar Adi Da Samraj; 2004; Dawn Horse Press, USA

The Essene Gospel of Peace, translated by Edmond Bordeaux Szekely, ©1975 by the author, San Diego CA USA

The Hippocrates Diet and Health Program, by Ann Wigmore; 191 pages; 1984

The Juiceman's Power of Juicing; by Jay Kordich

The Lifefood Recipe Book, by Annie and David Jubb; 162 pages; 2002

The Living Bible, Tyndale House Publishers, 1972

The Science of Eating Raw, by Swayze Foster

The Sunfood Diet Success System: 36 Lessons in Health Transformation, by David Wolfe; 624 pages; 2006.

The Yoga of Right Diet; by Adi Da Samraj; 88 pages; 2006; The Dawn Horse Press

Toxemia Explained, by J. H. Tilden, M.D.; 1935; 144 pages; try http://www.soilandhealth.org/02/0201hyglibcat/020103toxemia/020103 01.html

Vegan Health Coaching
—Los Angeles area: Marr Nealon marrnealon@gmail.com 818-554-0711 www.veganhealthcoaching.com

An Invitation to Health Professionals (or Those Wishing to Enter the Field of Natural Health)
Grand Medicine has produced several Online Eyology and Health Courses, including in the sciences of Physical Iridology, Personality Iridology, Sclerology, and Natural Medicine. These quality courses are available at www.eyology.com. To get a sense of the potency of Sclerology (e.g.) watch this one-hour video on the subject of Iridology and Sclerology in Clinical Practice: https://attendee.gotowebinar.com/recording/731794608451143936.

*More on Avatar Adi Da Samraj from a friend telling why he became a devotee of Adi Da Samraj. Gerald's website includes short video clips, interesting stories, and information about his book of stories compiled from 47 years with Adi Da Samraj. Check out his Website: www.storiesofthespiritualmaster.com. Also see many short videos of Adi Da on YouTube.

Artist / Author

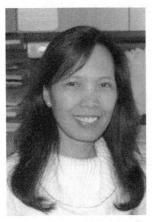

Nenita Sarmiento, BS, CPA

Ms. Sarmiento is Co-Director of Grand Medicine and the creative artist behind all GranMed publications and products. A top Eyologist and researcher, Nenita's energy and creativity plans, organizes, prepares, and manages hardware, software, materials, logistics, and technology at the GranMed lab and abroad. Her insistence on quality and integrity is our best help and sincerest critic.

Leonard Mehlmauer, ND (ret.)

Dr. Mehlmauer is Eyology professor, writer, and researcher at Grand Medicine in clinical practice since 1972. A now-retired Traditional Naturopath, he is author of acclaimed books, maps, essays, videos, and courses. His Sclerology manual, "*SCLEROLOGY—A New View of an Ancient Art*," has been praised by Bernard Jensen, DC (USA), Evgeny Velkhover, MD (Russia), Willy Hauser (Germany), and other top practitioners, and translated into several languages. His current work with *The GREAT Liquid Diet* is a team effort.

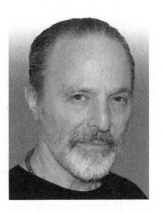

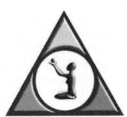

Made in the USA
Middletown, DE
08 April 2025

73962923R00205